Intensive Care: Advanced Concepts

Intensive Care: Advanced Concepts

Editor: Thomas Wood

MURPHY & MOORE
www.murphy-moorepublishing.com

www.murphy-moorepublishing.com

MURPHY & MOORE

Cataloging-in-Publication Data

Intensive care : advanced concepts / edited by Thomas Wood.
p. cm.
Includes bibliographical references and index.
ISBN 978-1-63987-325-8
1. Intensive care units. 2. Critical care medicine. 3. Emergency medicine. I. Wood, Thomas.
RA975.5.I56 I58 2022
362.174--dc23

Murphy & Moore Publishing,
1 Rockefeller Plaza,
New York City, NY 10020, USA

ISBN 978-1-63987-325-8 (Hardback)

Contents

Preface

Intensive care is a medical specialty that deals with the patients who require immediate medical support or whose lives are in immediate danger. The critical conditions that require immediate medical care are severe infections, cardio-vascular incidents, acute-respiratory infections, post-operative care, neurological problems, etc. Intensive care unit teams are made up of intensive care doctors, nurses and specialists who are responsible for providing critical care to patients with a variety of surgical, medical and trauma conditions. Every intensive care unit in a hospital has a different environment that reflects the special surgical and medical procedures being performed there. The various equipments used in intensive care units are heart monitor, artificial ventilators, dialysis machines, etc. Intensive care is an upcoming field of science that has undergone rapid development over the past few decades. This book explores all the important aspects of this branch of medicine in the present day scenario. It will provide comprehensive knowledge to the readers.

Various studies have approached the subject by analyzing it with a single perspective, but the present book provides diverse methodologies and techniques to address this field. This book contains theories and applications needed for understanding the subject from different perspectives. The aim is to keep the readers informed about the progresses in the field; therefore, the contributions were carefully examined to compile novel researches by specialists from across the globe.

Indeed, the job of the editor is the most crucial and challenging in compiling all chapters into a single book. In the end, I would extend my sincere thanks to the chapter authors for their profound work. I am also thankful for the support provided by my family and colleagues during the compilation of this book.

Editor

1

Aneurysmal Subarachnoid Hemorrhage

Adel E. Ahmed Ganaw, Abdulgafoor M. Tharayil,
Ali O. Mohamed Bel Khair, Saher Tahseen,
Jazib Hassan,
Mohammad Faisal Abdullah Malmstrom and
Sohel Mohamed Gamal Ahmed

Abstract

Aneurysmal subarachnoid hemorrhage (SAH) is a devastating neurological syndrome, which occurs at a rate of 3–25 per 100,000 population. Smoking and hypertension are the most important risk factors of subarachnoid hemorrhage. Rupture of cerebral aneurysm leads to rapid spread of blood into cerebrospinal fluid and subsequently leads to sudden increase of intracranial pressure and severe headache. Subarachnoid hemorrhage is associated with neurological (such as re-bleeding and vasospasm) and systemic (such as myocardial injury and hyponatremia) complications that are causes of high mortality and morbidity. Although patients with poor-grade subarachnoid hemorrhage are at higher risk of neurological and systemic complications, the early and aggressive management of this group of patient has decreased overall mortality by 17% in last 40 years. Early aneurysm repair, close monitoring in dedicated neurological intensive care unit, prevention, and aggressive management of medical and neurological complications are the most important strategies to improve outcome.

Keywords: albumin, aneurysmal subarachnoid hemorrhage, vasospasm, re-bleeding, hyponatremia, cardiac complication, coiling, clipping

1. Introduction

Subarachnoid hemorrhage (SAH) is a devastating disease and is associated with high mortality and poor outcomes among survivors, management by multidisciplinary team is associated with improved outcomes; however, intensive care management presents big challenge. Most of spontaneous SAH is due to the rupture of saccular aneurysm, the prevalence of intracranial saccular aneurysm by radiographic and autopsy series is 5%, about 20–30% of patients have several aneurysms [1].

Aneurysmal SAH (aSAH) occurs at a rate of 2–16 per 100,000 population, mostly occurring between 40 and 60 years of age; however, young children and elderly can be affected. The incidence of SAH is higher in women than men, which may be due to hormonal status. African Americans are at a higher risk of SAH than Caucasian Americans. Mortality rate is about 60% within first 6 months [2, 3].

2. Circle of Willis

The circle of Willis is an anastomotic structure. It is formed when the internal carotid artery enters the cranial cavity bilaterally and divides into the anterior cerebral artery and middle cerebral artery, and the anterior cerebral arteries are then united by an anterior communicating artery. These anastomoses form the anterior half of the circle (anterior circulation). Posteriorly, the basilar artery branches to give left and right posterior cerebral artery (posterior circulation). Posterior cerebral arteries join the internal carotid system anteriorly to complete the circle via posterior communicating arteries. **Figure 1** shows the common sites of cerebral aneurysm [4, 5].

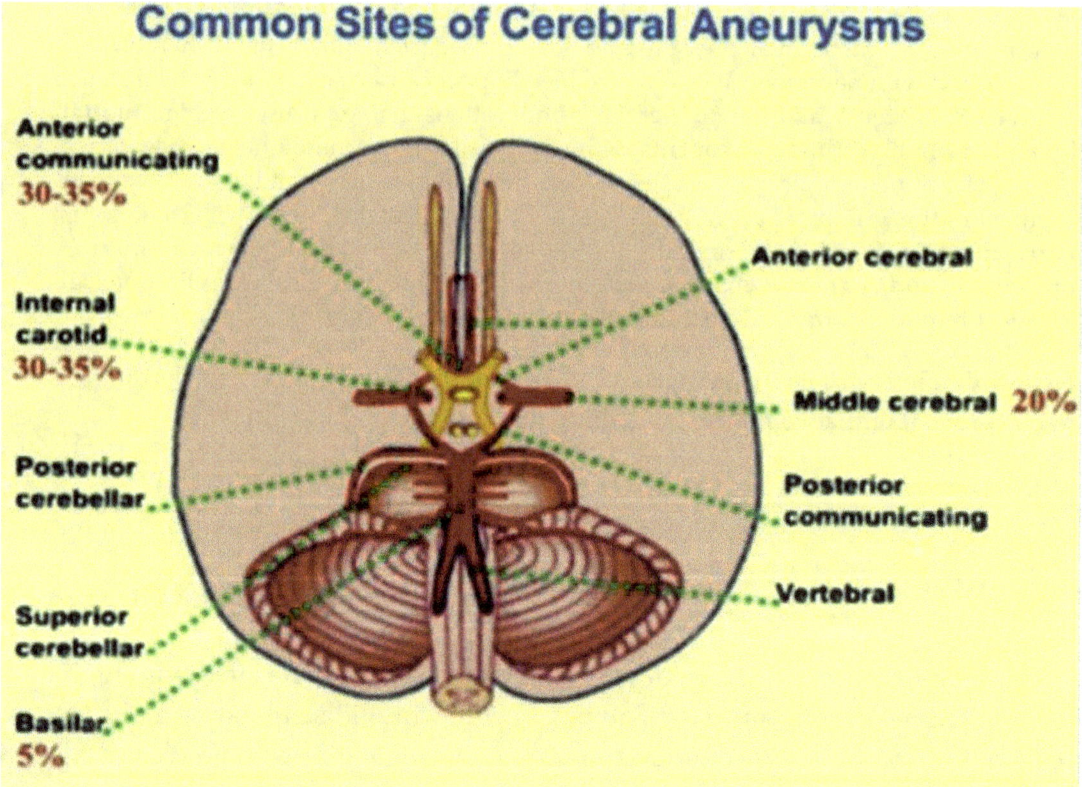

Figure 1. Common sites of cerebral aneurysm [5].

3. Etiology

Subarachnoid hemorrhage is defined as bleeding into the space between the arachnoid and pia mater of the meninges enclosing the brain (subarachnoid space). The most common reason for spontaneous (non-traumatic) SAH is the rupture of a cerebral aneurysm (85%) [5].

In about 15% of non-traumatic SAH, no bleeding cause is identified by digital subtraction angiography (DSA). In these scenarios, differentiation between perimesencephalic and non-perimesencephalic location of the SAH is very important to determine further therapeutic approach [3].

Perimesencephalic SAH (PMSAH) is defined by the absence of an aneurysmatic bleeding and the classic presence of blood within the perimesencephalic and prepontine cisterns [3].

Computed topography angiogram (CTA) and magnetic resonance angiography (MRA) have high sensitivity of excluding aneurysmal bleedings in PMSAH.

PMSAH has less complication and better prognosis than aneurysmal SAH.

Non-perimesencephalic is SAH without bleeding source in the baseline DSA, the chance of positive findings in a follow-up angiography fluctuated between 5 and 35%, that is why DSA should be repeated not before 3 weeks after the initial bleeding if there are no other therapeutic indications [3].

Non-traumatic SAH can be caused by various other non-aneurysmatic causes (**Table 1**), and the management of these cases must be performed according to the underlying cause [3].

Disease	Example
Infectious arterial vasculitis	Mycotic (infectious) aneurysm
	Meningovascular lues
	Lyme disease
	Gnathostomiasis (Gnathostoma spinigerum)
Immune vasculitis	Primary CNS angiitis
	Polyarteritis nodosa
	Wegener's vasculitis
	Churg-Strauss syndrome
	Behçet's disease
Other cerebrovascular diseases	Arteriovenous angioma
	Dural arteriovenous fistula
	Spinal arterial aneurysm
	Intracranial arterial dissection
	Venous sinus thrombosis
	Cerebral amyloid angiopathy
	Moyamoya disease

Disease	Example
Tumor	Intracranial und intraspinal tumor
Hematology	Sickle cell anemia
Drugs	Anticoagulants and thrombolytic therapy
Substance abuse	Cocaine

Table 1. Rare causes of non-traumatic SAH [3].

4. Risk factors

Most spontaneous SAHs result from the rupture of intracranial aneurysms; therefore, risk factors for aneurysm formation overlap with risk factors for SAH.

(1) Cigarette smoking: It is associated with 11-fold increased risk of SAH. Worldwide, it is the most important preventable risk factor, which has been proved in numerous cohort (relative risk, RR, of current smoking, 2.2) and case-control studies (odds ratio, OR, 3.1); cigarette smoking also hastened aneurysm growth rate [2, 3].

(2) Hypertension: It is a major risk factor for SAH and possibly for aneurysm formation and fatal aneurysm rupture. Treatment of hypertension may reduce the risk of aneurysmal SAH [6].

(3) Alcohol abuse: Excessive alcohol abuse raises the possibility for SAH independent of cigarette smoking, age, and history of hypertension [3].

(4) Genetic risk: The risk of SAH increases seven folds in first-degree relatives of patient; in addition, number of rare inherited conditions (Autosomal dominant polycystic kidney, Ehler-Danlos syndrome) are associated with cerebral aneurysm and SAH [2, 6].

(5) Use of sympathomimetic drugs such as (cocaine) [6].

(6) Female sex: This is believed to be due to estrogen deficiency (estrogen replacement therapy reduces the risk), so it is higher in postmenopausal women than premenopausal ones [3, 6].

(7) Antithrombotic therapy: It increases the severity of the hemorrhage, there are no data to prove whether antithrombotic therapy increases the risk of aneurysmal rupture or not [3, 6].

(8) Inflammation seems to play a vital role in the pathogenesis and growth of intracranial aneurysms. Prominent mediators include the nuclear factor k - light-chain enhancer of activated B cells (NF-κB), tumor necrosis factor, macrophages, and reactive oxygen species. Although there are no controlled studies in humans, 3-hydroxy-3-methylglutaryl coenzyme A reductase inhibitors (statins) and calcium channel blockers could impede aneurysm formation by the inhibition of NF-κB and other pathways [6, 7].

(9) Aneurysm size of 7 mm increases risk of rupture and subsequent SAH [6].

(10) Aneurysm morphology such as bottleneck shape and the ratio of size of aneurysm to parent vessels are associated with rupture of aneurysm [6].

(11) The risk of SAH increases in symptomatic patient with large unruptured cerebral aneurysm especially if it is located either on posterior communicating artery or on the vertebrobasilar system [6].

5. Pathophysiology

Smoking, chronic hypertension, and alcohol abuse lead to weakened arterial tunica media. Chronic exposure to intravascular shear stress leads to pouching of the weakened wall, especially in the vicinity of bifurcations where turbulent flow is prominent.

The aneurysmal rupture is directly proportional to the size of the aneurysm, which is rising from 0.05% in aneurysms less than 10 mm to 6% for those greater than 25 mm.

More than 80% of cerebral aneurysm arises from the anterior carotid circulation (anterior and posterior communicating and middle cerebral arteries), with only 10–20% arising from the posterior vertebrobasilar circulation [1, 2].

Subsequent to aneurysmal rupture, blood spreads quickly within cerebrospinal fluid (CSF), rapidly increasing intracranial pressure (ICP), this sudden increase in the ICP leads to severe headache, cerebral edema, and hydrocephalus. Bleeding usually lasts for a few seconds; however, re-bleeding is common and occurs within the first 24 h. The presence of blood and breakdown products of hemoglobin in the subarachnoid space is responsible for meningeal irritation, meningism, and vasospasm [2].

6. Clinical manifestation

Headache is the hallmark of aSAH in awake patient who describes it "as worst headache in their life," this headache has a sudden onset and immediately reaches maximal intensity (thunderclap headache). Sentinel headache is also reported by 10–43% of patients, which is minor headache, and it is symptoms of minor hemorrhage (sentinel bleed or warning leak). Most of these minor hemorrhages occur within 2–8 weeks before major hemorrhage [6, 8].

The headache may be associated with nausea and/or vomiting, stiff neck, photophobia, brief loss of consciousness, or focal neurological deficits (including cranial nerve palsies).

Seizures occur in about 26% of patients within the first 24 h of SAH, most of the time before medical care is accessed. It is common in presence of intracerebral hemorrhage, in hypertensive patients, and patient with middle cerebral or anterior communicating artery aneurysms [6].

7. Diagnosis

7.1. Non-contrast head CT scan

Non-contrast CT scan is the cornerstone of SAH diagnosis, it confirms the presence of blood clot in subarachnoid space in most of the cases if the scan is performed in the first 24 h, and it may also provide an idea of the cause of the bleeding and site of the aneurysm. In addition to that, it is useful in diagnosis of intraventricular and subdural hematoma [2, 6].

CT scan sensitivity is highest in the first 3 days (close to 100%) and progressively decreases over time to about 58% in the fifth day [6].

7.2. Lumbar puncture

The typical findings are an elevated opening pressure and presence of xanthochromia, which can last for 2 weeks after SAH. Xanthochromia represents hemoglobin degradation products in CSF and indicates that the blood has been in CSF for at least 2 h [6, 9].

7.3. Brain MRI

MRI has advantages over CT brain in detection of subacute subarachnoid hemorrhage (after 4 days), when head CT scan is negative and there is clinical suspicion of SAH, and possibly avoiding the need of lumbar puncture. The most important disadvantages are difficulty in scanning acutely confused ill patient, without sedation for at least 45 minutes, predisposing to motion artifact, and is expensive in comparison with CT [6].

7.4. Digital subtraction angiography (DSA)

Once diagnosis of SAH has been completed, the source of bleeding must be identified with angiographic studies. Digital subtraction angiography (DSA) is the gold standard for the detection of intracranial aneurysm and study of anatomical features of cerebral blood vessels [3, 6].

7.5. CT and MR angiography

Both CT and MR angiography are useful for screening and pre-surgical planning, they can detect aneurysms ≥3 mm with high degree of sensitivity; however, they are less sensitive than conventional angiography. CTA can be achieved immediately after the diagnosis of SAH by CT scan when the patient is still in scanner; CTA is more practical than MRA in acute setting. CTA is used as an alternative to conventional angiography in SAH patients, especially in acute setting and rapidly declining patient who needs emergent craniotomy for hematoma evacuation. CTA can substitute catheter cerebral angiography in older patient with degenerative vascular disease provided that the quality is excellent and investigation is performed cautiously. Negative CTA should be followed by two- and three-dimensional cerebral angiography in case of diffuse SAH [3, 6]. MRA is rarely indicated in SAH, because of limited routine availability, difficulty in scanning acutely sick patient, who is poorly compliant to commands, which can affect quality of the study, moreover MRA is time consuming and very expensive [6].

8. Grading of SAH

Hard work has been made for the development of scales to clinically grade patients with SAH, to assess the severity of initial injury, to guide treatment decision, to provide prognostic information regarding outcome, and to standardize patient evaluation for scientific study purposes. Since 1933, more than 40 grading systems have been proposed for patients with cerebral aneurysm. Currently, the most commonly used SAH grading scales are the Hunt and Hess scale, Fisher scale, Glasgow Coma Scale (GCS), and the World Federation of Neurological Surgeons (WFNS) scale [10].

8.1. World Federation of Neurosurgeons SAH Scale (WFNS)

In 1998, an expert judgment committee projected the WFNS scale, it was based on GCS and the presence of focal neurological deficit (**Table 2**). Numerous studies found direct association between WFNS grade and outcome [10].

WFNS scale	GCS	Motor deficit, aphasia±hemiparesis or hemiplegia
I	15	Absent
II	14–13	Absent
III	14–13	Present
IV	12–7	Present/absent
V	6–3	Present/absent

Table 2. World Federation of Neurosurgeons SAH scale.

8.2. Prognosis on Admission of Aneurysmal Subarachnoid Hemorrhage (PAASH)

PAASH is solely based on the GCS; it has excellent internal and external validity in regard to clinical outcome. In a study comparing prognostic accuracy of WFNS and PAASH, PAASH had a good prognostic value for patient outcome (**Table 3**) [3].

Scale	Grade	Criteria	Proportion of patient with poor outcome (%)
WFNS	I	GCS 15	14.8
	II	GCS 13–14 no focal deficits	29.4
	III	GCS 13–14 focal deficits	52.6
	IV	GCS 7–12	58.3
	V	GCS 3–6	92.7
PAASH	I	GCS 15	14.8
	II	GCS 11–14	41.3
	III	GCS 8–10	74.4
	IV	GCS 4–7	84.7
	V	GCS 3	93.9

Table 3. Two SAH grading scales with criteria per grade and relation with outcome [3].

8.3. The Hunt and Hess scale

The Hunt and Hess scale was projected in 1968 as an adjustment to an older system initially described by Botterell and colleagues in 1956. The scale was prepared to stratify the surgical risk and to help the surgeon on making appropriate decision in appropriate time. It is well known in the neuroscientific community; however, many of the terms used to define grades, such as drowsy, stupor or deep coma, headache (mild, moderate, severe), nuchal rigidity (slight vs. sever), are subjective and vague which makes this grading system neither reliable nor valid (**Table 4**) [3, 10].

Grade	Clinical description
I	Asymptomatic or minimal headache and slight nuchal rigidity.
II	Moderate to severe headache, nuchal rigidity, no neurological deficit other than cranial nerve palsy.
III	Drowsiness, confusion, or mild focal deficit.
IV	Stupor, moderate to severe hemiparesis, and possibly decerebrate rigidity and vegetative disturbances.
V	Deep coma, decerebrate rigidity, moribund appearance.

Table 4. Hunt and Hess scale.

8.4. Fisher scale

In 1980, the Fisher scale was projected to predict cerebral vasospasm after SAH (**Figure 2**), the scale quantifies the amount of blood seen on CT scan (**Table 5**). It was developed when imaging technology had roughly one-tenth of the resolution currently available. Subarachnoid

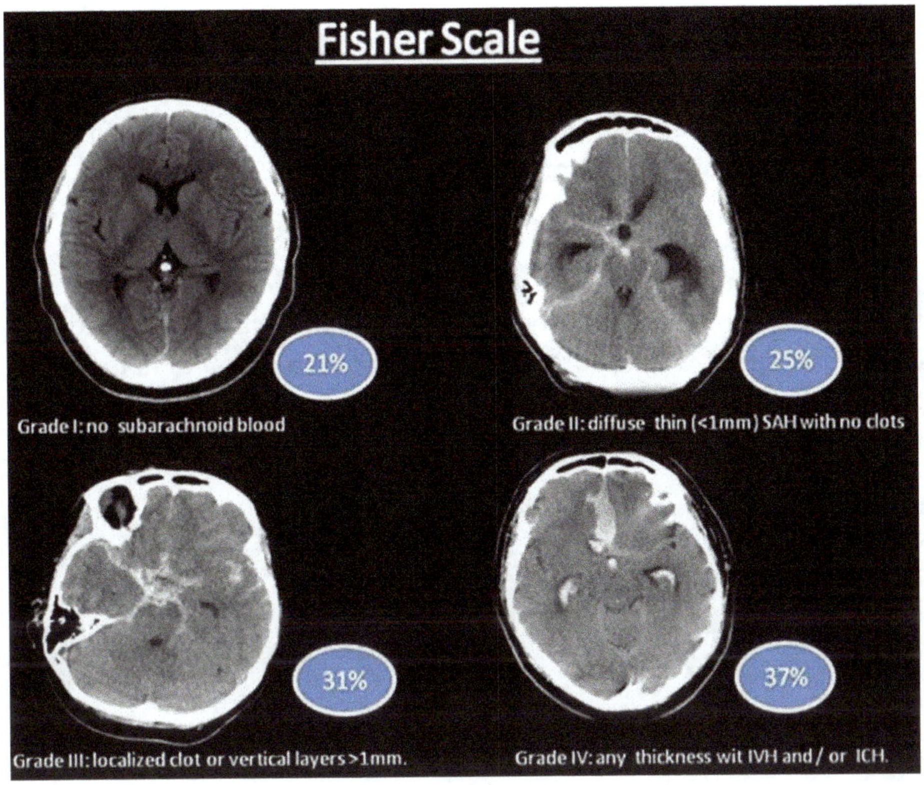

Figure 2. Scale grading system used to quantify the amount of subarachnoid hemorrhage and intraventricular hemorrhage (IVH). The percentages in the circles refer to the risk of vasospasm. Grades III and IV in the scale are the ones with the higher risk to develop "symptomatic vasospasm." Adopted with permission from Ref. [11].

Group	Blood on CT scan
I	No subarachnoid detected.
II	Diffuse or thin vertical layer <1 mm thick.
III	Localized subarachnoid clot and/or vertical layer >1 mm thick.
IV	Intraventricular or intra-parenchymal clot with diffuse or no SAH.

Table 5. Fisher grade scale.

clot less than 1 mm in true thickness is uncommon, as is the finding of no blood on admission CT scan, therefore, grades 1 and 2 were actually be quite uncommon [3, 10].

9. Complications associated with SAH

Complications of subarachnoid hemorrhage can be divided into CNS and systemic compli cations.

9.1. CNS complications

Re-bleeding, vasospasm, hydrocephalus, and seizures are the most important CNS complications of SAH. The high rates of mortality and morbidity after aneurysmal subarachnoid hemorrhage are mainly due to CNS complications.

9.1.1. Re-bleeding

Re-bleeding occurs at a rate of 4–13% in the first 24 h, maximal risk of re-bleeding is in the first 2–12 h, most of re-bleeding (73%) occurs within the first 72 h of initial hemorrhage. Re-bleeding is associated with very high mortality and morbidity, especially if it occurs in the first 12 h after the hemorrhage, the mortality rate reaches to 70% [6, 12].

Many factors are considered as predictor for re-bleeding:

Hunt-Hess grade on admission.

Maximal aneurysmal diameter.

High initial blood pressure.

Sentinel headache preceding SAH.

Longer interval from ictus to admission.

Ventriculostomy before aneurysmal treatment [6, 13].

Re-bleeding diagnosis is based on the deterioration of neurological status and appearance of new hemorrhage in CT scan. Early securing of the aneurysm is the treatment of choice to prevent re-bleeding; however, the optimum time for early intervention is unclear whether intervention within 24 h (ultra-early) is superior to intervention after 3 days [12].

The management of high blood pressure after SAH is still debatable due to the lack of evidence from randomized controlled trial. Data from observational studies propose that aggressive management of blood pressure reduces the risk of re-bleeding, however, at the expense of an increase in secondary ischemia. It looks acceptable but without strong evidence to stop all antihypertensive medications that the patients were taking, and treat hypertension only when it is extremely high. It is very difficult to give limits for extreme blood pressures, because extreme varies between patients and it is affected by many factors such as previous blood pressure, cardiac disease, patient age, and other factors [3].

European stroke organization guidelines for the management of intracranial aneurysm and subarachnoid hemorrhage recommended that the systolic blood pressure should be kept less than 180 mmHg in patients with unsecured aneurysm, till the aneurysm is secured with coiling or clipping. They also recommended keeping mean arterial pressure (MAP) above 90 mmHg when blood pressure is lowered [3].

Nicardipine is short-acting calcium channel blocker, used for smooth control of blood pressure [3, 6].

For patient with an unavoidable delay in obliteration of aneurysm, and great risk of re-bleeding, short-term (72 h) therapy with tranexamic acid or aminocaproic acid is advisable (provided there is no medical contraindication) to decrease the risk of early bleeding. The overall outcome did not noticeably improve in patients treated with tranexamic acid, in spite of a remarkable decrease in re-bleeding [3, 6].

In an uncontrolled study of 18 patients who received an intraoperative dose of Recombinant factor VIIa, no re-bleeding was reported; however, one case had deep venous thrombosis (DVT) and seven had thrombosis in upper extremity in association with peripherally inserted central lines. Currently, there is no evidence to support the use of recombinant factor VIIa [3].

9.1.2. Vasospasm

Vasospasm is luminal narrowing of large cerebral blood arteries after SAH, leading to cerebral ischemia. Vasospasm commonly occurs 3–5 days after initial hemorrhage, with peak vasoconstriction occurring between days 5 and 14; it usually resolves spontaneously after 21 days of SAH. It may manifest in many features such as reduced conscious level, focal neurological deficit, and simply nuchal rigidity; the exclusion of other causes, such as re-bleeding, hydrocephalus, sepsis, and metabolic derangement, is required to confirm the diagnosis [6, 14, 15].

Sometimes there is no correlation between severity of vasospasm and the symptoms of ischemia. There are patients with severe large artery spasm who never become symptomatic and others with quite modest spasm who develop infarction. Possibly various factors play important role in the development of ischemia and infarction, such as distal microcirculatory failure, poor collateral anatomy, and genetic or physiological variations in cellular ischemic tolerance. Vasospasm is confirmed angiographically in 70% of SAH patient, however it manifests as symptomatic spasm in 36% of all patients with SAH [6, 14, 15].

Age more than 80 years, smoking, hypertension, SAH clot volume (a higher Fisher's grade), location of aneurysm (vertebral artery, right sylvian fissure, pericallosal middle cerebral artery [MCA]), left ventricular hypertrophy, and treatment modality are the main risk factors for the development of cerebral vasospasm [15].

Digital subtraction angiography (DSA) is the gold standard diagnostic investigation to diagnose vasospasm (reduced arterial diameter). Computed tomography angiography (CTA) and MRI studies are alternative investigations to DSA [15].

Transcranial Doppler sonography (TCD) can be used at the bedside to aid the diagnosis of vasospasm. The TCD criteria for vasospasm include a mean flow velocity (MFV) greater than 120 cm/s, change in MFV value of more than 50 cm/s over 24 h, and Lindegaard ratio more than 3 (Lindegaard is a ratio derived from concurrent measurements of MFV in MCA and distal ipsilateral extracranial ICA). Diffusion-perfusion mismatch on MRI is an useful investigation for the identification of early stages of vasospasm. Increase in motor-evoked potential threshold more than 50 mA from the baseline value is an accurate indicator of vasospasm.

Inflammatory marker such as C-reactive protein has been investigated for its ability to predict vasospasm. In 93 SAH patients, postoperative and not preoperative C-reactive proteins were associated with vasospasm and poor outcome with a cut-off value of 4 mg/dL [15].

9.1.2.1. Pathophysiology of cerebral vasospasm

It is complicated. Various cascades in affected blood vessels and neurons are in play, they can be grouped into two categories.

9.1.2.1.1. Elevated intracellular calcium

After SAH, calcium influxes into smooth muscle and neuron is rapidly increased through N-methyl-D-aspartate receptor (NMDA) and voltage-gated calcium channels, moreover glutamate is increased and activates NMDA receptors, leading to further calcium influx in smooth muscle, high intracellular calcium concentration enhances binding of calcium to calmodulin. Calmodulin activates myosin light chain kinase (MLCK) to phosphorylate myosin, which induces myosin-actin interaction and smooth muscle contraction and blood vessels constriction [14].

In neuronal cells, increase in intracellular calcium leads to hyperactivation of enzymes, such as protease, endonuclease, phospholipase, which destabilizes cell body and membrane, leading to cellular injury and death [14].

9.1.2.1.2. Vasoactive compound and vessel wall injury

In days 3–5 after SAH, oxy hemoglobin—a red blood cell breakdown product—inhibits nitric oxide (physiologic vasodilator) and stimulates leukocytes to produce endothelin-1 (physiologic vasoconstrictor), resulting in potent vasoconstriction. Furthermore, breakdown of oxyhemoglobin leads to release of reactive oxygen species and iron which leads to oxidative damage to blood vessel walls [14].

In addition, production of vasoactive compounds after SAH, such as serotonin, norepinephrine, and angiotensin II, leads to potent vasoconstriction [14].

9.1.2.2. Treatment of cerebral vasospasm and cerebral ischemia

9.1.2.2.1. Nimodipine

It is L-type calcium channel blocker—it is the only drug that has been approved for SAH in European countries and the USA. It improves long-term neurological outcome if it is started on admission and administered for 21 days. The recommended oral dosage is 60 mg 4 hourly orally (maximum daily dose 360 mg). The role of nimodipine is based on general brain protective mechanism as there is no proof to suggest that it treats angiographically diagnosed vasospasm, and it also increases fibrinolytic activity and inhibits cortical spreading ischemia [2, 6, 12, 15].

Recently, biodegradable silica-based nimodipine implant was effectively used in the management of vasospasm. It is associated with higher nimodipine cerebrospinal fluid (CSF) to plasma ratio than traditional nimodipine [15].

The continuous intravenous infusion of nimodipine is not recommended as it is not superior to oral nimodipine and is associated with high incidence of hypotension especially in hypovolemic patient (an adequate systolic BP of 130–150 mmHg takes priority over nimodipine administration, and it should be stopped if a stable BP can't be maintained).

The recommended dose of Intravenous nimodipine is 1 mg/h in the first 6 h, then increased to 1.5 mg/h in next 6 h, then increased to 2 mg/h (maximum dose) [2, 6, 15].

9.1.2.2.2. Fasudil

It is Rho-kinase inhibitor, it decreases smooth muscle contraction and inhibits TNF-induced IL-6 release from C6 glioma cells, and it causes better angiographic reduction in vasospasm and better neurological outcome than nimodipine. Fasudil is approved for use in Japan and China but not in the USA or Europe [12, 15].

9.1.2.2.3. Triple-H therapy (hemodynamic augmentation therapy)

It is a combination of induced hypertension, hypervolemia, and hemodilution (HHH) to improve blood flow through narrowed cerebral blood vessels due to vasospasm. Triple-H has been for years used as a treatment of choice for the treatment of delayed cerebral ischemia, although the literature supporting its effectiveness and safety is lacking, in fact triple-H therapy is associated with an increase in the risk of systemic complications such as heart failure, pulmonary edema, and infections; therefore, the use of prophylactic triple-H therapy is not recommended [3, 12].

Angiographic vasospasm without a new neurological deficit should not be treated. The development of unexplained new neurological deficit or change in conscious level, immediate aggressive therapy should be started. The first step is a fluid bolus with normal saline to increase cerebral blood flow (CBF) in ischemic area, the goal is to maintain euvolemia. Hypervolemia and hemodilution do not increase cerebral oxygen delivery and might cause adverse events. If patients fail to respond completely to the fluid, management may undergo a trial of hypertension. Blood pressure is increased gradually with the use of a vasopressor. Neurological assessment should be repeated frequently in each blood pressure step (systolic blood pressure 180 mmHg / 190 mmHg / 200 mmHg), and the target should be based on neurological improvement. If the patient did not respond to induced hypertension (systolic blood pressure of 200–220 mmHg), a rescue cerebral angioplasty should be considered [12].

9.1.2.2.4. Balloon angioplasty

Cerebral angioplasty is indicated in symptomatic patient with cerebral vasospasm, who is not responding to hypertensive therapy, Prophylactic angioplasty is not recommended [2, 6, 12].

Cerebral angioplasty may lead to arterial dissection, rupture, thrombosis, infarction, hemorrhage, and reperfusion injury leading to cerebral edema [6, 15].

9.1.2.2.5. *Intra-arterial papaverine*

Up to 300 mg of papaverine per hemisphere is used for the treatment of distal vasospasm.

The main disadvantages of intra-arterial papaverine may require repeating, relatively short-acting, neurotoxic, seizures, blindness, coma, irreversible brain injury, arrhythmia, and hemodynamic instability refractory to treatment [2].

9.1.2.2.6. *Magnesium sulphate*

Currently, there is no evidence to support the use of magnesium sulphate ($MgSO_4$) prophylactically or as a treatment modality in delayed cerebral ischemia (DCI). In the Mash 2 Trial, $MgSO_4$ did not improve primary outcome. However, intrathecal and cisternal administration of $MgSO_4$ significantly decreased the severity of vasospasm without any reduction in incidence of DCI or functional outcome [3, 6, 15].

9.1.2.2.7. *Statins*

Recent meta-analysis reported no role of statin in SAH, and a larger phase 3 trial (Simvastatin in Aneurysmal Subarachnoid Hemorrhage [STASH]) failed to confirm any beneficial effect of statin for long- or short-term outcome and should not be used routinely in acute stage [6, 12, 15].

9.1.2.2.8. *Endothelin A-receptor antagonist*

Clazosentan (endothelin-1 receptor antagonist) had been presented to be associated with a dose-dependent decrease in the frequency of vasospasm in a phase IIb trial (Clazosentan to Overcome Neurological iSChemia and Infarct OccUrring after Subarachnoid hemorrhage [CONSCIOUS-1]) [6, 15].

Two further trials were carried out:

CONSCIOUS-2: A double blind, placebo-controlled trial, clazosentan was given at a rate of 5 mg/h for 15 days to patients treated with aneurysm clipping. There was statistically insignificant decrease in mortality and vasospasm-related morbidity [15].

CONSCIOUS-3: This study was double blind, placebo- controlled study to assess whether clazosentan reduced vasospasm-related mortality after securing aneurysmal SAH by endovascular coiling. The study was halted prematurely after completion of conscious-2 trial and failed to show any beneficial effect of clazosentan.

It is worth noting that patient who received clazosentan had more pulmonary complications, anemia, and hypotension than the placebo group [6, 15].

9.1.2.3. *Other miscellaneous treatments*

9.1.2.3.1. *Milrinone*

In a large case series based on the assessment of all subarachnoid hemorrhage patients diagnosed with delayed ischemic neurological deficit between April 1999 and April 2006, 88 patients were found to have received milrinone infusion for a median of 9.8 days. At 44.6 months, 75% of them had a good functional outcome. Because of obvious limitations in this study, further studies are warranted [15].

9.1.2.3.2. Stellate ganglion block

A small study included 15 patients who had refractory cerebral vasospasm after surgical clipping of aneurysm. Stellate ganglion block was performed using 10 mL of bupivacaine 0.5% on the side with maximum cerebral blood flow velocity. Neurological status, cerebral blood flow velocity, and pulsatility index were assessed before and 10 min, 30 min, 2 h, 6 h, 12 h, and 24 h after stellate ganglion block. The ipsilateral Middle Cerebral Artery (MCA) mean velocity was reduced with reduction in neurological deficit and improvement in GCS; because of obvious limitations in this study, further studies are required [15].

9.1.2.3.3. Albumin

Albumin 25% has been tried to improve outcomes in a pilot study (Albumin in Subarachnoid Hemorrhage trial). The incidence of vasospasm, DCI, and cerebral infarction was significantly reduced with high dose of albumin; however, this is still experimental and further studies are required to support this study [12, 15].

9.1.3. Hydrocephalus

Hydrocephalus is one of the common complications of SAH; it is either acute or chronic.

Acute hydrocephalus occurs in 15–87% of SAH patients as a result of obstruction of CSF flow by blood products or adhesion, some clinician avoid insertion of a ventricular drain in these cases immediately as half of them will recover spontaneously and there is a risk of re-bleeding and infection (meningitis and ventriculitis). Another approach recommended is to start immediate external ventricular drainage (keeping intracranial pressure between 10 and 20 mm Hg), especially when obstructive hydrocephalus is suspected or when the lumbar drainage is contraindicated (sever high intracranial pressure) [3, 6].

It has been recommended to apply lumbar drainage as a consecutive treatment of external ventricular drain (EVD) before shunting in cases with spontaneous intracerebral hemorrhage (ICH) when there is no blood in the third and fourth ventricles (communicating hydrocephalus). This option can be considered as an alternate approach to decrease the occurrence of permanent shunts, improve brain relaxation, and decrease risk of vasospasm; however, this approach may cause downward herniation in some cases such as supratentorial swelling and the development of hygroma. Currently no prospective clinical trial supports lumbar drain insertion either for spontaneous ICH or cases with SAH [3, 6].

Acute hydrocephalus increases risk of cerebral infarction and re-bleeding and eventually may worsen the mortality and morbidity secondary to cerebral infarction and re-bleeding [3, 6].

Chronic shunt-dependent hydrocephalus, which occurs in 8.9–48% of patients with SAH due to a decrease in CSF absorption at the arachnoid granulation, it is usually treated with shunt placement [3, 6].

Many factors are considered as predictor of hydrocephalus:

- Elderly.
- Intraventricular hemorrhage.
- Hypertension.
- Hyponatremia at presentation.
- Low Glasgow Coma Score at presentation.
- Antifibrinolytic agents.

9.1.4. Seizures

More than 26% of patients with SAH experience seizure-like episodes, the majority of such patients report the onset of these seizures occurring before medical care are accessed. There are variable risk factors for the development of early seizures, such as aneurysm in middle cerebral artery, thickness of SAH clot, hypertension, intracerebral hematoma, re-bleeding, cerebral infarction, and poor neurological grade. Routine use of anticonvulsants is associated with worsening of the cognitive function, delayed ischemia, fever, and vasospasm; however, it may be considered in patients with high risk of delayed seizure [3, 6].

9.2. Systemic complications associated with SAH

The high morbidity and mortality associated with SAH is not only due to neurological complications, non-neurological complications also play a major role in increasing mortality and morbidity rates [16].

9.2.1. Cardiac complications

Cardiac complications occur in about 50% of patients with SAH; it ranges from mild elevation in cardiac enzymes and electrocardiogram (ECG) changes to obvious clinical and echocardiographic pathology. Cardiac damage markers are associated with an increased mortality and poor outcome and DCI [16].

9.2.1.1. Pathophysiology

9.2.1.1.1. Mild myocardial injury

This is presented by mild elevation in serum cardiac troponin I (not reaching diagnostic threshold of MI). This elevation occurs in 20–68% of patients with SAH. The degree of neurological injury, as graded by the Hunt-Hess scale, is an independent predictor of myocardial injury in SAH patients. Serum troponin is a powerful predictor for cardiac and pulmonary complications, such as hypotension requiring vasopressor, left ventricular (LV) dysfunction, pulmonary edema, and DCI, especially in patient presenting with a high grade on WFNS.

Serum troponin is a more specific and sensitive indicator of myocardial injury than creatinine kinase-MB; therefore, serum troponin levels and trends must be monitored through serial measurements particularly in SAH patients with past history of cardiovascular disease [16].

9.2.1.1.2. Cardiomyopathy

Neurogenic stunned myocardium (NSM) is the most severe form of myocardial injury in SAH, it occurs in 20–30% of patients with SAH. The elevated level of sympathetic tone leads to calcium overload with reduced sensitization of contractile filaments to this cation, eventually causing myocardial depression. It is characterized by subendocardial contraction band necrosis.

Echocardiography shows abnormal LV contractility and abnormal wall motion, which are reversible but sometimes leads to cardiogenic shock [16].

CK-MB levels, female gender, and poor neurological grade are predictors of LV dysfunction.

Severe LV dysfunction decreases cardiac output (CO) and mean arterial pressure leading to reduction in cerebral blood flow (CBF). Furthermore, LV dysfunction may be associated with cerebral vasospasm and significant decrease in cerebral perfusion pressure therefore, optimization of heart function is critical to prevent progression of neurological dysfunction and to promote recovery in patients with SAH [2, 6, 16–18].

The use of inotropes such as dobutamine or milrinone may be required to optimize cardiac output (CO). In severe LV dysfunction, implementation of intra-aortic balloon pump may be required [2, 6, 16, 18].

9.2.1.1.3. ECG findings

It is common in SAH patients, particularly in the first 3 days of presentation, nearly 50–100% of SAH patients will show different forms of ECG changes such as ST segments changes, T wave changes, QTc prolongation, and Prominent U wave (**Table 6**) [16, 17].

Around 4–8% of SAH patients will have malignant arrhythmias such as ventricular tachycardia (VT), torsade de pointe, and asystole [16, 18].

ECG abnormality	Reported incidence (%)
ST-segment changes	15–51
Inverted or isoelectric T waves	12–92
QTc prolongation	11–66
Prominent U waves	4–47
Sinus bradycardia	16
Sinus tachycardia	8.5

Table 6. ECG changes after subarachnoid hemorrhage [17].

Management of arrhythmias in SAH patients depends upon the type of arrhythmia, clinical significance, and the patient's condition. As a first step, it is vital to assure satisfactory oxygenation and correct electrolyte abnormalities and metabolic disturbance.

The use of beta-blockers to treat cardiac tachyarrhythmia in SAH should be balanced against hypotension and decrease in cerebral blood flow (CBF). A new study concluded that the presence of arrhythmias is associated with poor outcome; in spite of this, no correlation was found between severity of cardiac arrhythmia and the site or the extent of intracranial hemorrhage on CT scan, neurological condition, or the location of ruptured malformation [6, 16, 18].

9.2.2. Electrolyte disturbance

The SAH is associated with different forms of electrolyte disturbances, such as hyponatremia, hypokalemia, hypocalcaemia, and hypomagnesaemia [6].

9.2.2.1. Hyponatremia

Hyponatremia is the most common clinically significant electrolyte derangement associated with SAH. It has an incidence ranging from 35 to 56 %, its diagnostic and therapeutic dilemma needs to be sorted to improve outcome of SAH patient [2, 16, 19].

Syndrome of inappropriate antidiuretic hormone secretion (SIADH) is the most common cause of hyponatremia; other causes are acute cortisol insufficiency, cerebral salt wasting syndrome (CSW), extreme fluid therapy, and/or diuretic therapy.

Kao et al. stated that 34.5% of severe hyponatremia were secondary to SIADH, whereas 23% were considered to be due to CSW. Noteworthy, the patients recruited in this study had more severe SAH than in the comparative studies, and the inclusion criterion was a plasma Na <130 mEq/L [19].

Irrespective of the cause, hyponatremia in SAH patients increases hospital stay, risk of vasospasm, and mortality rate.

The incidence of hyponatremia is associated with the location of aneurysmal rupture. Hyponatremia mostly occurs after rupture of anterior communicating artery (AComA). It was seen in 52.4% of patients with AComA; it may be because the hypothalamus is supplied by branch from AComA [19].

9.2.2.2. Causes of hyponatremia

SIADH is considered the most common cause of severe hyponatremia in SAH; it is secondary to excessive secretion of antidiuretic hormone as a result of stimulation of hypothalamus with traumatic or ischemic factor, causing increased water reabsorption in the distal convoluted tubule of the kidney, resulting in dilutional hyponatremia and fluid retention [19].

In CSW, the increase in urinary sodium excretion and urine output are due to abnormal release of atrial and brain natriuretic hormones, causing reduction in circulating blood volume, as well as extracellular fluid. Cerebral salt wasting syndrome can be treated with hypertonic saline solution which increases cerebral blood flow, brain tissue oxygen [19].

Clinically, it is very difficult to differentiate between SIADH and CSW syndrome, due to significant overlapping clinical findings between both syndromes: both syndromes are associated with brain lesions; have normal thyroid, adrenal, and kidney functions are hyponatremic, hypouricemic and have concentrated urines, high urinary sodium over 40 mEq/L, and high fractional excretion (FE) of urate. The only clinical difference is the state of their extracellular volume (ECV): being hypervolemic or euvolemic in SIADH and hypovolemic in CSW (**Table 7**) [20].

ECV assessment by usual clinical criteria is very difficult, not accurate to any degree [20].

Determination fractional excretion (FE) of urate is very helpful to differentiate between these syndromes, FEurate, normal 4–11%, has been constantly increased to >11% in both syndromes and has a distinctive relationship to serum sodium in both syndromes. In SIADH, correction of hyponatremia will normalize FEurate to 4–11% but in CSW syndrome FEurate consistently > 11% event after correction of hyponatremia (**Figure 3**).

This algorithm is useful only with normal glomerular filtration rate GFR, because FEurate can exceed normal values in patients with reduced glomerular filtration rate (GFR) [20].

Cortisol deficiency is one of the important causes of hyponatremia, which has not been well investigated in SAH patients because routine examination of adrenocorticotropic hormone (ACTH)/cortisol dynamic is not part of SAH work up [19].

Klose et al. and Parenti et al. investigated pituitary function post-SAH and found that between 7.1 and 12% of patients are cortisol-deficient at the time of presentation with SAH [20].

	SIADH	CSW
Plasma volume	↑ or ↔	↓↓
Water balance	↑ or ↔	Negative
Signs and symptoms of dehydration	Absent	Present
Central venous pressure	↑ or ↔	↓↓
Salt balance	Variable	Negative
Hematocrit	↔	↑ or ↔
Serum osmolality	↓↓	↓↓
Urine sodium	↑	↑↑
Urine volume	↓or ↔	↑↑
Plasma BUN/creatinine	↓↓	↑ or ↔
Treatment	Fluid restriction, hypertonic saline, furosemide, demeclocycline	Normal saline, hypertonic saline, fludrocortisone

Table 7. Difference between SIADH and CSW [21].

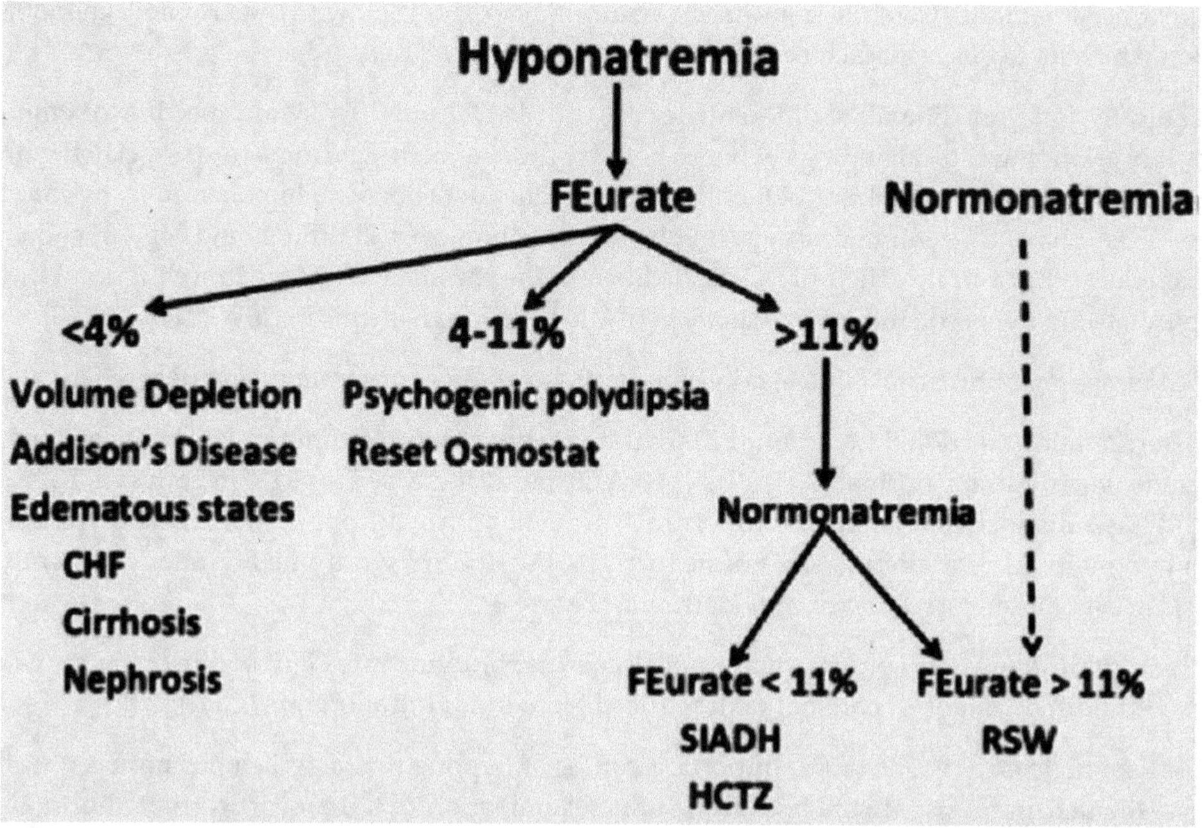

Figure 3. Algorithm for determining the cause of hyponatremia, using FEurate.

9.2.2.3. Treatment of hyponatremia

Patients with SAH should be closely monitored in an intensive care unit, preferably neurointensive care for at least 2–3 weeks post-SAH, to allow for close monitoring of signs and symptoms of delayed cerebral ischemia (DCI), cerebral vasospasm, as well as fluid and electrolyte balance on daily basis, which can help treating doctors in early detection and efficient management of hyponatremia. A daily follow-up of electrolyte is ideal and should be routine. If patients require intravenous hypertonic saline, sodium level should be checked every 4 h.

Urgent investigations of sodium level are mandatory if there are changes in mental status, massive fluctuation of fluid balance, and/or polyuria.

Rapid correction of hyponatremia can cause central myelinolysis and should be avoided, but insufficient correction of hyponatremia can result in brain edema, convulsion, and death [17, 20–22].

Fluid restriction to correct hyponatremia is associated with increased risk of cerebral vasospasm [19, 23].

Audibert et al. looked at the endocrinological response to severe SAH and found alterations in plasma level of numerous hormones such as aldosterone, renin, ADH, angiotensin, ANP, and BNP. However, these changes are noted during the first 12 days post-SAH. It is not practical to correctly and promptly get hormone levels, because their profile fluctuates frequently.

The expertise recommended that assessing bedside sodium and fluid balance is the best valuable and economical technique for avoiding hyponatremia in patients with SAH [17].

Traditionally, patients with SAH are maintained on sodium chloride-based fluids (i.e., 0.9% saline) for baseline and fluid replacement requirements, to avoid cerebral edema due to fluid shifts across a damaged blood-brain barrier [19].

The recent guidelines of the Neurocritical Care Society for the management of patients with SAH suggested avoiding large amounts of free water intake and fluid restriction to treat hyponatremia [19].

In addition, the guidelines of the American Heart Association recommend that volume contraction be replaced with isotonic fluids (Class IIa, Level B evidence) and that large volumes of hypotonic fluids should be avoided in patients with SAH. The guidelines, however, did not make recommendations on the composition of baseline fluid administration in SAH patients [17].

Recently, Lehmann et al. suggested balanced crystalloids and colloid solutions (those with electrolyte compositions similar to plasma) in SAH patients, which do not cause frequent hyponatremia or hypo-osmolality, also prevent electrolyte imbalance such as hyperchloremia, hyper osmolality, and extreme positive fluid balances associated with saline-based intravenous fluids [19, 24].

Fluid restriction to less than 500 mL/day is the treatment of choice in SIADH, although such approach may not be feasible in SAH, because fluid restriction can cause cerebral vasospasm and subsequently cerebral infarction. What's more, most of these patients are not fully conscious and require enteral feeding which results in a daily fluid intake of 1–2 L [19, 25].

Therapeutic options for water restriction include hypertonic saline solutions and albumin [19]. Hypertonic saline (2–3% solution) not only increases plasma sodium concentration efficiently and rapidly but also increases the risk of pulmonary edema and heart failure and neurological complications secondary to the increase in blood volume [19].

Fludrocortisone causes sodium retention, but it is associated with fluid overload and limited evidence of its effectiveness [19].

Vasopressin receptor antagonists such as conivaptan have been projected and trialed in small studies but have not become routine therapy, because harmful effect secondary to the rapid increase in plasma sodium (4–6 mEq/L) [19, 26].

Acute cortisol deficiency is typically corrected with administration of parenteral hydrocortisone, but the beneficial effect of hydrocortisone is still uncertain and further studies are required, because it is not clear whether corticosteroid therapy is effective in management of acute relative adrenal insufficiency after SAH [19, 27].

Overall, the management of hyponatremia in SAH patients necessitates additional investigation of treatment options that avoid fluid restriction, and further studies will help standardize ideal care.

9.2.3. Fever

Fever is one of the common medical complications of SAH and occurs in 70% of SAH patients. Fever may be due hypothalamic effect of the hemorrhage; it is associated with the severity of the injury, amount of hemorrhage, and development of vasospasm. Effective fever management may improve functional outcome. Paracetamol is the treatment of choice for fever. Active cooling is very effective but adverse effects of shivering may offset its benefit [6, 17].

It is worth noting that the infectious cause such as pneumonia needs to be excluded [17].

9.2.4. Anemia

Anemia is very common and is associated with poor outcome, due to compromising brain oxygen delivery. Correction of anemia and high hemoglobin value improve outcome after SAH. Current guidance recommends to keep hemoglobin concentration between 8 and 10 g/dL [17].

9.2.5. Thrombocytopenia and deep venous thrombosis (DVT)

Heparin-induced thrombocytopenia (HIT) is directly associated with the number of angiographic procedures have been performed. Patients with heparin-induced thrombocytopenia type II seems to be at high risk of thrombotic complications, vasospasm, and poor outcome.

Currently, it is uncertain whether there is practical means of avoiding HIT (as it is essential in angiographic procedures); however, it is vital to know this complication to avoid further heparin exposure and to use non-heparin substitute under the supervision of a hematologist.

DVT is relatively recurrent event after SAH, especially in immobilized patients [3, 6].

Table 8 and **Figure 4** summarize the incidence rate of non-neurological complications.

Complications	Incidence (%)
Fever	54
Anemia	36
Hyperglycemia	30
Hypertension	27
Hypernatremia	22
Pneumonia	20
Hypotension	18
Pulmonary edema	14
Hyponatremia	14
Life-threatening arrhythmia	8
Myocardial ischemia	6

Table 8. Non-neurological complications of subarachnoid hemorrhage [17].

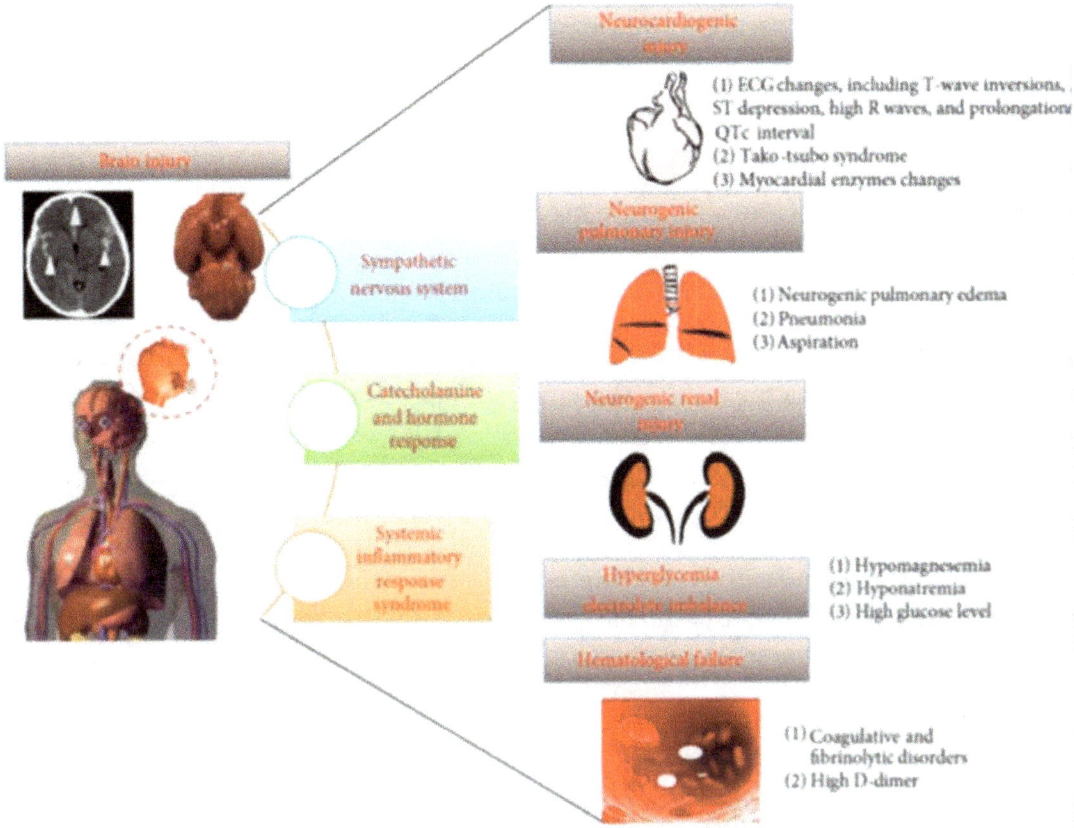

Figure 4. Harmful effects of SAH on extracerebral organs [28].

10. Surgical and endovascular methods for treatment of ruptured cerebral aneurysms

Ruptured aneurysms can be cured by microsurgical clipping or endovascular coiling.

Microsurgical clipping requires craniotomy to prevent re-bleeding of the aneurysm via insertion of a clip through its neck, thus isolating the aneurysm from circulation. This technique conveys a 98% certainty of elimination of the risk of rupture [29].

Endovascular coiling is the blocking of an aneurysm by an endovascular approach with electrically detachable platinum coils device which induces secondary thrombosis of the aneurysm [6]. The first published prospective randomized outcome study of surgical versus endovascular coiling, concluded that endovascular treatment results in clinical outcomes equal to that of surgical clipping.

Koivisto and co-worker (2000) published first prospective randomized outcome study of surgical versus endovascular coiling, they concluded that endovascular treatment results in clinical outcomes equal to that of surgical clipping [30].

The International Subarachnoid Aneurysm Trial (ISAT) is the first multicenter prospective randomized trial comparing the two options; the included 2143 patients with ruptured intracranial aneurysms were randomly assigned to clipping (1070) or coiling (1073). Primary outcomes included death or dependent living, and secondary outcomes included risk of seizures and risk of re-bleeding. Initially, 1-year outcomes concluded a fall in death and disability from 31% in the clipping arm to 24% in the endovascular arm, this difference was mainly driven by a reduction in the rate of disability among survivors (16% in the endovascular arm and 22% in the clipping arm) [6, 29, 30].

The risk of epilepsy and significant cognitive decline was also reduced in the endovascular group, but the occurrence of late re-bleeding was increased in endovascular group (2.9% after endovascular repair vs. 0.9% after open surgery) and only 58% of coiled aneurysms were completely obliterated compared with 81% of clipped aneurysms [6].

Although these results have affected the approach to patients with intracranial aneurysm in neurosurgical centers across the world, the study has been criticized due to the lack of generalizability, for example, posterior circulation aneurysms, which account for 8% of patients admitted with subarachnoid hemorrhage and up to 48% of ruptured aneurysms managed by endovascular coiling at some centers, made up only 2.7% of the ISAT study population [30].

Tahir et al. [29] concluded no significant difference in the clinical outcome of coiling and clipping of ruptured intracranial aneurysms; however, clipping is more cost effective than coiling.

Clipping is recommended for middle cerebral artery aneurysms (difficult to treat with endovascular technique) and patients presenting with an intraparenchymal hematoma >50 mL (high occurrence of critical outcome). Endovascular coiling is the preferred technique for patients presenting with vasospasm, elderly, poor clinical grade, and posterior cerebral aneurysms [6].

11. Time of surgical intervention

The most important strategy to reduce the risk of aneurysm rupture is early aneurysm repair, although evidence for best time of intervention is limited, it is uncertain whether ultra- early treatment (before 24 h) is better than aneurysm repair within 72 h (early). Recently published data analysis suggested that the surgical intervention can be done safely within 72 h after SAH. The American Heart Association/American Stroke Association recommend that "surgical clipping or endovascular coiling of the ruptured aneurysm should be performed as early as feasible in the majority of patients to reduce the rate of re-bleeding after SAH" (Class 1B). This recommendation is supported by the European Stroke Organization Guidelines for the Management of Intracranial Aneurysms and Subarachnoid Haemorrhage, which indicated that "aneurysm should be treated as early as logistically and technically possible to reduce the risk of re-bleeding; if possible it should be aimed to intervene at least within 72 hours after onset of first symptoms." There is ongoing study that only recruiting SAH with poor grade may help answer the question of whether intervention within 72 h (early intervention) is associated with better outcome compared with intervention within 4–7 days [12].

12. Prognosis and outcome

In spite of improvement in interventional and medical treatment of SAH, rupture of an aneurysm is still associated with significant high mortality rates (about 33%) and sever disability

(17%). In last decades, mortality rates decreased by 17%, and the chance to recover to independent state has increased by 1.5% per year. Severity of initial bleeding plays a vital role in the determination of mortality rate and functional outcome [3].

Age is another important factor: mortality rate increased three times if the patient was older than 80 years. Aneurysm size, site, history of hypertension, high systolic pressure, history of alcohol consumption, cigarette smoking are all important factors associated with poor outcome regardless the severity of SAH [3].

Complications such as re-bleeding, DCI, hydrocephalus, hyperglycemia, metabolic disturbances, cardiopulmonary complications, prolonged bed rest are associated with increased probability of poor outcome.

Small studies suggest that increased catecholamine levels in cerebrospinal fluid (CSF) are associated with early mortality or disability. Serum S100 is another marker of poor outcome after SAH [3].

13. Conclusion

Aneurysmal SAH is a devastating neurovascular disease associated with very high mortality and morbidity despite improvement in interventional and medical treatment due to multiple neurological and systemic complications, especially re-bleeding and DCI secondary to vasospasm. Age, smoking, alcohol consumption, hypertension, site and size of aneurysm are important factors associated with poor outcome. SAH needs multidisciplinary specialized care, best provided in high-volume centers to improve outcome.

Author details

Adel E. Ahmed Ganaw*, Abdulgafoor M. Tharayil, Ali O. Mohamed Bel Khair, Saher Tahseen, Jazib Hassan, Mohammad Faisal Abdullah Malmstrom and Sohel Mohamed Gamal Ahmed

*Address all correspondence to: adelganaw@yahoo.co.uk

Department of Anesthesiology, ICU and Perioperative Medicine, Hamad Medical Corporation, Doha, Qatar

References

[1] Vlak MH, Algra A, Brandenburg R, Rinkel GJ. Prevalence of unruptured intracranial aneurysms, with emphasis on sex, age, comorbidity, country, and time period: A systematic review and meta-analysis. Lancet Neurology. 2011;**10**:626

[2] Daniel C. Subarachnoid hemorrhage disease and anaesthetist. South African Journal of Anaesthesia and Analgesia. Vol 16 no 1(2010); 60-68

[3] Steiner T, Juvela S, Unterberg A, Jung C. European stroke organization guidelines for the management of intracranial aneurysms and subarachnoid haemorrhage. Cerebrovascular Diseases. 2013;**35**:93-112. DOI: 10.1159/000346087

[4] Kothandaraman U, Lokanadham S. Review on anatomy of cerebral arterial system—Clinical importance. Journal of Clinical and Biomedical Sciences. 2014;**4**(3):305-308

[5] Moss C, Wilson SR. Subarachnoid haemorrhage and anaesthesia for neurovascular surgery. Anesthesia and Intensive Care Medicine. 2011; 204-207.

[6] Sander Connolly E, Jr, Rabinstein Alejandro A, Ricardo Carhuapoma J, Derdeyn Colin P, Jacques D, Higashida Randall T, et al. Guidelines for the management of aneurysmal subarachnoid hemorrhage: Guidelines for healthcare professionals from the American heart association/American stroke association. Stroke. 2012;**43**:1711-1737

[7] Aoki T, Kataoka H, Shimamura M, Nakagami H, Wakayama K, Moriwaki T, et al. NF-κB is a key mediator of cerebral aneurysm formation. Circulation. 2007;**116**:2830-2840

[8] Evans RW, Dilli E, Dodick DW. Sentinel headache. Headache. 2009;**49**:599-603

[9] Czuczman AD, Thomas LE, Boulanger AB, Peak DA, Senecal EL, Brown DF, Marill KA. Interpreting red blood cells in lumbar puncture: Distinguishing true subarachnoid hemorrhage from traumatic tap. Academic Emergency Medicine. 2013;**20**:247

[10] Rosen DS, Macdonald LR. Subarachnoid hemorrhage grading scales. Neurocritical Care. 2005;**2**:110-118. DOI: 10.1385/

[11] Fernández TT, Capilla ME, *Morcillo CR*, Gonzalez RGG, Herrera I, Benassi GJM. Vasospasm After Subarachnoid Hemorrhage: Utility of Perfusion CT and CT Angiography on Diagnosis of Delayed Cerebral Ischemia. Spain: Department of Neuroradiology at Virgen de la Salud Hospital Toledo. ECR 2016/C-0298

[12] de Oliveira Manoel AL, Goffi A, Marotta TR, Schweizer TA, Abrahamson S, Macdonald LR. The critical care management of poorgrade subarachnoid haemorrhage. Critical Care. 2016;**20**:21. DOI: 10.1186/s13054-016-1193-9

[13] Naidech AM, Janjua N, Kreiter KT, Ostapkovich ND, Fitzsimmons BF, Parra A, et al. Predictors and impact of aneurysm rebleeding after subarachnoid hemorrhage. Archives of Neurology. 2005;**62**:410

[14] Chen T, Carter B. Role of magnesium sulphate in aneurysmal SAH management: A meta-analysis of controlled trial. Asian Journal of the Neurosurgery. 2011;**6**:1

[15] Ganne S, Rao U, Muthuchellappan R. Cerebral vasospasm: Current understanding. Current Opinion in Anesthesiology. 2016;**29**:544-551. DOI: 10.1097/ACO.0000000000000370

[16] Behrouz R, Sullebarger JT, Malek AR. Cardiac manifestations of subarachnoid hemorrhage. Expert Review of Cardiovascular Therapy. 2011;**9**(3):303307

[17] Highton D, Smith M. Intensive care management of subarachnoid haemorrhage 2C04,3C00, review article. The Intensive Care Society. 2013; 28-35

[18] Chatterjee S. ECG changes in subarachnoid haemorrhage: A synopsis. Netherlands Heart Journal. 2011;**19**:31-34. DOI: 10.1007/s12471-010-0049-1

[19] Marupudi NI, Mittal S. Diagnosis and management of hyponatremia in patients with aneurysmal subarachnoid hemorrhage. Journal of Clinical Medicine. 2015;**4**:756-767. DOI: 10.3390/jcm4040756

[20] Maesaka JK, Imbriano L, Mattana J, Gallagher D, Bade N, Sharif S. Differentiating SIADH from cerebral/renal salt wasting: Failure of the volume approach and need for a new approach to hyponatremia. Journal of Clinical Medicine. 2014;**3**:1373-1385. DOI: 10.3390/jcm3041373

[21] Cerdà-Esteve M, et al. Cerebral salt wasting syndrome. Review. European Journal of Internal Medicine. 2008;19:249-254.

[22] Gharaibeh KA, Brewer JM, Agarwal M, Fulop T. Risk factors, complication and measures to prevent or reverse catastrophic sodium overcorrection in chronic hyponatremia. American Journal of the Medical Sciences. 2015;**349**:170-175

[23] Tommasino C, Moore S, Todd MM. Cerebral effects of isovolemic hemodilution with crystalloid or colloid solutions. Critical Care Medicine. 1988;**16**: 862-868

[24] Lehmann L, Bendel S, Uehlinger DE, Takala J, Schafer M, Reinert M, Jakob SM. Randomized, double-blind trial of the effect of fluid composition on electrolyte, acid-base, and fluid homeostasis in patients early after subarachnoid hemorrhage. Neurocritical Care. 2013;**18**:5-12

[25] Bederson JB, Connolly ES, Jr, Batjer HH, Dacey RG, Dion JE, Diringer MN, et al. Guidelines for the management of aneurysmal subarachnoid hemorrhage: A statement for healthcare professionals from a special writing group of the stroke council, American heart association. Stroke. 2009;**40**:994-102

[26] Wright WL, Asbury WH, Gilmore JL, Samuels OB. Conivaptan for hyponatremia in the neurocritical care unit. Neurocritical Care. 2009;**11**:6-13

[27] Weant KA, Sasaki-Adams D, Dziedzic K, Ewend M. Acute relative adrenal insufficiency after aneurysmal subarachnoid hemorrhage. Neurosurgery. 2008;**63**:645-649

[28] Chen S, Li Q, Wu H, Krafft PR, Wang Z, Zhang JH. The harmful effects of subarachnoid hemorrhage on extracerebral organs: Review article. BioMed Research International. 2014;**2014**:12. Article ID 858496. DOI: http://dx.doi.org/10.1155/2014/858496

[29] Tahir ZM, Enam SA, Pervez AR, Bhatti A, ul Haq T. Cost-effectiveness of clipping vs. coiling of intracranial aneurysms after subarachnoid hemorrhage in a developing country. Surgical Neurology. 2009;**72**:355-361

[30] Molyneux AJ, Kerr RSC, Yu LM, Clarke M, Sneade M, Yarnold JA, Sandercock P. for the International Subarachnoid Aneurysm Trial (ISAT) Collaborative GrouISAT: Coiling or clipping for ruptured intracranial aneurysms? http://neurology.thelancet.com Vol 4 December 2005.

2

Intensive Care Unit Workforce: Occupational Health and Safety

Melek Nihal Esin and Duygu Sezgin

Abstract

There are many different work tasks and workplace hazards related to the ICU setting. The workplace hazards include the physical environment of the ICU, working conditions, psychosocial factors, ergonomic factors, biological factors and chemical factors that cause ICU workers to have health problems. The occurrence of occupational health problems in ICU workers not only leads to decreased job satisfaction and productivity but also increases absenteeism and burnout. Moreover, this situation adversely affects patient care and increases the cost of treatment. Recognising occupational hazards and risks arising from the work environment will assist in planning strategies to protect and promote health programmes for ICU workers. Understanding the importance of occupational health and safety practices by all institutions is a key factor to improve quality of life, work efficiency and work satisfaction of ICU workers.

Keywords: intensive care unit, ICU workforce, workplace hazards, occupational health, occupational safety

1. Introduction

This chapter presents information about occupational health and safety in the intensive care unit (ICU) settings. The reader is cautioned that ICU workers face many workplace hazards due to the complex nature of their work environment. Furthermore, this chapter aims to describe the occupational risks of ICU workers related to personal factors and to discuss prevention strategies related to this issue. Although traditional prevention strategies for occupational health and safety in the ICU are given, personal measures such as risk management and health promotion programmes for ICU workforce will also be provided.

2. Intensive care unit workforce

The health services provided in ICUs are carried out by a multidisciplinary team. The members of this team are intensivists, ICU nurses, pharmacists, dieticians, respiratory therapists, physiotherapists, occupational therapists, healthcare assistants and members of other professions [1, 2]. Other staff in secretarial and transportation services are in a position to support the ICU team [2].

The nursing staff in some countries may comprise distinct occupations such as nurses and nurse aids/assistants or technicians [3]. Nurses are the workforce in the ICU and are mostly involved in complex work tasks, such as medication management, organising the ICU environment, coordinating the work tasks between nursing staff and direct contact with patients while providing care, as well [3]. The working experience of the ICU nursing staff may vary with the hospital type and location. In the study done by Sevinç et al. [5], 30% of the ICU nurses had working experience of less than 1 year. In another study setting done in the United States, the mean age of ICU nurses was 46.5 [7]. Healthcare assistants are responsible for tasks related to patient care directly, inasmuch as they are the members of the ICU team that are most exposed to the physical workloads [3].

The work environment in the ICU setting poses many occupational hazards, especially for the female workforce. In recent years, the number of female intensive care medicine (ICM) specialists has increased. Studies show that the proportion of female ICM specialists in the United Kingdom and New Zealand in 2012 was 17% and 18%, respectively. On the other hand, majority of the nursing workforce in the ICUs consists of women. Although the nursing profession has become more popular for men in the recent years, female nurses in the clinical setting still have a slightly higher percentage than male nurses. Thus, the occupational hazards and challenges for female members of the ICU team must be considered during the risk assessment, hazard prevention and training processes as they might face higher risks due to pregnancy, motherhood and other conditions) [4].

Due to the fact that working conditions are hazardous in the ICU setting, nurses and other ICU workers transfer to other units in the hospitals after working there for a certain period. As in many other units in the hospitals, there are also shortages of staff in the ICU setting. Many studies show that inadequate numbers of the ICU staff have a negative impact on patient outcomes [5, 6]. However, not only the number of staff will prevent unexpected negative conditions of the patients, but also the work environment will improve patient outcomes [7].

The models advocating the improvement of patient outcomes and cost-effectiveness support having an intensivist present in the ICU setting, creating accurate job descriptions for all team members, developing procedures and providing continuous education to the staff [2].

3. The work environment in the ICU and the occupational hazards

The work environment is considered an important factor that affects the motivation and work satisfaction of employees. A productive and satisfying work environment is described as *"a multi-dimensional, integrated phenomenon"* and the importance of having all dimensions present in the work setting is stated by Schmalenberg and Kramer as *"an excellent work environment doesn't evolve from the presence of only a few desired processes. None of them optional, all are required."* [8].

The workplace environment must be considered carefully because of the fact that it can affect the motivation and capability of ICU workers to perform the tasks [9]. There is evidence about the impact of poor work environments on healthcare professionals and patient outcomes [7]. Negative outcomes for the ICU workforce can be related to job satisfaction and burnout. However, there are some other negative outcomes for the patients such as inadequate safety, impaired quality of care, medical errors and increased mortality [7].

The work environment in ICU is not only related to the physical environment, but also related to psychosocial settings [7]. The nature of a poor work environment is associated with a number of hazards and risks [10]. The terms "hazard" and "risk" are often used interchangeably which leads to confusion. Despite this, hazards in the workplace are described as "a potential source of harm or adverse health effect on a person or persons" [11, 12]. Additionally, the risks which arise from identified hazards are graded by combinations of severity and likelihood of harm [11, 13].

The ICU environment may cause a number of health risks in relation to occupational hazards. The workplace hazards include the **physical environment** of the ICU (*lighting, conditioning, noise, equipment, work space*), **working conditions** (*daily workload, working in shifts, standing for long hours, caring for patients with co-morbidities, inadequate income*), **psychosocial factors** (*dissatisfaction with work, workplace stress, frequently encountered deaths, interaction with families of patients, workplace violence*), **ergonomic factors** (*repositioning the patients* and *repeating movements such as pushing, pulling, elevating* and *bending*), **biological factors** (*being exposed to infectious organisms during invasive and non-invasive procedures*) and **chemical factors** (*being exposed to antiseptic and disinfectants or inhaling their gases*).

3.1. Physical environment

The physical environment of the ICU may contain various hazards likely to cause injuries to ICU workers. Those hazards are associated with mechanical factors, equipment, noise, light, heat and humidity. In the conditions where the physical characteristics of the workplace were not designed considering the needs and expectations of employees, it will result in decreased work performance of the employees and increased number of lost work days [14].

Mechanical hazards in the ICU include mobile equipment which is used to transfer patients, transported objects i.e. emergency trolleys, moving parts of objects, sharp edges of surfaces, falling objects, slippery surfaces, high pressure fluids and other items. ICU staff are more likely to sustain injuries caused by mechanical hazards inasmuch as they give care to patients in unstable conditions. A suitable workplace design, safety signs and risk measures should be applied to eliminate risks related to mechanical hazards in the ICU [15].

Intensive care units are one of the departments with the most advanced equipment in the hospital settings. With the aim of using that equipment effectively, it is important to design the bed spaces, monitor heights and drainage systems considering the architectural principles for the ICU standards so that healthcare personnel can have sufficient space to care for their patients [16, 17]. The environment of the ICU requires appropriate physical layout and workstation design. On the other hand, an inadequate patient room or bed space will make it difficult to interact effectively with the patient and provided equipment [9]. The architectural design of the ICU affects job satisfaction, the level of stress and well-being of the healthcare professionals working in the ICU setting. The ICU team members' experiences and opinions should be asked for before the architectural design of the ICU is made [17].

The equipment to improve the physical conditions might not have been developed yet for the specific needs in the ICU; on the other hand, it might be developed but not obtained by the facility (the hospital) or provided in some ICU setting [9]. The studies show that although in some ICU setting the staff are provided high technological equipment to prevent them from physical injuries and protect them from musculoskeletal disorders, they do not make use of the equipment reporting reasons such as the equipment being difficult to use (requiring complex work tasks or disinfection of the parts for every use) or being time-consuming [16].

The design of the ICU should prevent the distraction caused by the high level of noise in the ICU. It is also shown that noise may cause an increased stress level for the ICU staff [18, 38]. Moreover, it is also stated by the Occupational Health and Safety Administration that 20% of the workers may have a significant change in hearing if they are exposed to 90dBA noise for 8 h per day for 40 years [18].

Poor lighting in the ICU can cause discomfort while ICU workers are performing their daily tasks. Suitable lighting must consider the ideal level of lighting in different parts of the ICUs. Suitable lighting in the ICU varies as the lighting in the entrance and the waiting area is recommended to be 150 lx, circulation areas to be between 100 and 150 lx, and offices to be 750 lx. A direct interference with vision must be prevented and glare must be minimised. The nurse desks and monitoring areas should be located where light can be received in a 90° angle [12].

Heating and air conditioning in the ICUs are important physical conditions that affect the body temperature and cause heat stress in the ICU workers. Changes in the body temperature and heart rate along with sweating are known as the symptoms of the heat strain. This type of physiological strain indicates a cardiovascular response to the blood flow need. In the conditions where heat and ventilation in the ICU environment are not within ideal limits, the body starts to remove heat primarily by evaporation by sweating, the rate of which varies with air motion, humidity and type of clothing. The heat strain may primarily cause discomfort, but also induces heat-related disorders and acute musculoskeletal injuries [19]. The ideal temperature for workplaces is recommended as between 19° and 23°C but may vary in different settings [13].

Humidity is another factor in the working environment that affects workers' health. In conditions when humidity is low, it means the air is dry and can cause stuffy nose, dry and itchy skin, sore eyes, sore throat and flu-like symptoms in further cases. The relative humidity is stated as to be maintained between 40 and 70% [13].

3.2. Working conditions

Patients in ICUs receive continuous medical care 24 h a day from the ICU team. There are many different work tasks and related workload in the ICU setting. The influence of excessive workload in the ICU setting may result in a high level of stress, job dissatisfaction and physical injuries [20]. There is a direct correlation between the length of the shifts and the burnout due to excessive workload and fatigue. There are evidence and standards that consider the number of patients to be assigned to the ICU workforce. The evidence for the intensivist-to-patient ratios is ideally no higher than 1:14 inasmuch as it affects the staff well-being and patient care [21]. In a study investigating the clinical intensive care service, it was claimed that the paediatricians-to-patient ratio was 1:13, median working hours of the paediatricians were 60 h in a week, and indicated night shifts were 60 nights in a year [22]. The recommended nurse-to-patient rate is 1:1 for the critical patients with mechanical ventilation, and the maximum number of the patients to be assigned to a nurse is two according to the American College of Critical Care Medicine [23]. Those standards may vary with the national regulations in different countries. For example, the nurse-to-patient standard in Turkey is 1:4 for ICUs, not considering the dependency levels of the patients [5].

Studies in the literature show that there is a correlation between increased workload and increased medical errors and hospital infections [24]. Moreover, there is a relation between increased workload and death rates of the patients in the ICU. The excessive workload in the ICU setting is the main risk factor for hospital infections such as pneumonia, urinary tract infections, bloodstream infections, and surgical-site infections [25]. It is stated in the literature that when the ICU nurses give care to one patient above the recommended number, there is an increased risk for pulmonary failure by 53%, for nosocomial pneumonia by 7%, for unplanned extubation by 45% and for mortality rates by 9% [24]. In this context, the workload of the healthcare professionals in the ICU has crucial importance not only for causing occupational health problems, but also for patient safety issues [5, 24, 26].

The working characteristics in the ICU which require long work schedules lead to physical and mental fatigue [3]. Moreover, the long shifts (12 h and above) increase the errors and near misses, and decrease staff vigilance. As a further matter, the negative effects of shift work have been discussed for a long time, and are accepted as detrimental. It has a negative impact on individuals' health, such as disrupting the circadian rhythms, causing sleep disorders, causing increased risk of gastrointestinal tract disorders, increasing stress levels, altering activity and rest patterns and affecting the social and domestic life [27, 28]. Moreover, it disturbs the body's chemical and hormonal functions because of the fact that individuals working during the night are not able to benefit from the daylight. In many studies, it is discussed that working in night shifts for a long term increases the risk of breast cancer [29].

Nevertheless, the low salaries for healthcare professionals working in the ICU are not satisfying compared to the required working conditions [3].

3.3. Psychosocial factors

There are various psychosocial risk factors in ICU settings, such as high qualitative and quantitative demands, emotional demands, low job control, role conflicts, ambiguity, mobbing and physical violence, which affect ICU workers' well-being [30].

Intensive care units are stressful settings inasmuch as they require communicating with patients and their families facing the death and loss processes, coping with complex work tasks and adapting to busy work conditions [26]. The psychological hazards in the ICU may cause psychosocial burden, shifts in the mood, sadness, negative outlook towards life in general, irritation, loss of confidence and negative self-image [3]. Those negative conditions are related to symptoms of a high level of stress. Consequences of high levels of stress in the ICU can cause increased absence, lowered productivity, more accidents and physical injuries, higher job turnover and increased costs [30].

The ICU team members may encounter uncertainties, varied situations that require immediate action, high level of knowledge, psychomotor and cognitive skills and competences which may cause fatigue [3]. Lack of equipment and resources in the ICU may result in job dissatisfaction for the healthcare professionals working there [20]. In the studies done with anaesthesiologists and ICU nurses, it is found that overall nurses and the female anaesthesiologists consider the lack of resources as a cause for job dissatisfaction [2, 20].

Intensive care unit workers are responsible for many complex work processes in acute and chronic settings. There might be some role conflicts and ambiguity that result in decreased job control, misunderstanding and increased stress. However, in some cases, it is reported that physical aggression and physiological violence occur due to working in intense work conditions. Negative behaviours such as yelling, offending, ignoring, threatening or hiding important information can mean mobbing which are inadmissible for members of the ICU team. Being a victim of mobbing leads to physical and mental problems such as high level of stress, depression, eating disorders, addiction and suicide attempts [30].

The social hazards in the ICU setting are usually generated by working long shifts which require working at night and weekends. They may cause isolation from family relationships, social life difficulties, overall disinterest towards others, uncontrolled aggressiveness and difficulty in making decisions regarding personal life [3].

3.4. Ergonomic factors

Ergonomics are defined as the "laws of the work" and it primarily focuses on the physical aspects of the work. There are many force and energy requirements for work tasks in the ICU setting and there must be considerations of biomechanical rules and workplace adjustments to prevent ICU workers from musculoskeletal disorders [31].

Occupational musculoskeletal disorders not only occur in acute conditions but also may develop on account of cumulative micro traumas usually in relation to lack of *balance* of the body for tissue repair and adaptation to physical stress [32, 33].

Intensive care unit settings require physical loads on ICU workers during patient care [34, 35]. The physical hazards may cause ergonomic risks, which lead to musculoskeletal symptoms and disorders. Several conditions such as excessive and repetitive traumas while pushing and pulling heavy equipment, standing for long periods of time, not having adequate rest, manually lifting and moving partially or fully dependent patients in awkward, twisted or extremely bent positions requiring extreme muscular exertions must be considered as the major factors for musculoskeletal disorders [31, 34, 35]. The symptoms are mostly seen as pain in the leg, back, shoulder, neck and other parts of the body [3, 16].

In ICUs where the physical characteristics were not designed properly, healthcare professionals have a higher risk of musculoskeletal injuries due to repeated physical loads during patient care [34]. The ICU members with musculoskeletal symptoms are less productive because of pain and limited mobility, and they are likely to make consistent safety mistakes. Hence, they may also affect the health or endanger the safety of other members of ICU [31].

3.5. Biological factors

The ICU workers have increased risk related to biological hazards since they are exposed to infectious organisms during invasive and non-invasive procedures. Transmission of infectious agents can occur through blood and body fluids on equipment or their droplets' absorption by skin or mucosa through direct or indirect contact or lung penetration through the air. Intensive care unit work tasks and processes require direct or indirect contact with biological materials that results in illness and disease [13]. As in many other healthcare units, ICUs have the highest rate of needle stick injuries in the nursing workforce that can result in transmission of most common blood-borne infections such as Hepatitis B and C, other Hepatitis infections and HIV. Other infections can transmit to ICU workers by spreading through close contact and by droplets, such as tuberculosis and meningococcal meningitis [12, 36].

There are standard and transmission-based regulations in healthcare facilities to prevent infections occurring in the ICU workforce. Standard precautions include hand washing, respiratory hygiene and cough etiquette, waste management and decontamination, and appropriate use of personal protective equipment. Transmission-based interventions include airborne, contact and droplet precautions [13].

3.6. Chemical factors

The ICU workers face chemical hazards such as being exposed to antiseptic and disinfectants or inhaling their gases. During the work tasks and processes in the ICU settings, ICU workers can be exposed to surface cleaners, antiseptic solutions and anaesthetic gases such as formaldehyde. The exposure can occur through many routes, which commonly happens by penetration after lung inhalation, absorption by skin or mucosa contact through eyes or nose. They can cause inflammation or irritation on the part where contact occurred. Moreover, it can lead to dermatitis, allergic reactions (i.e. sneezing and rhinitis), asthma and cancer [13].

The effect of chemicals in the workplace can vary depending on some factors such as age, sex, ethnicity, genetics, immune system, nutrition, disease history, occupational history, previous exposures, other exposures to synergistic or antagonistic chemicals and recently used medications [12]. The occupational health and safety team in the hospital should keep records of all chemical agents which are being used in the ICU, and prepare emergency action plans in acute and chronic exposure cases.

4. Risks related to the ICU workers

4.1. Personal factors

There are some personal factors related to occupational diseases acquired by ICU workers. These factors can be summarised as ageing, inadequate physical condition, smoking and obesity.

The workforce in the ICU is ageing since the healthcare industry workforce is getting older in accordance with an increase in the retirement age requirements in all industries (around the world). In the United States, the average age of registered nurses is 46.8 [9]. The ageing workforce in the ICU might face increased risks for physical injuries and musculoskeletal disorders due to decreased muscular endurance and physical strength by age 50 and above [31]. Moreover, the workforce in the ICU is likely to have more chronic diseases with the ageing population [37].

The demographic characteristics of the society have changed in recent years. The body weight in certain populations is increasing rapidly. People's lifestyle is changing and it is leading to less healthy eating and having a more sedentary life. Obesity may cause many health problems such as back pain, osteoarthritis, diabetes mellitus, hyperlipidaemia, coronary heart diseases and other health conditions [37]. Considering the population trends, it has been shown that the body weight of ICU workers has also changed, and they are more likely to have obesity-related health problems and are at an increased risk of musculoskeletal injuries. Similarly, patients in the ICU have become heavier. Thus, this situation increases the risk of physical injuries of the ICU workforce while lifting or moving or transferring heavy patients [31].

4.2. Personal habits

The work tasks in the ICU setting require intense physical activity during the shift, even without lunch breaks or other breaks in some cases. Healthcare professionals who work in the ICU get fatigued after working for long hours. There are some personal habits that affect the level of physical or mental tiredness of the ICU workforce.

Studies have shown that regular physical activity prevents musculoskeletal disorders by maintaining flexibility of muscles and ligaments. According to this, ICU workers with a habit of regular physical activity have a decreased risk of physical injuries and musculoskeletal disorders [16, 38].

Intensive care unit workers might face sleeping disorders due to working night shifts. The high level of stress and physical tiredness after working for long hours might cause sleep disturbances in ICU workers [3]. Moreover, having inadequate sleep and rest increases the risk of unsafe practices and occupational accidents. It is shown in the studies that, there is a direct relation between sleep and level of attention [28].

Negative stress and poor balance between work and social life can cause careless dietary habits. A poor lifestyle implies a poor diet, which is not only related to eating too much or little, but also eating low-quality foods such as fast food and frozen food [13].

There is evidence about the correlation between an unhealthy lifestyle and decreased physical and mental abilities for work tasks [39]. Positive lifestyle such as having adequate sleep/rest, healthy eating habits and regular physical exercise affects job security and occupational quality [40].

4.3. Cognitive features

The cognitive features include individual differences, perceptions and decision making and human error. Individuals differ from each other by personality, reliability, perceptions and self-awareness. Moreover, some people are more likely to make errors [41]. It is shown in the literature that there is a correlation between cognitive failures and accidents [40].

The ICU setting has many different hazards, and the perceptions, decisions, and capabilities of the ICU workers are crucial to avoid the risks related to them. Decision making is an important factor that affects the level of risks and prevents accidents when an ICU worker makes the right decision at the right time. Individuals' competence is also important. Although some people are very capable of avoiding errors, their physical ability and willingness impact dealing with hazards [41]. However, cognitive features are directly related to occupational stressors so they can easily be changed [40].

There are some workplace interventions recommended to control and manage risks in the ICU setting, and most of these interventions are focused on behaviour change processes [16]. However, there are some individual factors affecting staff's behaviour change. Self-efficacy is the ability of individuals to accomplish tasks with barriers to change that they encounter during the process of behaviour change. It is related to the level of control of individuals over situations that affect their health [42].

In the conditions when the perceived self-efficacy level is high, the individual will realise the priority of the occupational health and safety principles to prevent work-related injuries or disorders while managing their work tasks [42].

There are some factors related to self-efficacy that affect the individual's behaviour change process negatively, such as decreased awareness of the benefits of the change and loss of interest or having a high level of perceived barriers to change (i.e. claiming to not have proper facilities for physical activity or complaining about time pressure while doing their work tasks) [42].

4.4. Occupational and health history

Risks arising from the previous workplace affect ICU workers' current health conditions. Some biological and chemical agents require a long period of time before causing any signs and symptoms while they are affecting the body functions. A detailed employment history provides information about the current occupational diseases and future health problems which might occur while performing in the ICU [10, 41].

Illnesses might have many causes such as ageing, lifestyle or genetic characteristics or viruses. Intensive care unit workers lose work days due to common illnesses i.e. symptoms of musculoskeletal disorders, headaches, dental issues, infectious diseases, gastric problems, among others. The health history of the ICU workers needs be recorded and comorbidities should be considered in relation to risk factors in the ICU [13].

5. Occupational health and safety practices in the ICU

The work tasks and processes in the ICUs are identified in a variety of guidelines prepared by the ILO (International Labour Organisation) and OSHA (Occupational Health and Safety Administration). The measures and practices related to protecting the ICU workers' health are identified in these guidelines. The measures and practices can be divided into two main topics such as workplace interventions and personal measures. Workplace interventions can be summarised as reducing the working hours and workload, designing and organising the work environment properly. Personal measures include staff training, providing risk management and health promotion programmes and other measures.

5.1. Workplace interventions

5.1.1. Reducing the working hours and workload

Changing work patterns and improving control strategies will result in decreased risks and reduced health deficits among ICU workers. Evidence shows that re-arranging working hours and workload results in reduced occupational health symptoms of the ICU workers. Improved working conditions, material and moral support, properly managed work shifts provide a safe environment in the ICU setting [40]. The occupational and safety team members have responsibilities to recognise workplace hazards and identify risks in the ICU setting that impact workplace practices and the workers' health status [10].

5.1.2. Designing and organising the work environment

A positive work environment is linked to improved patient and staff outcomes such as decreased hospital infections, death rates, and increased motivation and job satisfaction [43, 44].

The occupational health and safety team are involved in designing work equipment and ICU work process. Moreover, studies show that in situations where ICU workers' opinions were asked on the process of redesigning the unit, there was a significant increase in job satisfaction of staff and a dramatic reduction in turnover and absenteeism [10, 30].

5.1.3. Other interventions

Workplace interventions designed to prevent hazards and reduce related risks allow the occupational and safety team to implement strategies to improve safety culture in the ICU [44]. Safety culture is described as *"the product of individual and group values, attitudes, perceptions, competencies, and patterns of behaviour that determine the commitment of an organisation's health and safety management"* [45]. There is a direct connection between safety culture and trusted communication in the organisation. Moreover, increased perception of the importance of safe practices and sufficient confidence in preventive measures are remarked as the fundamentals of the safety culture [44]. Studies in this area show that perceptions of ICU safety are influenced by factors such as opinions of the management, working conditions, job satisfaction, team work climate, stress recognition, and safety climate [46]. Thus, workplace interventions to manage occupational risk factors should be focused on improving the safety culture of the ICU setting. After being established, the safety culture can be improved by initiating different intervention strategies [44]. The safety culture is known as a two-way system between the management's responsibilities and employees' commitment to their duties, which can only be established by key strategies: control, cooperation, communication and professional competence [13].

Designing safety checklists is another intervention that results in improved patient and workforce outcomes. A safety checklist aims to monitor safety performance and make improvements to work systems [38]. There are different aspects to creating safety criteria since they may be related to organisational, personal or professional characteristics. The safety hazards that threaten patient safety as well as health, well-being and safety of the ICU workforce must be stated on the checklists [38].

5.2. Personal measures

5.2.1. Staff training

Staff training interventions include prevention programmes related to physical, psychological, chemical, biological, ergonomic and other hazards in the ICU setting. In recent years, the importance of health promotion programmes is becoming more recognised as workplaces provide occupational health and safety (OHS) team members with access to a large group of people, who have good inter-communication and facilities to exchange information. Workplace health promotion activities enable OHS team members to participate in continuous assessment of the healthy lifestyle behaviours of ICU workers and to develop specific training interventions for them [10].

Occupational and safety practices should appreciate the biological, psychological, and social characteristics of individuals considering that interventions in the workplace will be integrated into adult life and health. The ability of the staff to participate in the training productively is an important factor that contributes to the effectiveness of the intervention. There are studies showing the benefits of on-work training programmes [16]. In this case, ICU professionals would not be requested to participate in staff training sessions when they need to rest after working long hours. Additionally, it is discussed in the literature that the on-work training sessions are more successful when they are model based or combined with multiple interventions [47–49].

Training should include different time periods such as orientation programmes when workers start working in the ICU (pre-employment examinations); periodical training; condition-based training where ICU workers need information about an unexpected or unusual situation (e.g. when they were caring for patients with an epidemic disease); return to work programmes for staff who have been absent after having a workplace accident or long-term leave from the ICU; and other programmes [10, 41].

5.2.2. Risk management

Risk management programmes comprise planning, applying and evaluating personal, physical and organisational interventions that aim to assess and decrease occupational risks to employees [50–52]. In recent years, many studies have been done with the aim of identifying high-risk tasks; creating and implementing solutions to reduce these risks in the workplace. There is legislation in many countries, for different work areas as well as ICUs to implement risk analysis and management programmes. Risk assessment involves the assessment of the severity and likelihood of harm which arises from identified hazards [11, 13]. Risk assessment can be made by using both qualitative and quantitative methods. However, in relation to legislations in many countries, a written risk assessment should be done including the risk control measures such as elimination of hazards, engineering controls, administrative controls and distribution of personal protective equipment [13]. Risk assessment and management interventions in the ICU should be performed as general and job-specific controls [31]. Therefore, safety hazards affecting the ICU workforce should be assessed individually, considering the work task–specific hazards that they might face. For example, in relation to biological risks, hazardous materials and wastes must be disposed safely. Continuous monitoring should be performed for persons who come into contact with biological materials by handling, manufacturing or storing them [13].

Work-related musculoskeletal disorders are one of the most common occupational health problems seen in ICU workers. The literature shows that evidence-based interventions used in ergonomic risk management programmes such as body mechanics training, ergonomic guidelines, exercise programmes, cognitive-behavioural interventions, social support programmes and workplace adjustments were found to be effective in terms of reducing the ergonomic risks to ICU workers [33, 47, 48, 50, 51, 53–57].

5.2.3. Health screening

Health screenings of ICU workers should be done regularly. A detailed history of previous employment and a comprehensive assessment of the current occupational diseases should be performed when the staff start working in the ICU setting (pre-employment examinations). Eventually, it should be followed by periodical screenings, condition-based screenings (e.g. when they were caring for patients with an epidemic disease) and return to work screenings for workers who had a workplace accident or a long-term leave from the ICU [10, 41].

5.2.4. Health promotion programmes

Occupational hazards and risk factors in the ICU are not only associated with the workplace setting, but are also related to personal habits such as smoking, not having a healthy diet or inadequate physical activity. Therefore, risks related to personal factors can only be managed by conducting health promotion programmes in their workplace. Health promotion programmes in the ICU are valuable interventions when they are used proactively, developed, and managed/monitored by experienced health professionals [9]. Health promotion activities (i.e. programmes aimed at diet management, weight control, physical activity or coping with stress) in the ICU should be developed considering the needs of ICU workers. For example, conditions related to high level of stress can be managed by improving coping skills. Those skills can be improved through stress management, problem solving, relaxation, and self-awareness trainings [13, 30]. However, a good health promotion intervention should be based on a model (i.e. Pender's Health Promotion Model; Prochaska's Trans-theoretic Model; Green's PRECEDE-PROCEED Model) [58]. According to these models, there are some factors such as past experiences, unsuccessful attempts to change, self-efficacy, social support, self-awareness and readiness to change that affect the positive results that may be achieved by workplace health promotion programmes [58–60].

5.2.5. Other measures

There are other monitoring and prevention programmes in relation to risks arising from hazards in the ICU setting. Different forms of prevention can be applied for varied risks as follows:

- Limitation of risk sources
- Limitation of ICU workers' reactions towards hazardous conditions
- Treatment of injuries and harm caused by hazards, including monitoring the long-term effects [30]

The aim of the preventative measures and interventions is to strengthen how ICU workers deal with physical, chemical, biological, psychosocial and ergonomic hazards. Another form of risk prevention is the optimisation of task content in connection with job rotation, job enlargement, job enrichment and creation of autonomous work groups (**Table 1**) [30].

Optimisation	Main focus/action
Job rotation	Move workers to different stations regularly
Job enlargement	Merge similar jobs into larger modules
Job enrichment	Group basic tasks and control elements together and assign workers to higher tasks
Creation of autonomous work groups	Create independent worker groups and give them the responsibilities of larger job fragments

Table 1. Optimisation of task content.

6. Conclusion

The ICU environment may cause a number of health risks in relation to occupational hazards. The workplace hazards include the physical environment of the ICU, working conditions, psychosocial factors, ergonomic factors, biological factors and chemical factors. The occurrence of occupational health problems in ICU workers not only leads to burnout and decreased job satisfaction, but also affects patient care and increases the cost of treatment. Workplace interventions and personal measures should be done in terms of reducing hazards and related risks in the ICU setting. Increased employee participation should be considered in all risk management, monitoring, and prevention programmes. The contribution of ICU workers in these programmes will improve the effectiveness of the interventions associated with reducing health risks in the ICU settings.

Author details

Melek Nihal Esin[1] and Duygu Sezgin[2*]

*Address all correspondence to: dusezgin@gmail.com

1 Public Health Nursing Department, Florence Nightingale Nursing Faculty, Istanbul University, Istanbul, Turkey

2 Department of Nursing & Midwifery, Education & Health Sciences Faculty, University of Limerick, Limerick, Ireland

References

[1] Durbin Jr CG. Team model: Advocating for the optimal method of care delivery in the intensive care unit. Critical Care Medicine. 2006 Mar 1;**34**(3):S12-S17

[2] Türkmen E, Sevinç S, İlhan M. Intensive care units in Turkish hospitals: Do they meet the minimum standards? Nursing in Critical Care. 2014 Jan 1;**21**:5

[3] Shimizu HE, Couto DT, Merchán-Hamann E, Branco AB. Occupational health hazards in ICU nursing staff. Nursing Research and Practice. 2011 Feb 7;**2010**:1-6.

[4] Hawker FH. Female specialists in intensive care medicine: Job satisfaction, challenges and work-life balance. Critical Care and Resuscitation. 2016 Jun;**18**(2):125

[5] Sevinç S, Türkmen E, İlhan M. The nursing workforce in critical care units in university and private hospitals in Turkey. Training. 2014 Apr 1;**15**:16

[6] Laschinger H. 14. Organisational and health effects of workplace empowerment in health care settings. The Innovation Imperative in Health Care Organisations: Critical Role of Human Resource Management in the Cost, Quality and Productivity Equation. 2012:**221**;221-222

[7] Ulrich BT, Lavandero R, Woods D, Early S. Critical care nurse work environments 2013: A status report. Critical Care Nurse. 2014 Aug 1;**34**(4):64-79

[8] Schmalenberg C, Kramer M. Essentials of a productive nurse work environment. Nursing Research. 2008 Jan 1;**57**(1):2-13

[9] Bhattacharya A, McGlothlin JD, editors. Occupational Ergonomics: Theory and Applications. Clark DR. Workstation Evaluation and Design. CRC Press; 2012 Mar 8. pp. 294, 302

[10] Sines D, Aldridge-Bent S, Fanning A, Farrelly P, Potter K, Wright J. Community and Public Health Nursing. John Wiley & Sons; 2013. pp. 192-193

[11] Health and safety essentials booklet. University of Limerick and NUI Galway, (nd) Ireland. p. 6

[12] Aw TC, Gardiner K, Harrington JM. Occupational Health (Pocket Consultant). 5th ed. USA: Blackwell Publishing; 2007. pp. 63-68, 73, 144

[13] Safety and Health at Work (QQI Level 5). Dublin: Nifast, Gill & McMillan; 2015. pp. 6-8, 54-58, 67-70, 77-78, 83-90

[14] Huisman ER, Morales E, Van Hoof J, Kort HS. Healing environment: A review of the impact of physical environmental factors on users. Building and Environment. 2012 Dec 31;**58**:70-80

[15] Koradecka, D, editor. Handbook of Occupational safety and health. In: Myrcha K, Gierasimiuk J, editors. Mechanical Hazards. USA: CRC Press; 2010. pp. 360-366

[16] Sezgin D, Esin MN. Predisposing factors for musculoskeletal symptoms in intensive care unit nurses. International Nursing Review. 2015 Mar 1;**62**(1):92-101

[17] Olausson S, Ekebergh M, Österberg SA. Nurses' lived experiences of intensive care unit bed spaces as a place of care: A phenomenological study. Nursing in Critical Care. 2014 May 1;**19**(3):126-134

[18] Bhattacharya A, McGlothlin JD, editors. Occupational ergonomics: Theory and applications. In: Grinshpun SA, Kim J, Murphy WJ, editors. Noise Exposure and Control. USA: CRC Press; 2012 Mar 8. pp. 792-793

[19] Bhattacharya A, McGlothlin JD, editors. Occupational ergonomics: Theory and applications. In: Bernard TE, editor. Occupational Heat Stress. USA: CRC Press; 2012 Mar 8. pp. 738-739

[20] Shidhaye RV, Divekar DS, Goel G, Shidhaye R. Influence of working conditions on job satisfaction in Indian anesthesiologists: A cross sectional survey. Anaesthesia Pain & Intensive Care. 2011 Jun 1;**15**(1):30-37

[21] Ward NS, Afessa B, Kleinpell R, Tisherman S, Ries M, Howell M, Halpern N, Kahn J, Members of Society of Critical Care Medicine Taskforce on ICU Staffing. Intensivist/patient ratios in closed ICUs: A statement from the Society of Critical Care Medicine Taskforce on ICU Staffing. Critical Care Medicine. 2013 Feb 1;**41**(2):638-645

[22] Radabaugh CL, Ruch-Ross HS, Riley CL, Stockwell JA, Conway Jr EE, Mink RB, Agus MS, Poss WB, Salerno RA, Vernon DD. Practice patterns in pediatric critical care medicine: Results of a workforce survey. Pediatric Critical Care Medicine. 2015 Oct 1;**16**(8):e308-e312

[23] Brilli RJ, Spevetz A, Branson RD, Campbell GM, Cohen H, Dasta JF, Harvey MA, Kelley MA, Kelly KM, Rudis MI, Andre AC. Critical care delivery in the intensive care unit: Defining clinical roles and the best practice model. Critical Care Medicine. 2001 Oct 1;**29**(10):2007-2019

[24] Kane RL, Shamliyan T, Mueller C, Duval S, Wilt TJ. Nurse staffing and quality of patient care. Evidence Report Technology Assessment (Full Report). 2007 Mar;**151**:1-15

[25] Daud-Gallotti RM, Costa SF, Guimarães T, Padilha KG, Inoue EN, Vasconcelos TN, Rodrigues FD, Barbosa EV, Figueiredo WB, Levin AS. Nursing workload as a risk factor for healthcare associated infections in ICU: A prospective study. PloS One. 2012 Dec 27;**7**(12):e52342

[26] Endacott R. Intensive Care Medicine. The continuing imperative to measure workload in ICU: Impact on patient safety and staff well-being. 2012; **38**(9):1415-1417

[27] Aveyard, D. How do 12-hour shifts affect ICU nurses? Kai Tiaki Nursing New Zealand. 2016 December;**22**(11):34-36.

[28] Koradecka D, editor. Handbook of occupational safety and health. In: Zuzewicz K, editor. Shift Work. USA: CRC Press; 2010. pp. 501-508

[29] Kamdar BB, Tergas AI, Mateen FJ, Bhayani NH, Oh J. Night-shift work and risk of breast cancer: A systematic review and meta-analysis. Breast Cancer Research and Treatment. 2013 Feb 1;**138**(1):291-301

[30] Koradecka D, editor. Handbook of occupational safety and health. In: Widerszal-Bazyl M, editor. Psychosocial Risk in the Workplace and its Reduction. USA; CRC Press: 2010. pp. 60-73, 77-80

[31] Bhattacharya A, McGlothlin JD, editors. Occupational ergonomics: Theory and applications. In: Longmate AR, editor. Ergonomic Control Measures in the Health Care Industry. USA: CRC Press; 2012 Mar 8. pp. 599, 601, 614-617, 623-624

[32] Dale AM, Jaegers L, Buchholz B, Welch L, Evanoff BA. Using process evaluation to determine effectiveness of participatory ergonomics training interventions in construction. Work. 2012 Jan 1;**41**(Supplement 1):3824-3826

[33] Côté JN, Ngomo S, Stock S, Messing K, Vézina N, Antle D, Delisle A, Bellemare M, Laberge M, St-Vincent M. Quebec research on work-related musculoskeletal disorders: Deeper understanding for better prevention. Industrial Relations/Relations Industrielles. 2013 Oct 1;**68**(4):643-660

[34] Freimann T, Merisalu E, Pääsuke M. Effects of a home-exercise therapy programme on cervical and lumbar range of motion among nurses with neck and lower back pain: A quasi-experimental study. BMC Sports Science, Medicine and Rehabilitation. 2015 Dec 4;**7**(1):31

[35] Ganiyu SO, Olabode JA, Stanley MM, Muhammad I. Patterns of occurrence of work-related musculoskeletal disorders and its correlation with ergonomic hazards among health care professionals. Nigerian Journal of Experimental and Clinical Biosciences. 2015 Jan 1;**3**(1):18

[36] Koradecka D, editor. Handbook of occupational safety and health. In: Dutkiewicz J, editor. Biological Agents. USA: CRC Press; 2010. pp. 386-388, 395-396

[37] Watkins D, Cousins J, editors. Public Health and Community Nursing: Frameworks for Practice. USA: Elsevier Health Sciences; 2009 Oct 23

[38] Bowie P, Ferguson J, MacLeod M, Kennedy S, de Wet C, McNab D, Kelly M, McKay J, Atkinson S. Participatory design of a preliminary safety checklist for general practice. British Journal of General Practice. 2015 May 1;**65**(634):e330-e343

[39] El Fassi M, Bocquet V, Majery N, Lair ML, Couffignal S, Mairiaux P. Work ability assessment in a worker population: Comparison and determinants of Work Ability Index and Work Ability score. BMC Public Health. 2013 Apr **8**;13(1):305

[40] Abbasi M, Zakerian A, Kolahdouzi M, Mehri A, Akbarzadeh A, Ebrahimi MH. Relationship between Work Ability Index and cognitive failure among nurses. Electronic Physician. 2016 Mar;**8**(3):2136

[41] Boyle T. Health and Safety: Risk Management. USA: Routledge; 2015 Sep 14.

[42] Larsson A, Karlqvist L, Westerberg M, Gard G. Identifying work ability promoting factors for home care aides and assistant nurses. BMC Musculoskeletal Disorders. 2012 Jan 11;**13**(1):1

[43] Vigorito MC, McNicoll L, Adams L, Sexton B. Improving safety culture results in Rhode Island ICUs: Lessons learned from the development of action-oriented plans. The Joint Commission Journal on Quality and Patient Safety. 2011;**37**(11):509-514

[44] Chaboyer W, Chamberlain D, Hewson-Conroy K, Grealy B, Elderkin T, Brittin M, McCutcheon C, Longbottom P, Thalib L. CNE article: Safety culture in Australian intensive care units: Establishing a baseline for quality improvement. American Journal of Critical Care. 2013 Mar 1;**22**(2):93-102

[45] Sorra JS, Nieva VF. Hospital Survey on Patient Safety Culture. Rockville, MD: Agency for Healthcare Research and Quality; September 2004. Prepared by Westat, under Contract 290-96-0004. AHRQ Publication 04-0041

[46] Sexton JB, Berenholtz SM, Goeschel CA, Watson SR, Holzmueller CG, Thompson DA, Hyzy RC, Marsteller JA, Schumacher K, Pronovost PJ. Assessing and improving safety climate in a large cohort of intensive care units. Critical Care Medicine. 2011 May 1;**39**(5):934-939

[47] Stigmar KG, Petersson IF, Jöud A, Grahn BE. Promoting work ability in a structured national rehabilitation program in patients with musculoskeletal disorders: outcomes and predictors in a prospective cohort study. BMC Musculoskeletal Disorders. 2013;**14**(1):1

[48] Rasmussen CD, Holtermann A, Mortensen OS, Søgaard K, Jørgensen MB. Prevention of low back pain and its consequences among nurses' aides in elderly care: A stepped-wedge multi-faceted cluster-randomized controlled trial. BMC Public Health. 2013;**13**(1):1088

[49] Lim HJ, Black TR, Shah SM, Sarker S, Metcalfe J. Evaluating repeated patient handling injuries following the implementation of a multi-factor ergonomic intervention program among health care workers. Journal of Safety Research. 2011;**42**(3):185-191

[50] Black TR, Shah SM, Busch AJ, Metcalfe J, Lim HJ. Effect of transfer, lifting, and repositioning (TLR) injury prevention program on musculoskeletal injury among direct care workers. Journal of Occupational and Environmental Hygiene. 2011 Jan 22;**8**(4):226-235

[51] Rivilis I, Van Eerd D, Cullen K, Cole DC, Irvin E, Tyson J, Mahood Q. Effectiveness of participatory ergonomic interventions on health outcomes: A systematic review. Applied Ergonomics. 2008 May 31;**39**(3):342-358

[52] Yildiz AN, Çaman ÖG, Nihal ES. Işyerinde sağliği geliştirme programlari. Ankara: TÜRK-İŞ; 2012

[53] Silverstein B, Clark R. Interventions to reduce work-related musculoskeletal disorders. Journal of Electromyography and Kinesiology. 2004 Feb 29;**14**(1):135-152

[54] Sato N, Sekiguchi M, Kikuchi S, Shishido H, Sato K, Konno S. Effects of long-term corset wearing on chronic low back pain. Fukushima Journal of Medical Science. 2012;**58**(1):60-65

[55] Bigos SJ, Holland J, Holland C, Webster JS, Battie M, Malmgren JA. High-quality controlled trials on preventing episodes of back problems: Systematic literature review in working-age adults. The Spine Journal. 2009 Feb 28;**9**(2):147-168

[56] Roelofs PD, Bierma-Zeinstra SM, van Poppel MN, van Mechelen W, Koes BW, van Tulder MW. Cost-effectiveness of lumbar supports for home care workers with recurrent low back pain: An economic evaluation alongside a randomized-controlled trial. Spine. 2010 Dec 15;**35**(26):E1619–E1626

[57] Calmels P, Queneau P, Hamonet C, Le Pen C, Maurel F, Lerouvreur C, Thoumie P. Effectiveness of a lumbar belt in subacute low back pain: An open, multicentric, and randomized clinical study. Spine. 2009 Feb 1;**34**(3):215-220

[58] Pender NJ, Murdaugh CL, Parsons MA. Health Promotion in Nursing Practice. USA: 6th ed. 2006.

[59] Gielen AC, McDonald EM, Gary TL, Bone LR. Using the precede-proceed model to apply health behavior theories. Health Behavior and Health Education: Theory, Research, and Practice. 2008;**4**:407-429

[60] Prochaska JO, Velicer WF. The transtheoretical model of health behavior change. American Journal of Health Promotion. 1997 Sep;**12**(1):38-48

3

Anesthesia and Intensive Care Management for Cardiac Transplantation

Massimo Baiocchi, Maria Benedetto,
Marta Agulli and Guido Frascaroli

Abstract

Patient management in heart transplant is quite complex and includes multiple steps from preoperative recipient evaluation to postoperative ICU treatment. Monitoring, anesthesia induction, and cardiopulmonary bypass weaning strategies are discussed. The success of the operation also depends on right heart support especially in case of pulmonary hypertension. Many details like fluid management, well-timed respiratory weaning, and primary graft dysfunction management can make the difference in terms of outcome. Pediatric heart transplants represent a small group of total cardiac transplant, but the differences in anatomy and physiology make the surgical and anesthesiological management more complex in unique scenario that requires a specific knowledge at different stages of growth, from newborn through childhood up to adulthood.

Keywords: anesthesia, intensive care, monitoring, inotropic drugs, mechanical support

1. Intraoperative management

Intraoperative management in heart transplant is quite complex and includes multiple steps from preoperative evaluation to ICU admission.

1.1. Preoperative evaluation

During this phase, we need to collect the consent from the patient after having explained to him all the possible complications coming from surgery, anesthesia, and ICU stay.

Above all, we need to know the background history of the patient, any previous issue with general anesthesia, allergies, difficult airway management, and any possible contraindication to the transplant itself [**Table 1**].

A multiorgan analysis must be taken into account:

- Neurological history: syncopal episodes, carotid stenosis, ischemic or hemorrhagic stroke, transitory ischemic attack.
- Respiratory history: smoke, COPD, spirometry, DLCO test.
- Cardiovascular history:
  1. origin of cardiomyopathy: dilated/hypertrophic/ischemic cardiomyopathy
  2. noncompaction left ventricle (LV), sarcoidosis, amyloidosis, and others
  3. arrhythmias: episodes of sudden cardiac death syndrome, implantation of an ICD
  4. right side catheterization: pulmonary artery pressures (PAP), pulmonary capillary wedge pressure (PCWP), pulmonary vascular resistances (PVR), results of reversibility test with enoximone, origin of pulmonary hypertension (prepost capillary)
  5. presence of prosthetic valves in situ
  6. home medications: oral anticoagulants, ace inhibitors, b-blockers, diuretics
- Renal history: chronic or acute renal failure, preoperative serum level of creatinine and urea, creatinine clearance, history of renal replacement therapy.
- Hepatobiliary history: a systemic portal venous congestion can often derive from chronic congestive heart failure. In this case, high levels of transaminases and bilirubin may occur and this may influence the pharmacological and hemodynamic management during anesthesia.

Absolute contraindications	Relative contraindications
Significant COPD (FEV1 < 1 L/min)	Age > 72 years
Fixed pulmonary hypertension	Active infections
PAPs >60 mmHg	BMI > 35 kg/m^2 or <18 kg/m^2
GTP > 15 mmHg	Creatinine clearance < 25 ml/min
PVR > 6 wood units	Active mental illness or psychosocial instability
Irreversible renal or hepatic dysfunction	Severe peripheral vascular disease
AIDS/malignancy/lupus	Diabetes mellitus with end organ damage

Table 1. Contraindications to heart transplantation.

- Metabolic history: surgical stress and corticosteroid therapy may dramatically increase glycemia levels and hyperglycemia may dramatically increase the lactate levels during and after surgery; this is the reason why we need to know if the patient has diabetes and plan a proper blood glucose control with continuous infusion insulin (usually 50 UI/50 ml gelatin starting with a speed of 2–3 ml/h, depending on glucose plasma levels, with a target of 80–150 mg/dl). Among metabolic disorders, hypothyroidism can be further impaired during and after heart transplantation because plasma levels of triiodothyronine are often decreased during long periods of cardiopulmonary bypass, so that it's important to plan an early replacement thyroid therapy.
- Preoperative fasting: the patient should fast from food at least 8 hours and from fluids 4–6 hours before the operation.
- Premedication: it's important to avoid any preoperative oversedation since hypoxia may increase the pulmonary vascular resistances (PVR). We usually do not exceed a dose of 10—15 drops per os of diazepam in adult patients before going to theater, but, if the patient is really critical, we avoid any premedication.

1.2. Recipient with pulmonary hypertension

Severe pulmonary hypertension in the recipient is one of the major contraindications to heart transplant [1, 2] due to high risk of right heart failure. When pulmonary hypertension persists up to 1 year from transplant, clinical outcomes and percentage of long-term survival are really poor [3]. For the above-mentioned reasons, a potential recipient must be evaluated with caution before being added to the waiting list. First of all, he needs to be sent for cath lab in order to evaluate his own pulmonary vascular resistances (PVR), mean pulmonary arterial pressure (m-PAP), pulmonary artery wedge pressure (PAWP), cardiac output (CO), cardiac index (CI), and the transpulmonary gradient (TPG).

This last equals the difference between mPAP and wedge pressure (TPG = mPAP – PAWP).

In case of high PVR (PVR > 3 wood units [WU]), it is important to perform the reversibility test with enoximone or dobutamine in order to quantify the reversibility degree of pulmonary hypertension. When postcapillary pulmonary hypertension (defined as mPAP ≥ 25 mmHg, PAWP > 15 mmHg and PVR > 3WU) is unresponsive to dobutamine reversibility test (i.e., PVR > 3 WU or mPAP > 35 mmHg with a TPG > 12 mmHg), a team made of cardiologists, anesthesiologists, and cardiac surgeons should seriously evaluate if the patient is suitable for receiving a new heart.

A preventive treatment with pulmonary vasodilators such as sildenafil should be considered since it has been shown to decrease the PVR in a period of few months [4].

A preventive treatment with sildenafil should also be considered when patients are scheduled for receiving an LVAD positioning as bridge to transplant, thanks to its effectiveness in long-term reduction of the PVR and major responsiveness to a further test with dobutamine [5].

2. Monitoring and induction of general anesthesia

Timing to get the patient ready to receive the new organ is crucial because the ischemia of the donor heart should be as short as possible to avoid the ischemia-reperfusion injury.

Everyone in the theater should wear sterile surgical gown, hat, mask, and sterile gloves for any procedure on the patient especially because he will go under immune deficiency. Once the patient is in the theater, he will be connected to multiparametric monitor, with the 12 lead ECG and oximetry probe. Two peripheral venous lines are placed (generally 18G for iv sedation and 14G for rapid fluid infusion), and an arterial catheter, generally 20G, is placed into the radial or humeral artery. When the patient is very unstable, an arterial catheter is placed in the left femoral artery, to estimate central to peripheral arterial pressure gradients. Placement of an arterial line can be very difficult in patients with previous implantation of LVADs as bridge to transplant, due to the absence of arterial pulse. In such situations, ultrasound guidance can be very helpful (see **Table 2**).

Induction of general anesthesia usually starts just with the final acceptance of the donor organ. Drugs used for general anesthesia should impact the less possible on hemodynamics. A rapid sequence induction is preferred since recipients are always very stressed and sometimes not present with an empty stomach [6].

Midazolam (10–15 mg) or etomidate (20 mg) are preferred to propofol for hypnosis, due to the less impact on hemodynamics. Opioids like fentanyl or sufentanil are preferred for the same reason ("stress-free anesthesia"), with an induction dose of 0.2–0.4 mcg/kg for sufentanil and 2–4 mcg/kg for fentanyl. Continuous infusion analgesia remifentanil is preferable for the less impact on renal function since it is metabolized by plasmatic esterase. This is particularly important in patients with low cardiac output and preexisting renal failure. Remifentanil will be turned off and replaced by morphine or tramadol (30 mg/die and 300 mg/die, respectively), before moving to the intensive care unit. Mean term muscle relaxant rocuronium (1 mg/kg) is usually the first choice for rapid sequence induction. Sometimes short-term cisatracurium

Device	Measure
PA radial	Invasive arterial pressure (peripheral)
PA fem	Invasive arterial pressure (central)
CVP	Central venous pressure
ECG	12 lead electrocardiography
SpO2	Oxygen saturation levels
PAC	(pulmonary artery catheter) PAPs, PAPm, PAPd, sVO_2
TEE	Biventricular function, shape of ventricular septum, filling, air etc.
NIRS	$ScvO_2$ correlation, adequate tissue perfusion, brain perfusion
LAP	LV filling pressure

Table 2. Standard monitoring.

besylate (0.15–0.2 mg/kg for induction and 1–2 mcg/kg/min for continuous iv infusion during surgery) is a good alternative since it is metabolized by ester hydrolysis and Hofmann reaction, so the duration of block is not affected by renal or hepatic function. During induction of general anesthesia, severe hypotension can occur, so that a fluid iv bolus ad availability of rapid onset vasoconstrictors as metaraminol, phenylephrine, noradrenaline should be ensured. Cardioplegia is not administered in the recipient during heart transplantation, so that the risk of related hemodilution is less than routine cardiac surgery. On pump, sevoflurane or iv 2% propofol infusion (4 mg/kg/h) are the options for maintenance of general anesthesia. Monitoring the depth of anesthesia with bispectral index (BIS) should be routinely adopted in order to decrease the risk of awareness. Once having put the patient asleep, central lines must be placed (queen central venous pressure [CVP] line and 8 Fr line for the pulmonary artery catheter [PAC]). The ideal site for puncture (blind or ultrasound-guided) is the left internal jugular vein (IJV), since the right one can be reserved for eventual postoperative biopsy (necessary to evaluate the level of graft rejection). When this is not possible (presence of ICD on the left side), we can adopt the right subclavian vein. Sometimes, when the preoperative renal function is really compromised, we can already place into the femoral or subclavian vein a catheter for continuous renal filtration afterwards. The PA catheter is flown through the 8 Fr line up to the right atrium, and then, once the new heart is placed, it will be advanced by the cardiac surgeon up to the superior right pulmonary artery. Vigilance calibration will be done immediately before weaning from the CPB.

3. CPB and weaning

If the graft is not carried out into the organ care system (OCS), the ischemic time is crucial and the risk of ischemic/reperfusion injury is proportionally high, with possible dramatic increase of blood lactate levels and decrease of the graft global function. This is the reason why we must ensure adequate glycemia control, urine output, and, in general, an optimal tissue perfusion during CPB. This means to guarantee an adequate oxygen delivery (DO_2), which means to keep MAPs about 60–80 mmHg and Hb levels at least about 8–9 mg/dL. When the aorta is unclamped, VF can occur (50% of patients). A shock delivery (10–30 J) followed by lidocaine bolus (when VF is refractory to electrical therapy) will take to resolution of the arrhythmia and return to sinus rhythm. In case of sinus bradycardia, temporary epicardial pacing will ensure adequate heart rate (100–110 bpm). Due to limited muscular mass, the ability of the right ventricle (RV) to increase contractility is limited and a temporary pacing at about 110 bpm will increase RV output and will overpace possible arrhythmias. Surgeons will also place a left atrial catheter for continuous measurement of the left atrial pressure (LAP) as an indicator of the left ventricle performance and stiffness. This value, together with CVP, PAPs, MAPs, and SvO2, will influence the posttransplantation hemodynamic management. Throughout this period, it will be mandatory to ensure adequate MAPs and diastolic pressure to allow adequate coronary perfusion, while maintaining medium-low preload pressures (CVP < 12 mmHg, LAP/PCWP < 12 mmHg). The biventricular assessment with transesophageal echocardiography should be done simultaneously.

Pharmacological tools for CPB weaning will include the following [**Tables 3** and **4**]:

- Isoprenaline at low-moderate dose (0.02–0.04 mcg/kg/min): it is the first choice in heart transplantation due to the positive chronotropic effect; it helps to guarantee a heart rate of 100–110 bpm. If it does not work, do not go beyond 0.04 mcg/kg/min, in order to avoid hypotensive effects. In this case, switching to atrial pacing is the best choice.
- Adrenaline (0.02–0.2 mcg/kg/min): it provides inotropic support to the new heart, especially to the right ventricle, which is the one more at risk of failure.
- Milrinone (0.2–0.5 mcg/kg/min) or other phosphodiesterase inhibitors (enoximone at 5–8 mcg/kg/min): they increase contractility especially of the right ventricle, while decreasing pulmonary vascular resistances. They both increase intracellular levels of cAMP, but they also decrease the systemic vascular resistances (SVR), so that the patient may benefit from low-moderate noradrenergic support in addition. If systemic peripheral resistances are really low, selective pulmonary vasodilators, aimed to decrease RV afterload without affecting peripheral resistances, are a better choice: inhaled nitric oxide (iNO) at 20–40 ppm [9, 17]) or aerosolized prostaglandins (iloprost 20 mcg/15 min, repeated after 4 hours).

  Possible side effects of these selective inhalation drugs are inhibition of platelet activation and aggregation and inhibition of leucocyte adhesion.
- Levosimendan (0.1–0.2 mcg/kg/min) has also been reported to reverse low cardiac output after heart transplantation [10], although its use has not been shown to reduce cardiac surgery mortality [11].

After having unclamped the aorta and before weaning from CPB, about 1 hour of assistance to the new heart is provided. During this period, an adequate temperature is achieved (36–36.5°C measured by nasopharyngeal temperature probe). Vigilance calibration is performed by providing Hb levels and SvO_2 from gas analysis; it gives results about the indexed cardiac output, pulmonary vascular resistances, and systemic peripheral vascular resistances, indexed on the patient weight. PAPs are shown on the monitor together with CVP, LAP, MAPs, and ECG. The PAVR (pulmonary artery vascular resistance) equals: PAVR = [80 × (mean pulmonary artery pressure – pulmonary + capillary wedge pressure)/cardiac output] (normal value 100 dynes/cm^{-5}).

The TPG (transpulmonary gradient) equals: TPG = mPAP – PCWP (normal value 6 mmHg).

A TPG > 15 mmHg is considered at high risk to develop early postoperative RV dysfunction [7]. The reason for RV dysfunction development may be found in the background of the donor heart. Especially when young and comparably small, it may not easily adapt to the already existing pulmonary hypertension in the recipient. Furthermore, as a result of a long ischemia and CPB time, with ischemia-reperfusion injury, RV dilates, becomes ischemic, and further reduces its own contractility. In this case, we need to adjust the amount of inotropes, chronotropes, and pulmonary vasodilators given, basing also on transesophageal echocardiography that can show the biventricular systolic-diastolic function and fluid responsiveness. Once the patient is stable and the heart rate is appropriate, we can start ventilation and slowly decrease the pump flow until 0.5–1 L/min. At that point, we come out from bypass. During CPB weaning, the heart should be loaded with caution because RV is very sensitive to distension. Echocardiographic parameters to asses the RV behavior will be RVFAC (fractional area change), leftward shift of

Sustain SVR and arterial pressure (if necessary)	Norepinephrine vasopressin
Maintain DO_2 level 272 ml/min/m^2	Raise in pump flow Raise Hb level Raise O_2 sat Decrease body temp
Support graft	Milrinone (0.2–0.5 mcg/kg/min) Dopamine (4–6 mcg/kg/min) Epinephrine (0.05–0.25 mcg/kg/min)
Hb level	11 g/dl
Maintain regular rhythm and A-V synchrony 110 bpm	K^+/Mg^+ Pacing Isoprenaline (0.02–0.04 mcg/kg/min)
Pacing with 110–120 bpm	Increase of HR increases CI, avoid overload
Reduce PVR (if necessary)	iNO (20–40 ppm) Inhalatory iloprost (10–20 ng) Inhalatory milrinone (5 mg) for 15 min
Slowly reduce CPB flow (careful monitoring CVP, TEE, LAP)	Check/change drug infusion rate Check chamber filling Check contractility

Table 3. Practice guide to wean from CPB.

Drug	Average dosage	Advantages	Side effects
Epinephrine	0.05–0.25 mcg/kg/min	Support RV overload	Tachycardia, arrhythmias, raise O_2 demand
Norepinephrine	Up to 0.15 mcg/kg/min	Contrast vasodilatation	Increase PVR
Levosimendan	0.1–0.2 mcg/kg/min	Support RV overload	Vasodilation
Milrinone	0.2–0.5 mcg/kg/min	Support RV overload	Arrhythmias, raise O_2 demand, vasodilation
Vasopressin	2.5–5 U/h	Contrast vasodilatation	Increase SVR impair forward flow of LVAD
i-NO	20–40 ppm	Reduce PVR (if not fixed)	
i-Milrinone	5 mg/15 min	Reduce PVR (if not fixed)	
i-Iloprost	20–30 mcg/15 min	Reduce PVR (if not fixed)	
Methylene blue	0.5–2 mg/kg	Contrast vasodilation	

Table 4. Inotropes/vasoactive: average therapeutic dosage to support hemodynamics.

Inotropic score	Dopamine (μg/kg/min) + dobutamine (μg/kg/min) + 100 × epinephrine (μg/kg/min)
Vasoactive inotropic score (modified by Davidson et al. with inclusion of vasoactive medication	IS + 10 × milrinone (μg/kg/min) + 10 × vasopressin (U/kg/min) + 100 × norepinephrine (μg/kg/min
Vasoactive inotropic score plus levosimendan	VIS + 10 × levosimendan (mcg/kg/min)
Poor clinical outcome	VIS 20–24 (in the first 24 h) + VIS 15–19 (in the subsequent 24 h)

Table 5. Inotropic score.

IAS (interatrial septum) or "fluttering" of IVS (interventricular septum) during end-diastole, TAPSE(tricuspid annular plane systolic excursion), and MPI (myocardial performance index).

Basic ventilation strategies to reduce pulmonary artery resistances such as hyperoxia and moderate hyperventilation are mandatory. Ventilation should be set at 60–100% FiO_2, 6–8 ml/kg TV (tidal volume), and low-moderate PEEP (5–6 cmH_2O), after recruitment maneuver, with the intention to prevent lung atelectasis [12].

Chest closure can be very critical for hemodynamics. In some rare cases (i.e., 2.5%), primary graft failure can occur [13], and it is responsible for more than 30% of early deaths after cardiac transplantation. Clinical onset of primary graft failure is with hypotension, low cardiac output, high preload pressures (PVC, LAP, and wedge pressure), and biventricular failure. When necessary, a temporary IABP (intra-aortic balloon pump), as first step, and then peripheral (femoral vein-femoral artery) or central (left atrium, right atrium, aorta) VA-ECMO (venous-arteriosus extracorporeal membrane oxygenation) should be taken into account, whenever hemodynamics remain unsatisfactory despite high inotropic support (**Table 5**) [14].

4. Fluid management

Fluid management should be "goal directed," that is, guided by the above-mentioned hemodynamic and echocardiographic parameters, and with the aim to avoid a fluid overload, which is very harmful for the lungs and the right ventricle, while providing adequate intravascular space filling. This should be done via balanced colloids and crystalloids in order to avoid electrolyte disorders and hyperchloremic hyperkalemic metabolic acidosis. Adequate oxygen delivery is ensured by maintaining the hemoglobin level around 10–11 g/dL and an adequate plasma oncotic power is ensured by giving the right amount of albumin.

5. Anticoagulation and hemostasis

To go on CPB, we need to provide an appropriate anticoagulation via unfractionated heparin (300–400 U/kg). A value of ACT at least of 480 s is enough to start the extracorporeal circulation. In case of low response to a full dose of heparin, we can achieve an adequate ACT by administering antithrombin III (AT3), especially when AT3 plasma levels are less than 70%. From 0.5 to 5% of patients with end-stage heart disease can develop HIT (heparin-induced thrombocytopenia), due to repeated heparin exposures related to the placement of IABP, LVADs, or frequent catheter procedures. Alternative anticoagulation, with direct thrombin inhibitors (bivalirudin and argatroban), [8] is recommended in such patients. At the end of organ implantation, once the aortic and right atrium cannulas are removed, we need to guarantee an appropriate heparin reversal with protamine (50 mg of protamine every 50 mg of heparin). We also give the patient 2 g of tranexamic acid at the induction of general anesthesia and 2 g (25–50 mg/kg) with protamine in association with 1 g of gluconate calcium, to avoid hyperfibrinolysis and replace calcium deficiency. Severe bleeding is not a rare condition especially in patients with previous heart surgery. Particularly, in patients with LVADs as bridge to transplant, severe bleeding can often occur due to the large wound area and pretreatment with multiple anticoagulants and platelet inhibitors. If hemostasis is insufficient and the patient is still bleeding, we need to check for coagulation disorders via ROTEM (i.e., hyperfibrinolysis, coagulation factor deficiency, and hypofibrinogenemia) or via TEG and correct the specific deficiency (prothrombin complex concentrate for clotting factor deficiency or fibrinogen concentrate for hypofibrinogenemia). We prefer this approach instead of large dose of fresh frozen plasma, in order to avoid TACO (transfusion-associated circulatory overload), TRALI (transfusion-related lung injury), immune modulation, and increased risk of infections.

6. Intensive care management

Almost 90% of heart transplants are due to ischemic or dilatative cardiomyopathy and men over 40 years of age are the most involved. They all need a special care and a multimodal approach, even because not only cardiovascular balance but also respiratory care, fluid management, and immune system modulation impact on the overall survival.

6.1. ICU admission

Patients incoming from the operating room have to be placed in an isolated single bed room to avoid contamination, since they will undergo immunosuppressive therapy. Everyone in contact with them must wear mask, cup, and sterile gown and do routine sterile hand washing. Invasive hemodynamic monitoring, including systemic arterial pressure, right atrial pressure, pulmonary artery pressure through the PAC, and left atrial pressure, should be immediately reconnected in the room.

Twelve lead ECG at the arrival is mandatory to check heart rhythm disorders. Bradyarrhythmias and supraventricular arrhythmias are the most frequent and should be related to inotropic and chronotropic support, hypovolemia, and electrolyte disorders. If atrial fibrillation occurs, an acute rejection should be considered and a 500 mg bolus of methylprednisolone should be administered, eventually followed by amiodarone (300 mg iv bolus in 30 min) for pharmacological cardioversion and rate control. In case of failure of pharmacological cardioversion, we can try electrical cardioversion. Sinus bradycardia can be treated with low-dose isoprenaline (0.01–0.04 mcg/kg/min), adrenaline (0.01–0.04 mcg/kg/min), and/or temporary atrial pacing, in order to ensure a heart rate about 100–110 bpm. In case of severe AV block, a sequential pacing is required. Anyway, if the patient is still pacing dependent after 2 weeks from the operation, implantation of a permanent pace maker should be considered. Then, you can proceed to request chest X-ray to check the lungs, endotracheal and nasogastric tube position, chest drains, and intravascular devices (CVP line, PAC, and pacing wires) and send for laboratory tests including standard coagulation, renal and liver function, platelets, red blood cell and white blood cell counts, troponin I, CK, albumin, viral markers, thyroid markers, and glycaemia. Blood samples should be sent for good practice also for coagulation tests (ROTEM or TEG) in case of excessive bleeding. A plan for immunosuppressive therapy (methylprednisolone, thymoglobulins, etc.) must be provided in collaboration with specialist immunologist and cardiologist. Antibiotic therapy must be tailored on the background history of donor and/or recipient.

7. Hemodynamic management

Hemodynamic stability, after heart transplant, may be impaired by several pathophysiological processes, including autonomic denervation, with subsequent chronotropic and inotropic failure, ischemia reperfusion injury, metabolic acidosis, and volume depletion. To support such effects, several endpoints must be taken into account:

7.1. Intravascular volume optimization

A goal-directed therapy is the ideal way to ensure adequate fluid filling. It means using the above-mentioned hemodynamic parameters coming from invasive monitoring and from echocardiographic evaluation, to be guided in the fluid replacement. Once the need of fluids is clear, the physician should decide the most ideal fluid in order to avoid peripheral organ oncotic damage (i.e., hyperoncotic kidney failure from hydroxyethyl starches [15]); hyperchloremic hyperkalemic acidosis, which can impact itself on kidney function; and fluid overload into the interstitial space. Crystalloids have a less oncotic power than colloids; however, albumin can cross the pulmonary capillary membrane, if damaged, and anyway it can recirculate through the pulmonary barrier 24 hours from the administration: then balanced crystalloids and balanced colloids (albumin solution at 5 or 20%) should be given at the right per kilo amount and the fluid responsiveness should be tested while they are given.

7.2. Narrow monitoring of hemodynamic parameters

During the recovery period (approximately 7–14 days), a narrow monitoring of hemodynamic and vital parameters is mandatory: IBP, CI, CO, ISVRI, IPVR, PAPs, HR, SvO_2, LAP/PCWP, TPG, SpO_2, ECG, body temperature, urine output, and lactate levels.

Target values are: CVP $\leq$ 12 mmHg, MAP > 65 mmHg, LAP 8–12 mmHg, SvO_2 over 65%, HR about 100–110 bpm, urine output > 1.5 ml/kg, and lactate < 2 mmol/L.

7.3. Pharmacological support

The goal is to ensure adequate CO, avoiding excessive increase of cardiac preload and afterload, while maintaining adequate heart rate. Chronotropic support is achieved through low-moderate dose of isoprenaline or by atrial-sequential external pacing. Inotropic effect is achieved through moderate-high dose of adrenaline and, when necessary, with phosphodiesterase inhibitors as milrinone that also decreases peripheral vascular resistances. Other pharmacological tools that are aimed to control arterial ventricle coupling are nitroglycerin and sodium nitroprusside, very helpful to decrease the afterload of the left ventricle and increase cardiac output, when used together with an inotropic drug. In case of preexistent pulmonary hypertension, inhalation of nitric oxide and imbrication with sildenafil can help to reduce pulmonary vascular resistances [14]. In the further postoperative course, addition of an upstream therapy including ace inhibitors, b-blockers, or calcium antagonists may be helpful as cardiac protection.

7.4. Support the right ventricle of the donor heart

The donor heart, particularly the right ventricle, in case of preexisting precapillary or post-capillary pulmonary hypertension, has to fight with high afterload [**Table 6**]. The preexisting conditions may be impaired in case of coexisting hypoxia or hypercapnia, prolonged extracorporeal circulation, and donor ischemia with consequent ischemia-reperfusion injury, blood transfusion, and protamine administration. Right ventricular failure may be challenging and really impacts on the overall survival of transplanted patients [18].

Early PA pressure monitoring at the time of CPB weaning is fundamental and has to be continued in the early postoperative period. The first aim in hemodynamic management of the graft is to offload the right ventricle, decreasing PA pressures and pulmonary vascular resistances while ensuring an adequate RV contractility. Inhaled nitric oxide at 20–40 ppm is a rapid onset tool to decrease PA pressures. It seems to improve early clinical outcomes in heart transplanted patients, but literature is still lacking in terms of overall survival [9].

This is the reason why it is often used preventively during weaning from the CPB. Alternatively, the prostacyclin analog iloprost (6 × 5–10 mcg) can be given.

After the very early postoperative period, inhaled nitric oxide can be substituted by the phosphodiesterase-5 inhibitor sildenafil at the dosage of 20 mg × 3/die via NG tube with very small effects on the systemic pressures, avoiding also the rebound phenomena coming from the discontinuation of inhaled nitric oxide therapy. Sildenafil has also been shown to decrease PA pressures during inhalation of nitric oxide, since they seem to activate different regulatory mechanisms of the vascular tone [19, 20]. Inotropic support of the RV should be guaranteed by moderate-high dose of adrenaline (0.05–0.1 mcg/kg/min) or low-moderate doses of phosphodiesterase inhibitors as milrinone (0.2–0.3 mcg/kg/min).

Clearly, while supporting the right ventricle, we need to ensure adequate oxygenation, avoid hypercapnia, maintain adequate lung recruitment by PEEP (not over 6 cmH_2O), and guarantee a negative fluid balance in order to reduce the preload and optimize the afterload [**Table 6**]. If all these maneuvers are not sufficient, we have to consider a temporary mechanical right ventricle support via peripheral VA-ECMO.

Monitor by PAC	CVP, MPAP, PCWP, CO, SvO_2
Mechanical ventilation	PaO_2 100 mmHg, pCO_2 30–35 mmHg, pH 7.5. Adequate peep level (5–10 cm H_2O) to recruit lung and optimize PVR
Restricted fluid therapy	Monitoring filling pressure CVP 10–12 mmHg, PCWP 12–15 mmHg
	Monitoring LVEDV, RVEDV by echocardiography
Inotropes to support RV contractility	Epinephrine 0.02–0.25 mcg/kg/min
Inodilator	Milrinone 0.2–0.5 mcg/kg/min
	Levosimendan 0.2 mcg/kg/min ± norepinephrine (up to 0.15 mcg/kg/min) to maintain right coronary perfusion pressure
iNO	5–40 ppm
Phosphodiesterase V inhibitor	Revatio 3 × 20 mg p.o.
Systemic vasodilators	Sodium nitroprusside, prostacyclin PGI_2 analogon iloprost (2 ng/kg/min)

Table 6. Pulmonary artery hypertension monitoring and right ventricular dysfunction prevention.

In case of concomitant LV insufficiency and signs of systemic hypoperfusion (with raising of LAP/PCWP and sudden reduction of CO, CI, and SvO_2), we will need to increase the inotrope support and try to compensate the peripheral vasoconstriction with peripheral vasodilators as nitroprusside, when the MAPs allow to do that, in order to reduce left ventricle afterload and facilitate the ejection. The conditioning with inodilators as levosimendan [10] can be very helpful and, in case of massive peripheral vasodilatory response, it can be compensated with mean dosage of noradrenaline to ensure adequate MAPs. When this is not enough, an additional support with IABP should be considered, but, when insufficient, a central or peripheral VA-ECMO will be placed. The simultaneous presence of the IABP will help avoid pulmonary edema by reducing the afterload of LV.

7.5. Avoid metabolic acidosis and monitor acid-base balance and kidney function

A patient undergoing heart transplant comes from a long period of low cardiac output, so the kidney dysfunction is often preexisting.

In the immediate postoperative period, urinary output may decrease for several reasons including intravascular volume depletion and kidney damage coming from long lasting extracorporeal support or from the use of unbalanced solutions for fluid challenge. In addition, a high use of colloidal molecules may damage directly the renal tubules with a process called "osmotic-nephrosis." If urine output is <0.5 ml/kg/h despite optimization of blood pressure, preload and CO, and use of standard diuretics (furosemide or torasemide), and the patient develops kidney failure with serum urea >200 mg/dL or hyperkalemia, kidney replacement therapy becomes mandatory.

We prefer early application of continuous venovenous hemofiltration (CVVH) for a complete hemodynamic and fluid rebalancing. In case kidney replacement therapy is necessary in a long-term postoperative period, the change is made to intermittent dialysis (three times weekly).

7.6. Consider echocardiography as a main tool, together with PAC, to guide hemodynamic management, inotropic support, and fluid challenge

At first, we may exclude significant pericardial collection, assess left ventricle diastolic function of the new performing heart, related to its stiffness and hypertrophy, and think about which wedge pressure we are expected to find [21]. If the systolic function of the new heart is failing, we should exclude an acute graft rejection. Regarding the right ventricle, we must know the recipient preoperative pulmonary vascular resistances, if pre- or postcapillary pulmonary hypertension persists and if it is reversible with phosphodiesterase inhibitors.

RV dysfunction is identified early with a dilation of the right chambers, alteration of interventricular septum movement, and appearance of tricuspid valve insufficiency.

8. Respiratory weaning

A patient undergoing heart transplant should remain under mechanical ventilation until hemodynamic stability is ensured, lactate levels are stable, and immunosuppressive therapy is started. To protect the lungs, we have to limit peak pressures and use low tidal volumes (6 ml/kg) with adequate PEEP level (at least 3–5 cmH_2O).

However, disadvantages coming from permissive hypercapnia on the pulmonary vascular resistances and right ventricle afterload, myocardial function, and renal blood flow loads must be taken into account [16]. As a consequence, there are no universal evidences, but the choice must be tailored for the patient. The only certainty is we must avoid hypercapnia, hypoxia, and PEEP over 10 cmH_2O and keep peak pressure under 35–40 cmH_2O.

During mechanical ventilation, inhaled nitric oxide can be administered in order to reduce right PA pressures, pulmonary vascular resistances, and then right ventricle afterload, especially in the first 24 hours from CPB weaning at the maximum dosage of 20–40 ppm [17, 18]. Once mechanical ventilation is discontinued, inhaled nitric oxide can be substituted by iv or oral pulmonary vasodilators as sildenafil. The weaning criteria do not differ from those used in normal cardiosurgical patients, and the goal is the same: maintain adequate analgesia and sedation levels and wean the patient from the mechanical ventilation as soon as possible. If this is not possible, due to unstable hemodynamics, high inotropic score, respiratory failure, or neurological issues, a percutaneous dilatation tracheostomy will be packaged without further delay (within the first 5–7 days of mechanical ventilation).

Once the patient is awake and self-breathing and the LAP line is removed (generally 24–48 hours from surgery), the patient will need physiotherapy and mobilization.

Early feeding is important. It is initially given via NG tube (25–30 kcal/kg/day) and then self-feeding is achieved once there is no more gastrointestinal paresis.

9. Infection control

Standard prophylaxis is due to cefuroxime 2 g iv every 6 hours in the first 24 hours from heart transplantation (the first two boluses are given in the operating room, at the induction of general anesthesia and once CPB is started). The amount of antibiotic given in the ICU should be tailored for the patient's creatinine clearance, especially if the patient is not under renal filter. Further extension and change of antibiotic therapy should depend on microbiological results of the donor and on microbiological samples of the recipient once admitted in the ICU. Furthermore, in case of redo-operation with existing wound infection, the patient will receive vancomycin and meropenem as standard medication and vancomycin plasma levels should be tested daily. Obviously, due to the immunosuppressive therapy, transplanted patients are very prone to infections. Delivery of care should be done in sterile conditions and, besides standard iv antibiotic therapy, topical antifungal medications should be given in the early postoperative period.

10. Immunosuppressive therapy

A specific team is taking care of immunosuppressive therapy. It starts with 500 mg iv bolus of solumedrol at the CPB weaning. Once admitted in the ICU, the patient will receive 125 mg bolus of solumedrol every 8 hours, with a specific descending dose scheme.

Antithymocyte globulines (1.5 mg/kg iv) are usually given 4, 24, and 48 hours after the end of the transplantation. They will be adjusted based on eventual presence of high body temperature, bleeding, and thrombocytopenia. There are several possible immunosuppressive agents that will be tailored for the patient such as tacrolimus, cyclosporin A, everolimus, and mycophenolate.

11. Graft dysfunction

An international consensus conference in 2014 has classified the graft dysfunction into primary graft dysfunction (PDG) and secondary graft dysfunction (SGD). The first one occurs 24 h from heart transplant and can involve the left, the right ventricle, or both, with different degrees of dysfunction. Typical signs are severe deficit of systolic function, low cardiac output, and high filling pressures without evidence of acute graft rejection or cardiac tamponade. The SGD has a specific reason such as acute rejection, pulmonary hypertension, or surgical complications. Risk factors to develop PGD may be related to the recipient, donor, or technical factors [22].

Donor-related risk factors may be:

- Age (increased risk of 20% every decade)
- Sex (nearly doubled risk with female)

Recipient-related risk factors may be:

- High vasoactive or inotropic support (doubled risk)
- Uncontrolled diabetes (doubled risk)

Technical risk factors are:

- Warm ischemic time (= explant time + implant time); implant time was found to be a strong predictor of PGD.
- Resternotomy (it has been identified as a risk factor for severe PGD due to adherences and tissue fibrosis that can extend the explant time and increase the risk of infections).
- Prolonged CPB time, with subsequent systemic inflammatory response, vasoplegia, clotting and platelet dysfunction, leukocyte activation, free oxygen radical release, and larger amount of blood products given.

All these factors can increase the ischemic-reperfusion injury and the overall mortality [23].

The first step to treat a PDG is vasoactive and inotropic support. If it were not sufficient, an intra-aortic balloon pump (IABP) placement may help.

In case of very severe PGD, an extracorporeal membrane oxygenation (ECMO) becomes the only emergency treatment.

11.1. Anesthesia and intensive care management

11.1.1. For cardiac transplantation in pediatrics

Pediatric heart transplant represents a small subgroup (14%) of total cardiac transplant where the differences in anatomy and physiology make the surgical procedure and the management more complex and creates a unique scenario [24].

The management of pediatric patients undergoing cardiac transplantation differs from the adult patients because it requires a specific knowledge of physiology and physiopathology at different stages of growth, from the newborns through childhood up to adulthood.

This heterogeneous population with a wide range of age, genetic disorders, anatomical anomalies, and symptoms can be classified in four different groups based on the different etiology: 1—CHD (congenital heart disease); 2—DCM (dilated cardiomyopathy); 3—RETX (retransplant); 4—OTHER (**Table 7**) [25]; each of these has specific features.

11.1.2. Preoperative evaluation

The preoperative evaluation is an essential step in order to better analyze both the cardiac pathology and the possible related comorbidities.

Category (abbreviation)	Diagnoses in category
Congenital heart disease (CHD)	Congenital heart defects: HLHS-unoperated, with surgery, without surgery, valvular heart disease
Dilated cardiomyopathy (DCM)	Dilated myopathy due to alcohol, familiar, idiopathic, myocarditis, viral, postpartum, etc.
Retransplant (RETX)	Due to acute rejection, coronary artery disease, etc.
Other (OTHER)	Arrhythmogenic right ventricular dysplasia, cancer, coronary artery disease, myopathy-ischemia, hypertrophic cardiomyopathy, etc.

Table 7. Diagnosis for pediatric heart transplant.

Main preoperative features and examinations that must be considered are:

- Type of heart disease (CHD, DCM, RETX, and OTHER)
- Right heart catheterization (RHC): pulmonary artery pressure (PAP), pulmonary capillary wedge pressure (PCWP), pulmonary vascular resistances (PVR), and pulmonary hypertension etiology. Unfortunately, most patients with congenital heart defects have high PVR because of pulmonary vascular disease. However, the presence of systemic-to-pulmonary shunts, intra-pulmonary shunting, and caval pulmonary circulation does not allow a correct assessment of PVR. For these patients, RHC should be performed at 3–6 month interval in adult patients but is not advocated as routine surveillance in children unless a clinical change is noted [26].
- Numbers and types of previous operations (sternotomy and thoracotomy).
- Cyanotic congenital heart disease (secondary erythrocytosis, hyperviscosity, and coagulation deficit).
- Panel reactive antibody (PRA) identifies sensitized patients. It may be elevated in patients with allograft patch or with multiple redo-operations, due to the multiple transfusions. It may result in an increased risk of acute rejection [27].
- Variable anatomic substrates (isomerism, issues of situs, MAPCAs, aberrant right or left subclavian artery, and persistence of left superior vena cava).
- Previous venous or arterial thromboembolism (central venous catheter thrombosis).
- Previous neurological history: syncope, previous stroke, and cerebral arteriovenous malformation.
- Respiratory insufficiency: smoke, chronic obstructive pulmonary disease (COPD), anatomical anomalies of the pulmonary vessels, and presence of bronchial or pulmonary stents.
- Arrhythmias and previous ICD implantation.
- Liver disease: an evaluation of the patient's liver profile is extremely important. Chronic heart failure and in particular the univentricular heart physiology can lead to a liver dysfunction.

Fontan-associated liver disease (FALD) is a liver dysfunction due to a chronic elevated central venous pressure, low cardiac output, persistent hypoxemia, and intrahepatic venous thrombosis. FALD can be expressed in different stages, from moderate hepatic congestion up to liver cirrhosis with portal hypertension. In several cases, liver function is preserved or is only slightly altered, with high international normalizer ratio (INR), low factor V levels, and elevated factor VIII levels [28].

- Kidney disease: acute or acute-on-chronic renal dysfunction.
- Coagulation anomalies may be present as result of chronic anticoagulation, liver disease, or as a result of cyanotic congenital heart disease (reduced levels of coagulation factors II, V, VII, IX, and X, accelerated fibrinolysis, and fibrinogen alterations).
- Gastrointestinal disorders: necrotizing enterocolitis in newborns or protein losing enteropathy (PLE), which is an excessive protein loss through the gastrointestinal tract that can be present after Fontan operation (even if its origins are poorly understood) [29]

12. Intraoperative management

The anesthetic management should consider that these patients have a poor cardiac reserve and that the premedication, general anesthesia, and the surgical manipulation after the sternotomy can lead to a destabilization of the hemodynamics.

Antibiotic therapy differs according to age and weight and background of both the donor and recipient (**Tables 8** and **9**).

Immunosuppression is started 1 hour before going to the operating room: thymoglobulin 1 mg/kg/12 h and methylprednisolone 7–10 mg/kg (max. 125 mg).

Premedication is performed, according to clinical condition, with low doses of benzodiazepines (midazolam 0.3–0.5 mg/kg orally or rectal in neonate) avoiding excessive sedation and consequently hypercapnia.

It is well known that in newborns and infants, placing an invasive monitoring before induction of anesthesia is not always possible; therefore, it is essential to have a noninvasive monitoring before starting the drug administration.

General anesthesia is induced by inhalation of sevoflurane/desflurane in newborns and infants and by intravenous injections of midazolam 0.3–0.5 mg/kg, fentanyl 2–4 mcg/kg, rocuronium 1 mg/kg, and propofol 2–4 mg/kg in adults and children. Moreover, for continuous infusion of the anesthesia, propofol 4–6 mg/kg/h in adults, while midazolam 0.2 mg/kg/h and fentanyl 2 mcg/kg/h in newborns and children are recommended. After induction, hydrocortisone 10–20 mg/kg is infused.

In all patients, regional cerebral monitoring is achieved with the use of near infrared spectroscopy (NIRS).

Newborn < 1200 g	20 mg q 12 h
Newborn ≥ 1200 g < 7 days of life	20 mg q 12 h
Newborn ≥ 1200 gr > 7 days of life	20 mg q 8 h
Infants and children	100 mg/kg/24 h in 3 doses

Table 8. Antibiotic therapy (cefazolin).

Newborn < 1200 g	5 mg q 12 h
Newborn = 2000 g < 7 days of life	5 mg q 12 h
Newborn = 2000 g > 7 days of life	5 mg q 8 h
Newborn > 2000 g < 7 days of life	5 mg q 8 h
Newborn > 2000 g > 7 days of life	5 mg q 6 h
Infants and children	15/40 mg/kg/24 h in 3–4 doses
In case of allergy to beta-lactams, clindamycin is administered.	

Table 9. Antibiotic therapy (clindamycin).

Different conditions may complicate the venous central catheter placing as: anatomical variables, possible occlusion due to previous repeated catheterizations, and previous positioning of central lines. In these cases, the echo-guided assistance is recommended. In smaller patients or in occluded jugular/subclavian veins, femoral veins can be also used. The sizing of the catheter and the numbers of lumens used depend on the weight and age of the patients. When possible, a pulmonary artery catheter (PAC) must be placed into the superior vena cava and then correctly repositioned by the cardiac surgeon before removing the aortic cross-clamp. In newborns and infants, placing PAC may be problematic or impossible due to the size of the patient. In these cases, it is possible to use the central venous oxygen saturation ($SCvO_2$) as a surrogate of SVO_2 even if the results are controversial [30].

As an alternative, the left atrial pressure (LAP) can be monitored with the insertion of a catheter through the right superior pulmonary vein.

Transesophageal echocardiography (TEE) is always recommended for a correct evaluation of biventricular function, after the CPB weaning, accordingly with the patient's weight.

After induction of the anesthesia, the ventilation management requires extreme attention since the hypoxia and the hypercapnia can increase PVR leading to a low cardiac output syndrome. In case of hypotension, before infusing, a bolus of colloid is essential to secure the correct ventilation, avoiding respiratory acidosis.

The majority of patients with CHD undergoing cardiac transplantation are reoperation candidates, so it is important to put into account long operative times, due to dissection of the adhesions and complex reconstruction of the anatomy.

12.1. CPB and weaning

CPB management can be extremely complex and differs according to the patient's weight and age. The main aim is to maintain a correct medium arterial pressure (MAP) and a correct DO_2/VO_2 ratio.

Sometimes, this is difficult to be achieved, due to the possible presence of anatomical extra-cardiac shunts. The dose of unfractionated heparin for the CPB is 200 U/kg in newborns and infants or 300 U/kg in the child and adult, in order to have an ACT > 400 s. In case of reduced response to heparin, administration of ATIII at a dose of 100 mg/kg is recommended. Furthermore, in case of HIT or low response to heparin, direct thrombin inhibitors are administered (bivalirudin and argatroban) as in adult patients. After the aortic cross-clamp is removed, methylprednisolone is administered with the dose of 7–10 mg/kg (max. 125 mg/kg).

Weaning from CPB always requires inotropic support and the right ventricular failure is a possible complication, characterized by restrictive pattern that can be managed by inhaled nitric oxide (5–40 ppm) and inotropic support (milrinone 0.3–0.75 mcg/kg/min, adrenaline 0.02–0.1 mcg/kg/min, and isoprenaline 0.1–1 mcg/kg/min) in order to vasodilate the pulmonary circulation improving biventricular contractility and providing a chronotropic effect if bradycardia occurs. It is extremely important to keep normal PVR by providing a proper ventilation, avoiding hypoxia and maintaining normocapnia.

Once the patient has been weaned form CBP, the vigilance or $SCvO_2$ can monitor the hemodynamic profile and biventricular function can be evaluated with echocardiogram.

However, in case of poor CO, despite maximal inotropic support and correct ventilation, we should consider the support via an extracorporeal membrane oxygenation (ECMO).

12.2. Anticoagulation and hemostasis

At the end of CPB, heparin is antagonized with a ratio 2:1 or 1:1 with protamine based on the ACT values. Antifibrinolytic agents are administrated at the dosage of 50 mg/kg (25 mg/kg after general anesthesia induction and 25 mg/kg at the end of CPB). Severe bleeding is not uncommon in pediatric population. Main reasons of postoperative bleeding are previous heart surgery, cyanotic congenital heart disease, immature coagulation system, and excessive hemodilution due to the disproportionate ratio of CPB circuit volume to patient blood volume, especially in newborns and infants. Correct coagulation management is always achieved through ROTEM.

12.3. Intensive care

During the postoperative intensive care course, close monitoring of hemodynamic parameters, inotropes, ventilation, and acid base balance is required to predict pulmonary hypertension, biventricular failure, and LCOS. Normalization of the oxygenation and ventilation is the primary goal in these patients and ventilation support must be discontinued as soon as possible. The antibiotic therapy will be set according to microbiological surveillance. Immunotherapy during the postoperative course is managed by the cardiologist as follows: methylprednisolone, thymoglobulin, tacrolimus, and mycophenolate.

12.4. Peculiar problems

In the postoperative setting, the main problems for pediatric patients are comorbidities related to chronic decompensation and univentricular physiology.

- Cyanotic congenital heart disease: patients with long standing hypoxemia often develop severe alteration of whole blood viscosity and alteration of coagulation profiles with high risk of postoperative bleeding [31].
- Plastic bronchitis: it is a rare complication of univentricular physiology characterized by the formation of exudative airway casts that can occlude airways and cause respiratory failure. The etiology is still not well identified, but it seems to relate to an increased central venous pressure or lymphatic drainage alterations [32].
- Protein losing enteropathy (PLE): it is defined as a possible complication of the univentricular circulation. It can arise after the Fontan operation (5–15% of the patients) [33]. It is characterized by the abnormal loss of proteins into the enteral lumen, which results in hypoproteinemia and hypoalbuminemia. This leads to an increase of lymphatic drainage and a dilation of intestinal lymphatic system with an impaired fat absorption resulting in steatorrhea. Moreover, the hypoproteinemia may result also in ascites, peripheral edema, and pleural/pericardial effusion. Therapy consists of diuretics, corticosteroids, and albumin supplementation.

Abbreviations

BIS	bispectral index
CI	cardiac index
CO	cardiac output
COPD	chronic obstructive pulmonary disease
CPB	cardiopulmonary bypass
CVC	central venous catheter
CVP	central venous pressure
CVVH	central venovenous hemofiltration
DLCO	carbon monoxide lung diffusion
ECMO	extracorporeal membranous oxygenation
HIT	heparin-induced thrombocytopenia
IABP	intra-aortic balloon pump
ICD	implantable cardioverter defibrillator

ISVR	indexed systemic vascular resistance
LAP	left atrial pressure
LV	left ventricle
LVAD	left ventricular assist device
NGT	nasogastric tube
NO	nitrogen oxide
OCS	organ care system
PAC	pulmonary artery catheter
PAP	pulmonary arterial pressure
PCWP	pulmonary capillary wedge pressure
PEEP	positive end expiratory pressure
PPM	parts per millions
PGD	primary graft dysfunction
PVR	pulmonary vascular resistance
RAP	right atrial pressure
RV	right ventricle
SIRS	systemic inflammatory response syndrome
SVR	systemic vascular resistance
TACO	transfusion-associated circulatory overload
TPG	transpulmonary pressure gradient
TRALI	transfusion-associated lung injury
TV	tidal volume
VAD	ventricular assist device
WU	wood unit

Author details

Massimo Baiocchi*, Maria Benedetto, Marta Agulli and Guido Frascaroli

*Address all correspondence to: massimo.baiocchi@aosp.bo.it

Anaesthesiology and Intensive Care Unit, Cardiothoracic and vascular Department, Policlinico S. Orsola University Hospital, Bologna, Italy

References

[1] Mehra MR, Kobashigawa J, Starling R, et al. Listing criteria for heart transplantation: International Society for Heart and Lung Transplantation guidelines for the care of cardiac transplant candidates – 2006. The Journal of Heart and Lung Transplantation. 2006;**25**:1024-1042

[2] Miller WL, Grill DE, Borlaug BA. Clinical features, hemodynamics, and outcomes of pulmonary hypertension due to chronic heart failure with reduced ejection fraction: Pulmonary hypertension and heart failure. JACC: Heart Failure. 2013;**1**:290-299

[3] Lundgren J, Soderlund C, et al. Impact of postoperative pulmonary hypertension on outcome after heart transplantation. Scandinavian Cardiovascular Journal. 2017; **51**(3):172-181

[4] de Groote P, El Sri C, Fertin M. Sildenafil in heart transplant candidates with pulmonary hypertension. Archives of Cardiovascular Diseases. 2015;**108**(6-7):375-384. DOI: 10.1016/j.acvd.2015.01.013

[5] Micha Z, Pacholewicz J, Copik I. Mechanical circulatory support is effective to treat pulmonary hypertension in heart transplant candidates disqualified due to unacceptable pulmonary vascular resistance. Kardiochir Torakochirurgia Pol. 2018;**15**(1):23-26

[6] Waterman PM, Bjerke R. Rapid-sequence induction technique in patients with severe ventricular dysfunction. Journal of Cardiothoracic Anesthesia. 1988;**2**:602-606

[7] Stobierska-Dzierzek B, Awead H, Michler RE. The evolving management of acute right-sided heart failure in cardiac transplant recipients. Journal of the American College of Cardiology. 2001;**38**:923-931

[8] Levy JH, Winkler AM. Heparin-induced thrombocytopenia and cardiac surgery. Current Opinion in Anaesthesiology. 2010;**23**:74-79

[9] Benedetto M, Romano R, et al. Inhaled nitric oxide in cardiac surgery: Evidence or tradition? Nitrix Oxide. 2015;**49**:67-69

[10] Weis F, Beiras-Fernandez A, Kaczmarek I, et al. Levosimendan: A new therapeutic option in the treatment of primary graft dysfunction after heart transplantation. The Journal of Heart and Lung Transplantation. 2009;**28**:501-504

[11] Landoni G, Lomivorotov VV, Alvaro G, et al. Levosimendan for hemodynamic support after cardiac surgery. The New England Journal of Medicine. 2017;**25**:2021-2031

[12] Koster A, Diehl C, Dongas A, et al. Anesthesia for cardiac transplantation: A practical overview of current management strategies. Applied Cardiopulmonary Pathophysiology. 2011;**15**:213-219

[13] Kirk R, Edwards LB, Kucheryavaya AY, et al. The registry of the International Society for Heart and Lung Transplantation: Fourteenth pediatric heart transplantation report-2011. The Journal of Heart and Lung Transplantation. 2011;**30**:1095-1103

[14] Costanzo MR, Taylor D, Hunt S, et al. The International Society of Heart and Lung Transplantation guideline for the care of heart transplant recipients. The Journal of Heart and Lung Transplantation. 2010;**29**:914-956

[15] Rioux JP, Lessard M, De Bortolli B, Roy P, Albert M, Verdant C, et al. Pentastarch 10% (250 kDa/0.45) is and independent risk factor of acute kidney injury following cardiac surgery. Critical Care Medicine. 2009;**37**(4):1293-1298

[16] The Acute Respiratory Distress Syndrome Network. Ventilation with lower tidal volumes as compared with traditional tidal volumes for acute lung injury and the acute respiratory distress syndrome. The New England Journal of Medicine. 2000;**342**:1301-1308

[17] Ardehali A, Hughes K, Sadeghi A, Esmailian D, Marelli D, et al. Inhaled nitric oxide for pulmonary hypertension after heart transplantation. Transplantation. 2001;**72**:638-641

[18] Kaul TK, Fields BL. Postoperative acute refractory right ventricular failure: Incidence, pathogenesis, management and prognosis. Cardivascular Surgery. 2000;**8**:1-9

[19] Atz AM, Lefler AK, Fairbrother DL, Uber WE, et al. Sildefanil augments the effect of inhaled nitric oxide for postoperative pulmonary hypertensive crises. The Journal of Thoracic and Cardiovascular Surgery. 2002;**124**:628-629

[20] Ghofrani HA, Wiedemann R, Rose F, Schermuly RT, et al. Combination therapy with oral sildenafil and inhaled iloprost for severe pulmonary hypertension. Annals of Internal Medicine. 2002;**136**:515-522

[21] Erb JM. Role of echocardiography in intensive care treatment of patients after heart transplantation or implantation of a ventricular assist device. Intensivmedizin und Notfallmedizin. 2006;**43**(5):431-443

[22] Kobashigawa J, Zuckermann A, et al. Report from a consensus conference on primary graft dysfunction after cardiac transplantation. The Journal of Heart and Lung Transplantation. 2014;**33**(4):327.40

[23] Avtaar Singh SS, Banner NR, et al. ISHLT primary graft dysfunction incidence, risk factors and outcome: A UK National Study. Transplantation. 2018;**5**

[24] Pediatric heart transplantation. Journal of Thoracic Disease. 2015;**7**(3):552-559

[25] The Registry of the International Society for Heart and Lung Transplantation. Nineteenth pediatric lung and heart-lung transplantation report—2016; Focus theme: Primary diagnostic indications for transplant. The Journal of Heart and Lung Transplantation. 2016;**35**(10):1196-1205

[26] The 2016 international society for heart lung transplantation listing criteria for heart transplantation: A 10-year update. Journal of Heart and Lung Transplantation. Jan 2016;**35**(1): 1-23. DOI: 10.1016/j.healun.2015.10.023

[27] Heart transplantation in children for end-stage congenital heart disease. Seminars in Thoracic and Cardiovascular Surgery. Pediatric Cardiac Surgery Annual. 2014;**17**:69-76

[28] Fontan-associated liver disease: Implications for heart transplantation. Journal of Heart and Lung Transplantation. 2016;**35**(1):26-33

[29] StrategFontan-associated protein-losing enteropathy and heart transplant: A pediatric heart transplant study analysis. Journal of Heart and Lung Transplantation. 2015; **34**(9):1169-1176

[30] Fiberoptic monitoring of central venous oxygen saturation (Pediasat) in small children undergoing cardiac surgery: Continuous is not continuous. Version3. F1000Research. 2014 Jan 23 [revised 2014 Jun 13];**3**:23. DOI: 10.12688/f1000research.3-23.v3. eCollection 2014

[31] Cyanotic congenital heart disease (CCHD): Focus on hypoxiemia, secondary erythrocytosis, and coagulation alterations. Pediatric Anaesthesia. 2015;**25**:981-989

[32] Plastic bronchitis in patient with Fontan physiology: Review of the literature and preliminary experience with Fontan conversion and cardiac transplantation. World Journal for Pediatric and Congenital Heart Surgery. 2012;**3**(3):364-372

[33] Strategies to treat protein-losing enteropathy. Pediatric Cardiac Surgery Annual of the Seminars in Thoracic and Cardiovascular Surgery. 2002;**5**:3-11

4

Fat Embolism Syndrome

Syed Abdul Rahman, Arif Valliani and

Arshad Chanda

Abstract

Fat embolism syndrome (FES) is a clinical syndrome characterized by signs and symptoms resulting from fat emboli and typically occurs after trauma, orthopaedic surgeries and non-traumatic conditions like acute pancreatitis. Literature reports an incidence of FES of up to 19% in prospective studies. Fat embolism refers to the presence of fat globules in pulmonary microcirculation and is often asymptomatic. The clinical syndrome of FES is characterized by systemic manifestations resulting from fat emboli which may manifest with a triad of lung, brain, and skin involvement in about 24–72 hours of asymptomatic period. The pathophysiology of fat embolism syndrome remains unclear. Two theories have been hypothesized: mechanical(disruptive) and biochemical(production of toxic metabolites). Universal agreement on the definition of FES is lacking. FES presents with nonspecific signs and symptoms;common to other critical illnesses and is often a diagnosis of exclusion. The clinical criteria proposed by Gurd and Wilson are popular. Biochemical tests and imaging may be of value in supporting the diagnosis. Treatment for FES is essentially supportive care in ICU. Principles of treatment include maintenance of adequate oxygenation, ventilation, hemodynamics, and organ perfusion. It may be prevented by early fixation of large bone fractures.

Keywords: fat embolism syndrome (FES), long bone fractures, clinical criteria, imaging studies, supportive care, early fixation

1. Introduction

The term "fat embolism" (FE) is often loosely used to describe both fat embolization (of insignificant clinical relevance) and the clinical syndrome of fat embolism syndrome (FES) [1].

The term "fat embolism" may be defined as the presence of fat globules in the pulmonary microcirculation irrespective of its clinical relevance, while the clinical syndrome of FES is characterized by the clinical signs and symptoms (systemic manifestations) resulting from fat emboli [2] and must be differentiated from the pathophysiological phenomenon of fat embolization [3].

2. History

Fat embolism was described as early as 1862 by Zenker. Warthin [4] opined that fat embolism from traumatic lipemia was not rare and the most frequent cause of death following long bone fractures in the absence of infection.

More data on FES came forth in the early twenty-first century from wounded soldiers involved in armed conflict across the world. A series of 1000 combats injured in the World War II reported the incidence of FES to be 0.8%. In Vietnam, cases of arterial hypoxemia among wounded soldiers were attributed to FES and also reported a few classic presentations of FES [3].

3. Pathophysiology

The pathophysiology of development of fat embolism syndrome is still unclear. However, two theories were hypothesized for its mechanism: mechanical and biochemical. Either the disrupted fat globules from bone marrow or adipose tissues enter into the bloodstreams (mechanical) or any sequel that leads to the production of toxic metabolites in the blood (biochemical) can give rise to a conundrum of clinical features that characterize the fat embolism syndrome. It is also likely that either the mechanisms exist in tandem or one gives rise to the other in the production of FES.

3.1. Mechanical theory

In the twentieth century, it was suggested that following a trauma, fat particles from the bone marrow and adipose tissues enter into the disrupted venules and travel to the pulmonary circulation or enter into the systemic circuit via arteriovenous shunts. The echocardiographic finding of echogenic material passing into the right heart during an orthopedic procedure contributed to this mechanical theory [5].

3.2. Biochemical theory

However, the mechanical theory does not explain the development of FES after a delay of 2–3 days postinjury. There are many biochemical mechanisms involved in the progression of fat embolism syndrome; the most widely accepted is the release of free fatty acids into the plasma following trauma, sepsis, and/or systemic inflammation. Acute phase reactants, like C-reactive proteins, lead to lipid agglutination that tend to cause Acute respiratory distress syndrome (ARDS) in animal models, dysfunction of cardiac contractility and increase in plasma lipase concentration, which are the features of FES. These free fatty acids migrate to other organs, causing multiorgan failure [6]. This theory also helps in understanding the development of nontraumatic fat embolism syndrome.

4. Incidence

Fat Embolism is common in trauma patients, particularly those with pelvic or long bone fractures [3]. Most literature reporting incidence of FES involves orthopedic or trauma patients with retrospective studies reporting an incidence of below 1%, while prospective studies have reported a much higher incidence of 11–19% [7]. Autopsy studies reported a much higher incidence of Fat embolism. One study demonstrated pulmonary fat emboli in 82% of trauma patients at autopsy [8]. Up to 67% of trauma patients without clinical features of fat embolism syndrome were shown to have circulating fat globules [3].

Fat emboli with a diameter of more than 20 μm have been shown to occur in up to 90% of patients with long bone fractures. Another study concluded that more than 90% of patients with long bone fractures had embolism with fat droplets more than 20 μm in diameter [9].

Gurd proposed that the clinical syndrome of fat embolism can be differentiated from a mere presence of fat emboli at autopsy in patients with no prior clinical features. Gurd suggested that a distinction can be made between the clinical syndrome of fat embolism and demonstration of fat embolism on autopsy with no prior clinical features of the syndrome [10].

Bulger et al. studied the incidence of FES at a level I trauma center over a 10-year period, reporting an incidence of 0.9% among patients with long bone fractures [11]. More recent data from the National Hospital Discharge Survey in USA looking at 21,538,000 patients with long bones and pelvic fractures reported a diagnosis of FES in 0.12% of the patients [12].

5. Etiology and risk factor

The development of FES is frequently associated following an orthopedic trauma, with highest occurrence in closed and/or multiple long bone fractures, particularly of lower limb bones like femur. Aggressive nailing of the medullary canal poses increased risk of FES. Vigorous nailing of medullary cavity during intramedullary nailing and increase in gap between nail and cortical bone puts the patient at high risk of developing FES [6].

Furthermore, younger populations of 10–40 years and men more often than women are at high risk. Fat embolism has been reported in other nontraumatic conditions like pancreatitis, liposuction, bone marrow transplant, sickle cell disease, and liver disease. Nontraumatic causes of fat embolism syndrome include bone marrow transplant, pancreatitis, liposuction, alcoholic liver disease, and sickle cell crisis [13].

6. Clinical features

The phenomenon of fat embolism (fat droplets in circulation) is often undiagnosed in clinical practice. The clinical syndrome of FES tends to present with signs and symptoms similar to other critical illness and is mostly a diagnosis of exclusion. Fat embolism, which is a mere presence of fat emboli in circulation, may frequently go undiagnosed [10], while fat embolism syndrome presents with nonspecific clinical features common to other critical illnesses and is often a diagnosis of exclusion.

The fulminating form may present with sudden cardiovascular collapse and right ventricular failure subsequent to pulmonary and systemic fat embolization. More often, it is characterized by a more gradual onset of hypoxemia, neurological symptoms and a petechial rash about 12–36 hours after an injury [7].

Fat emboli could travel through the systemic vasculature resulting in a multiorgan disease involving lungs, brain, skin, retina, kidneys, liver, and heart.

The most common manifestations among patients with FES are of pulmonary system. Pumonary manifestations though of varying severity are the most common finding in patient with fat embolism syndrome. Bulger et al. reported hypoxemia in 96% of the cases, and 44% of the patients with FES required mechanical ventilation [11]. Patients may develop dyspnea and tachypnea and a more severe syndrome indistinguishable from Acute respiratory distress syndrome (ARDS) may develop.

Nonspecific neurological symptoms including lethargy, restlessness or a decrease in Glasgow Coma Scale (GCS) may suggest cerebral edema subsequent to FES [14]. Severe neurological deterioration with cerebral edema has been reported with FES [15].

Skin involvement characterized by a petechial rash manifests in up to 60% of patients and usually affects oral mucous membranes, neck and axilla skin folds and conjunctiva. Dermal manifestations with a petechial rash pathogonomic of FES usually involves the conjunctiva, oral mucous membranes and skin folds of the neck and axillae and occuring in up to 60% of patients with FES [7].

7. Diagnosis

7.1. Gurd's and Wilson's criteria

Universal agreement on a standard definition of FES is lacking. There is a lack of universally accepted definition of FES [3]. The major and minor criteria proposed by Gurd and Wilson (**Table 1**) in 1970 are still popular [10]. It required one major criterion plus four minor criteria's in addition to fat macroglobulinemia for a diagnosis of FES.

7.2. Schonfeld's criteria

Other authors later adapted these criteria and proposed the combinations of major and minor features needed for a diagnosis. Schonfeld et al. proposed (**Table 3**) a quantitative measure to diagnose FES; a score of more than 5 is required to diagnose FES [3].

7.3. Lindeque's criteria

Lindeque proposed criteria for diagnosis of fat embolism syndrome based on respiratory changes alone [16]. A positive diagnosis of FES was proposed if atleast one of the criteria are met (**Table 2**).

1. Major criteria
   a. Petechial rash
   b. Respiratory insufficiency
   c. Cerebral involvement
2. Minor criteria
   a. Tachycardia
   b. Fever
   c. Retinal changes
   d. Jaundice
   e. Renal signs
   f. Thrombocytopenia
   g. Anemia
   h. High ESR
   i. Fat macroglobinemia

Table 1. Gurd's and Wilson's criteria (with permission from Dr. Nissar Shaikh) [6].

	Scores
Petechiae	5
X-Ray chest diffuse infiltrates	4
Hypoxemia	3
Fever	1
Tachycardia	1
Tachypnea	1
Confusion	1

Table 2. Lindeque's criteria (with permission from Dr. Nissar Shaikh) [6].

Sustained $pO_2 < 8$ kpa
Sustained $pCO_2 > 7.3$ kpa
Sustained respiratory rate > 35 per min, in spite of sedation
Increase work of breathing, dyspnea, tachycardia, anxiety
Schonfeld's criteria
Petechiae 5
Chest X-ray changes (diffuse alveolar infiltrates) 4
Hypoxaemia (Pao2 < 9.3 kPa) 3
Fever (>38°C) 1
Tachycardia (>120 beats min−1) 1
Tachypnoea (>30 bpm) 1
Cumulative score >5 required for diagnosis

Table 3. Schonfeld's criteria (with permission from Dr. Nissar Shaikh) [6].

8. Investigations

Diagnosis must be made on the basis of clinical findings but biochemical changes may be of value to support in diagnosis.

In the initial stages, a blood gas analysis is imperative, which will show hypoxia with paO_2 of less than 60 mmHg and hypocapnia within the first 24–48 hours. Also, there will be an unexplained increase in the pulmonary shunt fraction and an alveolar to arterial oxygen tension difference. These are highly suggestive of a diagnosis of FES.

Nonspecific findings include anemia, thrombocytopenia, hypofibrinogenemia and high erythrocytes sedimentation rate. Cytological examination of urine, blood, sputum, and pulmonary capillary blood may detect fat globules in patients with FES; however, these tests are rarely done in the immediate period as they lack sensitivity and their absence does not rule out fat embolism [6].

8.1. Imaging studies

8.1.1. Chest X-ray

Various nonspecific findings have been reported on chest X-ray though none of them is diagnostic. Numerous radiological findings have been described but none is diagnostic of fat embolism syndrome. The chest X-ray is often normal initially but in some patients bilateral fluffy shadows can be seen with worsening respiratory insufficiency (**Figure 1**).

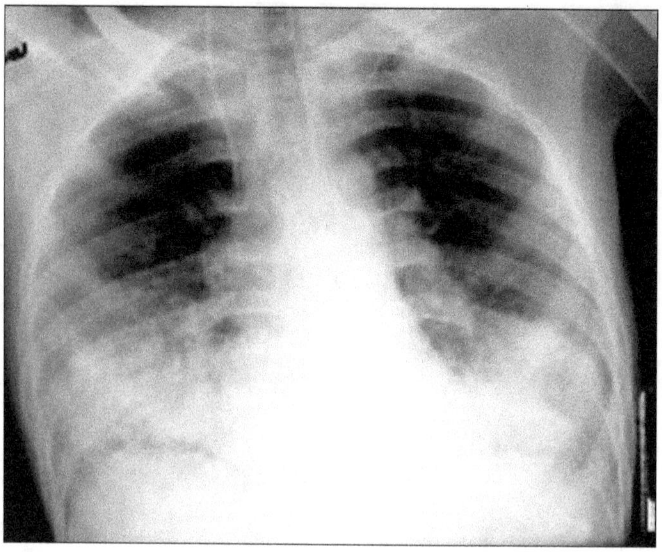

Figure 1. AP radiograph of the chest showing bilateral basal air space-filling lesions (consolidation in a patient of FES) (with permission from Dr. Nissar Shaikh) [6].

8.1.2. Ventilation – perfusion scan (V/Q)

V/Q scans may demonstrate a mottled pattern of subsegmental perfusion defects with a normal ventilatory pattern.

8.1.3. CT – computerized tomography chest and head

Spiral CT scan of the chest may show focal areas of ground glass opacification with interlobular septal thickening. Normal findings or diffuse petechial hemorrhages of white matter may be seen on CT scan of brain. CT Head may be normal or reveal diffuse white-matter petechial hemorrhages consistent with microvascular injury. This will also rule out other causes for deterioration in consciousness level (**Figure 2**).

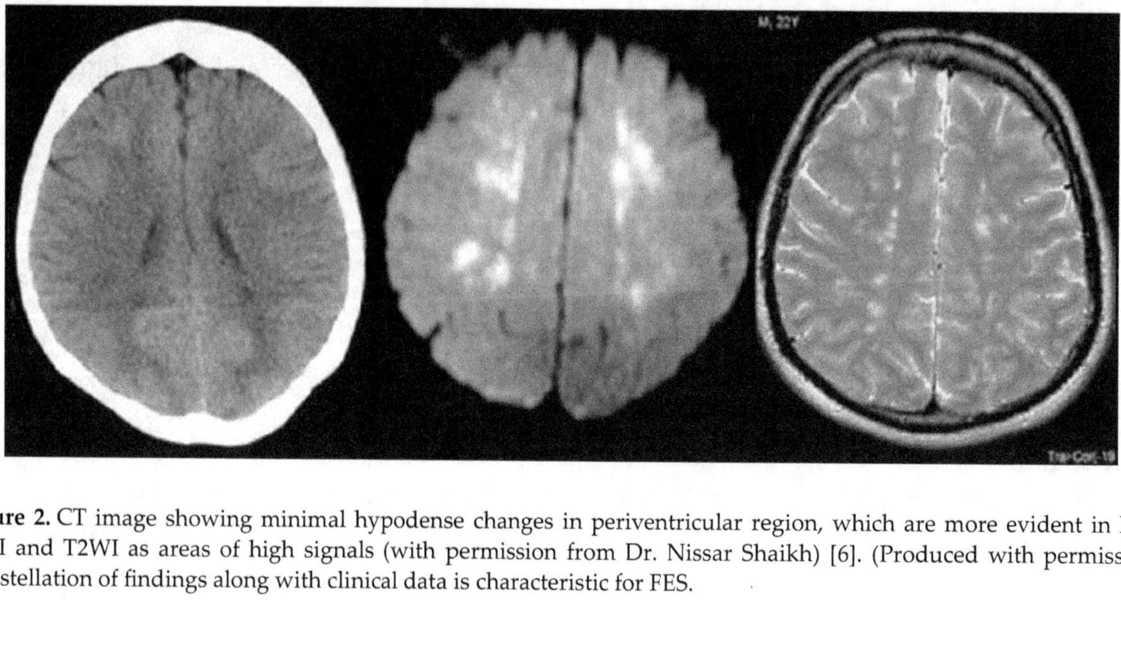

Figure 2. CT image showing minimal hypodense changes in periventricular region, which are more evident in MRI DWI and T2WI as areas of high signals (with permission from Dr. Nissar Shaikh) [6]. (Produced with permission) Constellation of findings along with clinical data is characteristic for FES.

8.1.4. MRI of brain

It may reveal high-intensity T2 signal which correlates with the degree of neurological impairment found clinically.

9. Treatment

Treatment is largely supportive care in a unit equipped with intensive care capabilities. Maintaining adequate oxygenation, ventilation, and organ perfusion are the essential goals of treatment. Principles of treatment include maintenance of adequate oxygenation and ventilation, hemodynamics, and perfusion. Correction of hypoxemia to maintain normal oxygen tension may require simple measures like oxygen supplementation or mechanical ventilation and Positive end expiratory pressure (PEEP) depending on the clinical context. Shock in patients with FES can worsen the lung injury and hence restoration of intravascular volume with balanced salt solutions or albumin is often required. Albumin administration not only expands the intravascular volume but may also mitigate the extent of lung injury as a result of its binding with fatty acids. Vasopressors to maintain the hemodynamics may be required. It has been proposed that heparin by enhancing lipase activity may augment the clearance of lipids from blood circulation. Treatment modalities including corticosteroids and anticoagulation have unfortunately not been shown to improve the morbidity or mortality. Other medications including alcohol and dextran have also been shown to be ineffective [2, 6].

10. Prognosis

Fat embolism occur in around 90% of all trauma patient, but FES accounts for less than 5% of patients having long bone fracture [17, 18]. The unstable form of FES presents as acute respiratory failure, cor pulmonale, and/or embolic event, leading to death within a few hours of injury. This is seen more often among high-risk patients and those with a background of multiple comorbidities.

It is hard to predict the extent of FES as it is often subclinical and the outcome of patients are generally favorable [6]. Mortality rate is less than 10% at present as there have been significant improvements in supportive care. Neurological deficits and pulmonary manifestations usually resolve completely over time [18].

11. Prevention

Studies have shown early fixation of fractures involving long bones is important in decreasing the incidence of fat embolism syndrome and may prevent it [6, 19, 20]. Preventing significant increase in intraosseous pressure in orthopedic surgeries may reduce embolization of fat droplets and thereby reduce the incidence of FES. It has been suggested that plate fixation and external fixation results in less emboli and less severity of lung injury than surgical fixation with intramedullary nailing [6]. Prophylactic use of corticosteroids may have a beneficial effect in preventing fat embolism syndrome [21]. Wong et al. suggested monitoring with continuous pulse oximetry in patients with long bone fractures for early identification of desaturation [22]. This would allow early initiation of appropriate oxygen supplementation and other measures, possibly reducing the systemic complications of fat embolism syndrome [6].

Author details

Syed Abdul Rahman, Arif Valliani and Arshad Chanda*

*Address all correspondence to: drarshadchanda@yahoo.com

Surgical Intensive Care Unit, Hamad Medical Corporation, Doha, Qatar

References

[1] Robinson CM. Current concepts of respiratory insufficiency syndromes after fracture. The Journal of Bone and Joint Surgery (Br). 2001;**83**(B):781-791

[2] Kosova E, Bergmark B, Piazza G. Fat embolism syndrome. Circulation. 2015;**131**:317-320

[3] Talbot M, Schemitsch EH. Fat embolism syndrome: history, definition, epidemiology. Injury. 2006;**37**(Suppl 4):S3–S7

[4] Warthin AS. Traumatic lipemia and fatty embolism. International Clinics 4:171, 1913

[5] Sulek CA, Davies LK, Enneking FK, et al. Cerebral microembolism diagnosed by transcranial Doppler during total knee arthroplasty: Correlation with transesophageal echocardiography. Anesthesiology. 1999;**91**(3):672-676

[6] Sheikh N. Emergency management of fat embolism syndrome. Journal of Emergencies Trauma and Shock. 2009;**2**(1):29-33

[7] Mellor A, Soni N. Fat embolism. Anaesthesia. 2001;**56**:145-154

[8] Eriksson EA, Pellegrini DC, Vanderkolk WE, et al. Incidence of pulmonary fat embolism at autopsy: an undiagnosed epidemic. The Journal of Trauma and Acute Care Surgery. 2011;**71**(2):312-315

[9] Weisz G. M. Fat embolism. Current problems in surgery. Chicago (Ill.): Year Book Publisher Nov. 1974

[10] Gurd AR, Wilson RI. The fat embolism syndrome. The Bone and Joint Journal. 1974;**56**B (3):408-416

[11] Bulger EM, Smith DG, Maier RV, et al. Fat embolism syndrome: A 10-Year Review. Archives of Surgery. 1997;**132**(4):435-439

[12] Stein PD, Yaekoub AY, Matta F, et al. Fat embolism syndrome. The American Journal of the Medical Sciences.2008;**336**(6):472-477

[13] Akhtar S. Fat embolism. Anesthesiology Clinics. 2009;**27**(3):533-550

[14] Kwiatt ME, Seamon MJ. Fat embolism syndrome. International Journal of Critical Illness and Injury Science. 2013;**3**(1):64-68

[15] Meeke RI, Fitzpatrick GJ, Phelan DM. Cerebral edema and fat embolism syndrome. Intensive Care Medicine. 1987;**13**:291-292

[16] Lindeque BG, Schoeman HS, Dommisse GF, et al. Fat embolism and the fat embolism syndrome. A double-blind therapeutic study. The Journal of Bone and Joint Surgery (Br). 1987;**69**(1):128-131

[17] Palmovic V, McCarroll JR. Fat embolism in trauma. Archives of Pathology. 1965;**80**(6): 630-635

[18] Habashi NM, Andrews PL, Scalea TM. Therapeutic aspects of fat embolism syndrome. Injury. 2006;**37**(Suppl 4):S68-S73

[19] Behrman SW, Fabian TC, Kudsk KA, et al. Improved outcome with femur fractures: Early vs. delayed fixation. The Journal of Trauma. 1990;**30**:792-797

[20] Svennisngsen S. Prevention of fat embolism syndrome in patients with femoral fractures-immediate or delayed operation fixation. Annales Chirugiae et Gynaecologiae. 1987;**76**(3):163-166

[21] Bederman SS, Bhandari M, McKee MD, Schemitsch EH. Do corticosteroids reduce the risk of fat embolism syndrome in patients with long-bone fractures? A meta-analysis. Canadian Journal of Surgery. 2009;**52**:386-393

[22] Wong MW. Continuous pulse oximeter monitoring for inapparent hypoxemia after long bone fractures. The Journal of Trauma. 2004;**56**(2):356-362

5

Abdominal Compartment Syndrome: What is New?

Abdulgafoor M. Tharayil, Adel Ganaw,
Syed Abdulrahman, Zia M. Awan and
Sujith M. Prabhakaran

Abstract

Intra-abdominal hypertension (IAH) and abdominal compartment syndrome (ACS) are continuation of the same pathological and physiological processes that are largely unrecognized in critical patients. From an era of indistinct definitions and recommendations, this condition has been studied extensively and experts have come forward with clear definitions and recommendations for management. IAH is graded in four grades and ACS is IAH above 20 cm H_2O with new organ dysfunction. IAH/ACS can present as acute, hyperacute, or chronic and aetiologically can be classified into primary, secondary and tertiary. It affects various body systems including respiratory, cardiovascular, central nervous, gastrointestinal, renal and hepatic systems adversely and results in deleterious consequences. Management of IAH/ACS is based on the evacuation of intra-luminal and extra-luminal contents, improving the abdominal wall compliance. There are various surgical techniques recommended for preventing the development of IAH/ACS and mitigating the negative consequences. New medical therapies such as octreotide, tissue plasminogen activator, melatonin and vitamin C are being investigated and non-pharmacological methods such as continuous negative abdominal pressure (CNAP) have been introduced recently but are still experimental and not recommended for routine use.

Keywords: intra-abdominal hypertension (IAH), abdominal compartment syndrome (ACS), open abdomen

1. Introduction

Intra-abdominal hypertension (IAH) and abdominal compartment syndrome (ACS) are largely unrecognized conditions but prevalent in ICU patients. It is a continuum of varying degree of increase in intra-abdominal pressure (IAP) ranging from IAH to ACS. Most studies evaluating the incidence of ACS have been performed in trauma patients, with estimates of incidence varying considerably. While the largest study [1] ($n = 706$) reported an incidence of ACS of 1%, two smaller though observational studies [2, 3] ($n = 128$ and 188) reported a higher incidence of ACS of 9–14%. The incidence of intra-abdominal hypertension (IAH) is not well reported in the literature. The wide variation in the reported incidence may be attributed to differences in diagnostic criteria employed in studies.

2. Definitions

There was an era of indistinct and variable definitions of IAH/ACS with variable methods of measurement of intra-abdominal pressure (IAP) until the World Society of Abdominal Compartment Syndrome (WSACS) was formed and they formulated definitions, standardized measurement methodology and provided management guidelines.

Intra-abdominal pressure: Intra-abdominal pressure (IAP) is the steady state pressure concealed within the abdominal cavity (**Figure 1**) [4]. An IAP of 5–7 mmHg is considered normal for most critically ill patients. IAP is directly related to body mass index (BMI) [5].

Abdominal perfusion pressure: Abdominal perfusion pressure (APP) is calculated by subtracting IAP from the mean arterial pressure (MAP): APP = MAP − IAP. Elevated intra-abdominal pressure reduces blood flow to the abdominal viscera. A target APP of at least 60 mmHg is correlated with improved survival among patients with IAH and ACS [6].

Intra-abdominal hypertension: Intra-abdominal hypertension (IAH) is defined as a sustained intra-abdominal pressure ≥12 mmHg (**Figure 1**) [7, 8]. This value was established arbitrarily. Intra-abdominal pressure can be further graded as follows:

Grade I = IAP 12–15 mmHg
Grade II = IAP 16–20 mmHg
Grade III = IAP 21–25 mmHg
Grade IV = IAP > 25 mm Hg

Hyper-acute IAH refers to elevation of the intra-abdominal pressure lasting only seconds due to any strenuous physical activity, sneezing, coughing, laughing, straining, or defecation, etc.

Acute IAH refers to elevation of the intra-abdominal pressure that develops over hours, which occurs usually due to surgical causes. Sub-acute IAH refers to elevation of the intra-abdominal pressure that develops over days usually due to medical conditions.

Chronic IAH refers to elevation of intra-abdominal pressure that develops over months (pregnancy) or years (morbid obesity)]. Chronic elevation of IAP usually does not result in ACS unless it is superimposed on acute or sub-acute IAH.

Abdominal compartment syndrome: ACS is defined as a sustained intra-abdominal pressure >20 mmHg (with or without APP <60 mmHg) that is associated with new organ dysfunction [4, 7, 8].

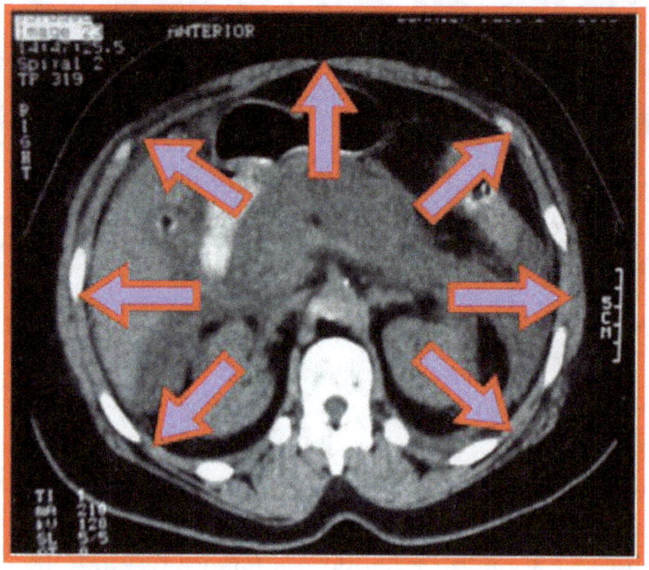

Figure 1. Intra-abdominal pressure (from: https://www.slideshare.net/drabdulgafoormt/intraabdominal-hypertension).

ACS can be classified as primary and secondary.

Primary ACS is due to injury or disease in the abdominopelvic region. This could be intra-luminal or extra-luminal causes. Extra-luminal causes could be any pathology causing intra-abdominal collections outside the bowel lumens e.g. abdominal trauma, hemoperitoneum and pancreatitis. IAH/ACS can also develop due to intra-luminal pathology like intestinal obstruction, gastroparesis, pseudocolonic obstruction and pseudomembranous colitis (**Figure 2**), etc.

Secondary ACS refers to conditions that do not originate in the abdomen or pelvis (e.g. fluid resuscitation, sepsis, and burns).

Recurrent ACS defines a condition in which ACS develops again following previous surgical or medical treatment of primary or secondary ACS [9].

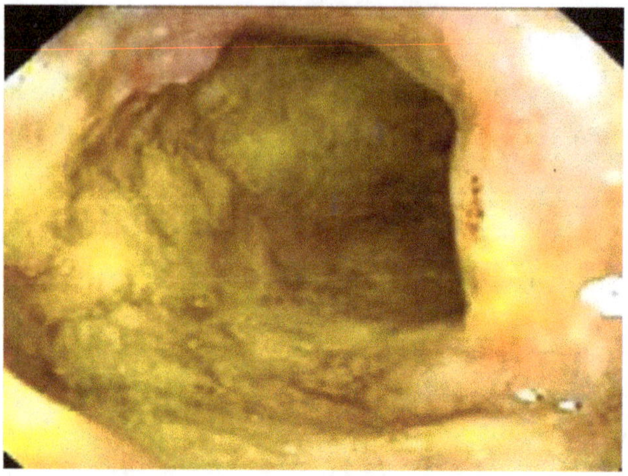

Figure 2. Pseudomembranous colitis due to clostridium difficile causing ACS [49].

3. Physiological consequences of IAH/ACS

ACS is not just an abdominal condition but rather a systemic problem that has tremendous impact on all organ systems including, but not limited to, cardiovascular system, respiratory system, central nervous system, renal system and hepatobiliary system.

Cardiovascular system: IAH/ACS results in cephalad movement of diaphragm that in turn can cause depression of ventricular compliance and contractility [10]. Another impact of IAH is reduced venous return from lower extremities that results in reduced preload and stagnation of blood in lower extremities causing deep vein thrombosis (DVT) [11].

Pulmonary system: Increased peak inspiratory and mean airway pressures induced by high IAP in mechanically ventilated patients can cause alveolar barotrauma. Associated with reduced chest wall compliance and reduced spontaneous tidal volumes, this cause arterial hypoxemia and hypercarbia. Pulmonary infection is also more common among patients with IAH [12]. According to animal studies, these effects are mediated through compression of the lung leading to atelectasis, oedema, increased intrapulmonary shunt fraction, decreased gas transfer and increased alveolar dead space [13].

Renal system: Kidney is affected by IAH/ACS by two ways: by direct compression of renal vein and by increased renal vasoconstriction caused by renin angiotensin induced by the decrease in preload.

The renal filtration gradient (FG) can be considered as the net force across the glomerulus. It is the gradient between the glomerular filtration pressure (GFP) and the proximal tubular pressure (PTP). In the presence of IAH, PTP is same as IAP. GFP is equivalent to the mean arterial pressure (MAP), and thus GFP can be estimated as MAP minus twice the IAP. Thus, the impact of IAP on the renal function and urine production is much greater than that caused by changes in MAP. So oliguria manifest is one of the first visible signs of IAH [14].

Filtration gradient: glomerular filtration pressure – proximal tubular pressure.

$$\begin{aligned} FG &= GFP - PTP \\ &= (MAP - IAP) - PTP \\ &= (MAP - IAP) - IAP \\ &= MAP - 2 \times IAP \end{aligned} \quad (1)$$

Hence, when IAP is doubled, filtration gradient will be decreased by four-folds. Oliguria generally develops at an intra-abdominal pressure of approximately 15 mmHg, while anuria usually develops at an intra-abdominal pressure of approximately 30 mmHg [15]. Because of impairment in renal perfusion, the urine sodium and chloride concentrations are usually decreased. Along with increased plasma renin activity, aldosterone concentration and antidiuretic hormone concentration are also increased to more than twice their baseline levels, which has tremendous impact on the renal function [16].

Gastrointestinal system: The gut is very sensitive to increase in IAP as the primary organ is exposed to high IAP, which can occur at IAP as low as 10 mmHg [17]. At 20 mmHg of IAP mucosal perfusion pressure of the gut is decreased [18] and at 40 mmHg celiac and superior mesenteric blood flow are reduced [19]. IAH also impairs venous flow from the intestine by compressing intestinal veins and causes intestinal oedema. This increases intra-abdominal pressure further, as a vicious cycle [20]. This leads to worsened hypo perfusion, bowel ischemia, decreased intra-mucosal pH and lactic acidosis [21]. Hypoperfusion of the gut may result in loss of the mucosal barrier, leading to bacterial translocation, sepsis and multiple system organ failure. Bacterial translocation has been shown to occur at IAP of only 10 mmHg in the presence of haemorrhage [22].

Hepatic: Liver is affected by IAH by reducing its ability to clear lactate even with adequate cardiac output and blood pressure and this can occur with IAP as low as 10 mmHg [23].

Central nervous system: The effect of IAH on intracranial pressure (ICP) range from transient increases during the short-lived elevation of intra-abdominal pressure that occurs with coughing, defecating or emesis to sustained elevation during persistent elevation of IAH. This can lead to a critical decrease in cerebral perfusion pressure (CPP) [24]. Decompressive laparotomy was found to decrease ICP drastically in a case of ACS as reported by Bloomfield et al. [25].

4. Diagnosis

Physical examination was found to be neither sensitive nor specific for the diagnosis of IAH/ACS with a sensitivity of 56%, specificity of 87%, positive predictive value of 35%, negative predictive value of 94% and accuracy of 84% [26]. Imaging studies such as chest X-ray, ultrasound abdomen and CT scan are not useful to diagnose IAH/ACS efficiently but can give some clue to the possibility, such as elevated diaphragm, basal atelectasis, inferior venae caval compression, tense infiltration of the retro peritoneum that is out of proportion to peritoneal disease, massive abdominal distension, direct renal compression or displacement, bowel wall thickening or bilateral inguinal herniation [27].

Various techniques have been described for IAP measurement using intra-vesical, intragastric or inferior venae caval catheters. WSACS has standardized intra-vesical (urinary bladder) pressure measurement as the gold standard for measurement of IAH/ACS [28]. This was done through puncturing the aspiration port of Folley's catheter or attaching a three-way stopcock and connecting it to a manometer, but nowadays a closed system has been developed which avoids the puncturing and ensures sterility (**Figure 3**). The pressure is measured at end-expiration in the supine position after ensuring that abdominal muscle contractions are absent. The transducer should be zeroed at the level of the mid-axillary line. WSACS has also standardized the amount of saline to be instilled as up to 25 ml. However, as a downside, the bladder pressure may be inaccurate in the presence of intra-peritoneal adhesions, pelvic hematomas, pelvic fractures, abdominal packs or a neurogenic bladder [29].

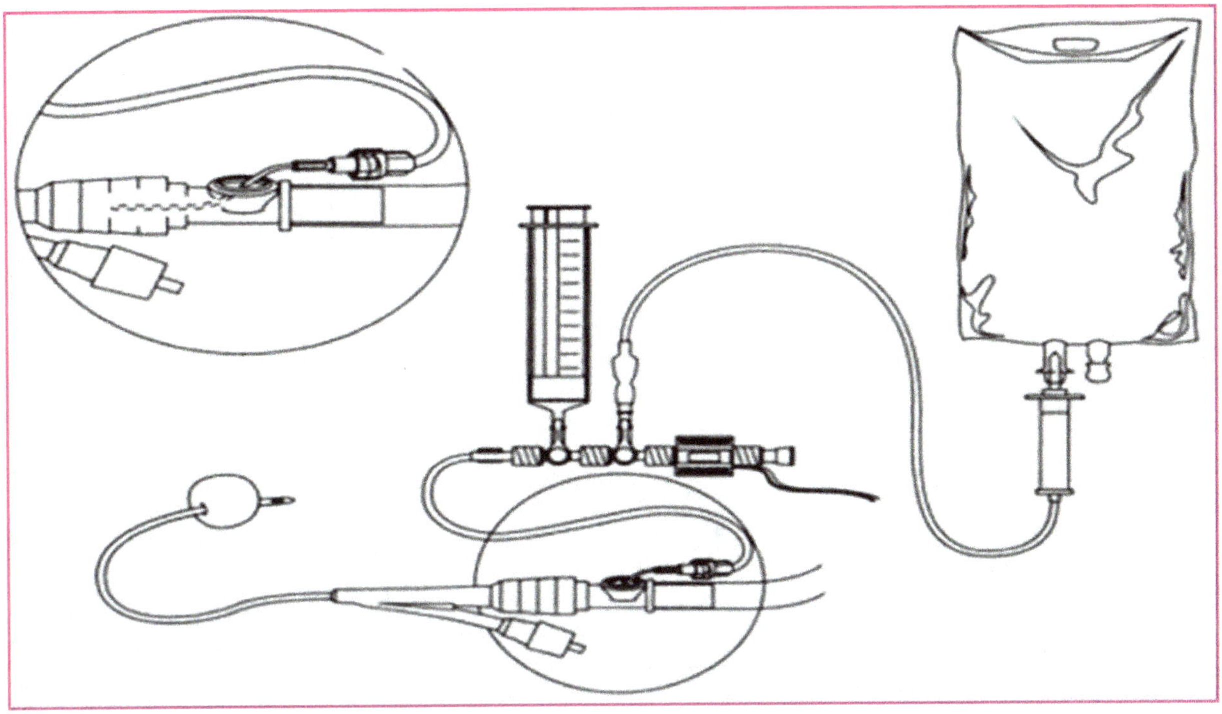

Figure 3. Closed system for intra-abdominal pressure monitoring (adapted from: Roberto et al. [50]).

5. Management of IAH/ACS

Surgical decompression is the definitive management of IAH/ACS but supportive medical therapy should be attempted before resorting to this. WSACS has provided algorithm for management of IAH/ACS (**Algorithms 1** and **2**). Nowadays, the trend is more towards less invasive management such as abdominal wall escharotomy in burns [30] or percutaneous drainage of intra-abdominal collections [31].

Principles of supportive care are [32] as follows:

1. *Evacuate intra-luminal contents*: nasogastric and rectal drainage.
2. *Drain extra-luminal collections*: evacuate hemoperitoneum, ascites, intra-abdominal abscess and retroperitoneal hematoma.
3. *Improve abdominal wall compliance*: supine position, adequate analgesia, sedation and sometimes muscle paralysis.

Many of IAH/ACS patients will need ventilatory support and should have a lung protective strategy like low tidal volume, pressure limitation, permissive hypercapnea, use of positive end expiratory pressure (PEEP) and use of muscle relaxants in indicated patients.

Aggressive fluid resuscitation is one of the risk factors for the development of ACS. As these patients are haemodynamically unstable initially, they receive large amounts of crystalloids with resultant bowel oedema and development or aggravation of ACS. Liberal use of colloids

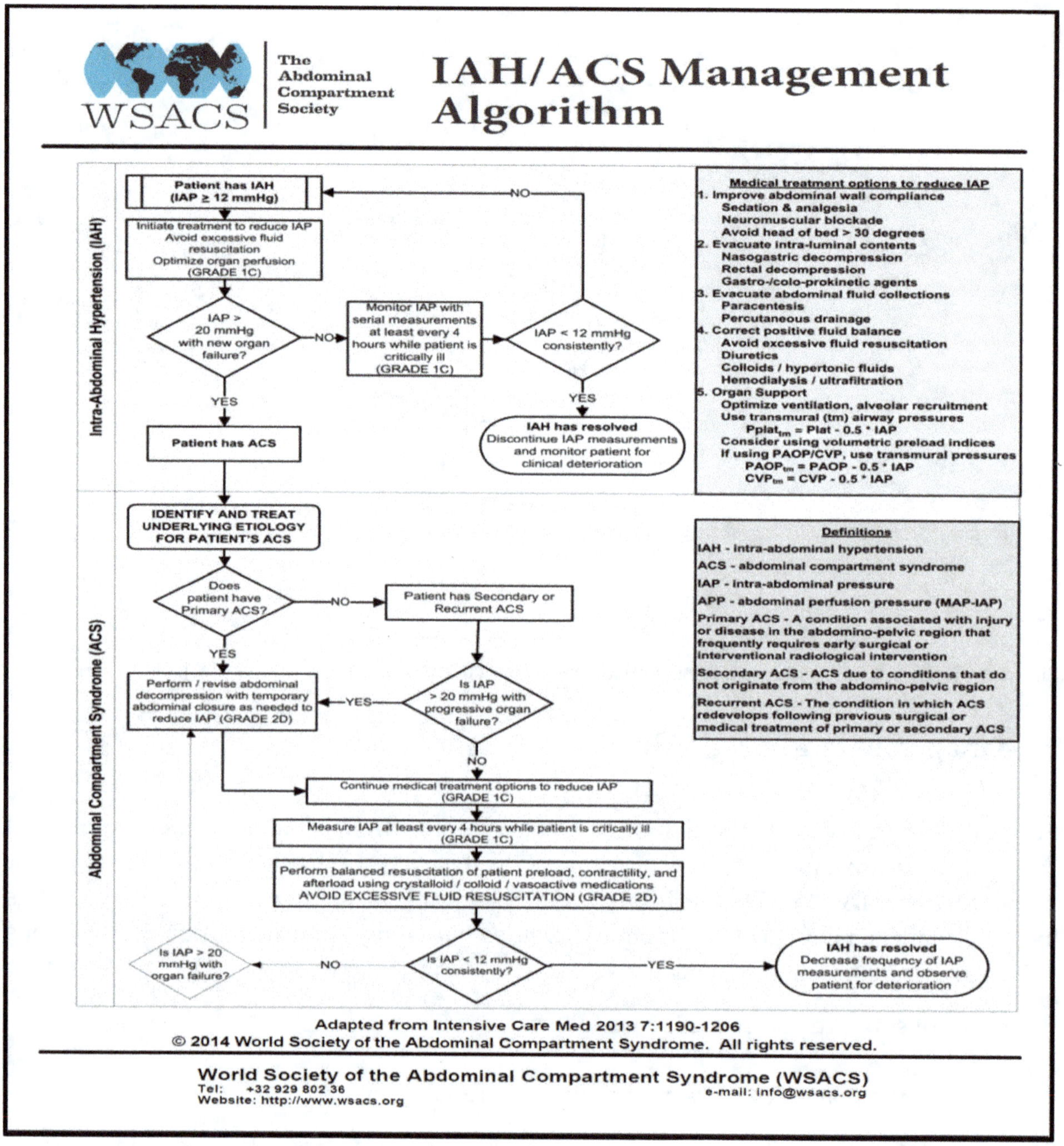

Algorithm 1. Management of IAH/ACS by WSACS: Adapted from World Society of the Abdominal Compartment Syndrome (WSACS) website: http://www.wsacs.org.

has not yet proved to prevent this. But on the other side optimum fluid resuscitation can prevent some negative aspects of ACS such as reduced cardiac output, renal blood flow, urine output and visceral perfusion.

Decompressive laparotomy is the definitive treatment for ACS. Many surgeons resort to decompression when the IAP is above 25, but a lower threshold would be better in terms of organ saving. An approach based on abdominal perfusion pressure (APP) rather than IAP would be more logical, and a threshold APP of 50 mmHg was found to correlate with mortality [33].

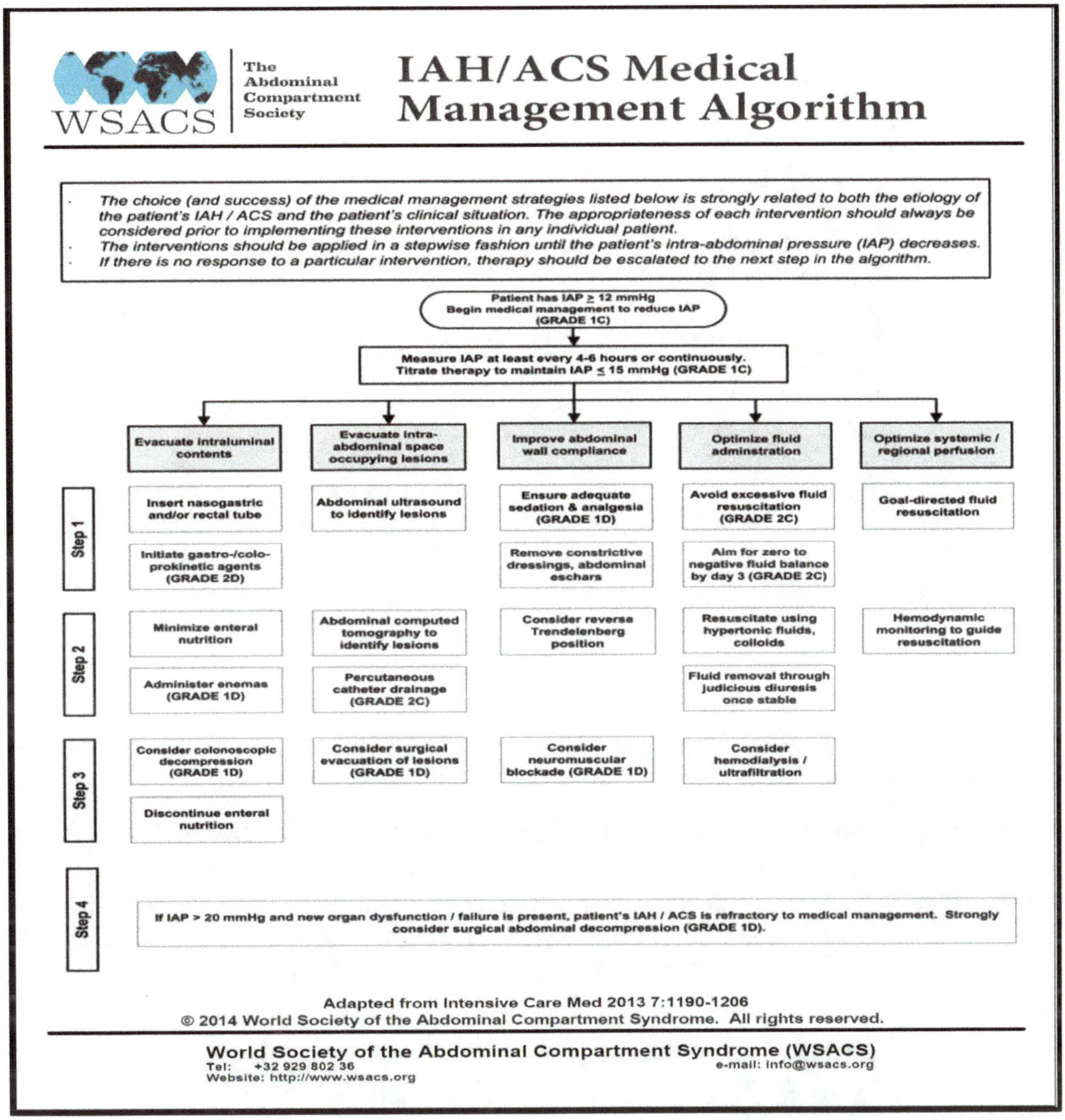

Algorithm 2. Medical management of IAH/ACS by WSACS: Adapted from World Society of the Abdominal Compartment Syndrome (WSACS) website: http://www.wsacs.org.

An open abdomen approach after decompression with temporary closure methods is commonly used by most surgeons to prevent recurrent ACS.

There are different methods for managing open abdomen (OA). Abdomen can be closed with temporary abdominal closure using various techniques, which should be later followed by interval abdominal closure, by bringing the edges of the abdominal fascia together primarily (primary closure) if possible technically. If technically not feasible, OA can be closed either using a functional closure or simple coverage [34]. Negative pressure techniques like vacuum-assisted closure (VAC) (**Figure 4**), patch technique (e.g. Whittmann patch, polytetrafluoroethylene patch),

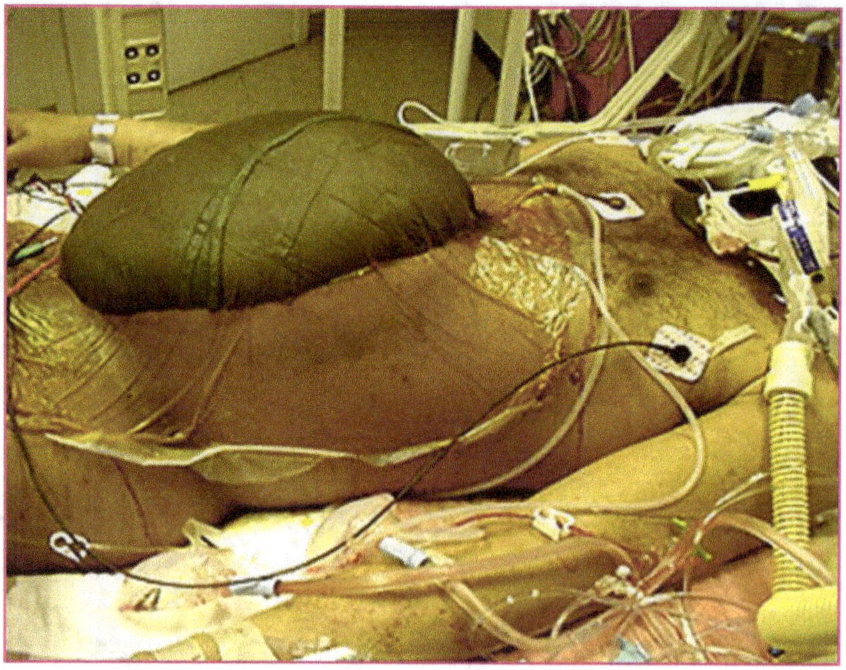

Figure 4. Vacuum-assisted closure (from: https://www.slideshare.net/drabdulgafoormt/intraabdominal-hypertension).

silo technique (e.g. Bagota bag) (**Figure 5**) and skin-only technique using towel clips are some methods used in the management of open abdomen. Each technique has its own advantages and disadvantages and description of that is beyond the scope of this chapter.

Closure of abdomen after the ACS also utilizes different methods such as STAR (staged abdominal repair), component separation and planned ventral hernia. An international consensus conference on open abdomen in Trauma [35] concluded that open abdomen (OA) in trauma is advisable at the end of damage-control laparotomy, especially in the presence of swelling of viscera, for a second look if there are vascular injuries or gross contamination of

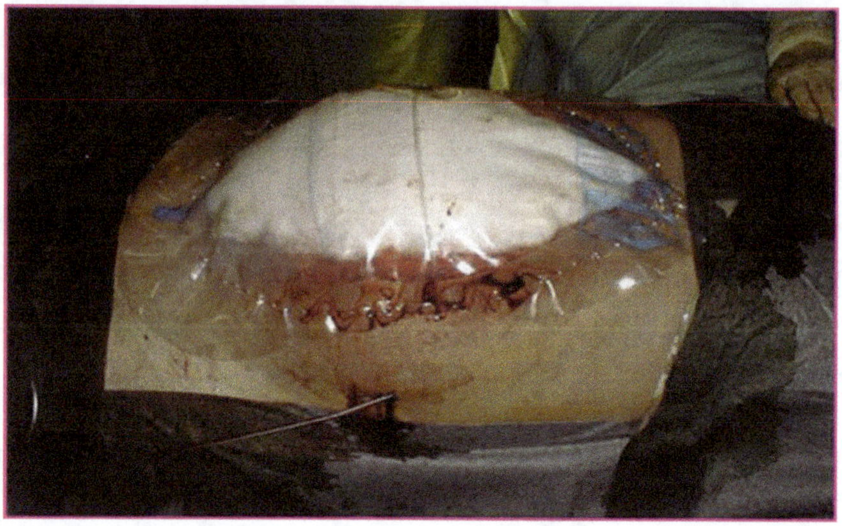

Figure 5. Bagota bag closure (from Huang et al. [51]).

the peritoneal cavity, or if there is loss of abdominal wall, and in cases of failure of medical treatment of abdominal compartment syndrome, but early closure is mandatory to prevent complications such as fistulae formation and frozen abdomen. A review by Sugrue M, opined that the key to optimizing outcome in ACS is early abdominal closure within 7 days because failure to do so increases morbidity, mortality and fistulae formation [36].

6. Recent insights

In a recent experimental study, Leng et al. [37] indicated that mitochondrial Ca^{2+}uptake 1 (MICU1)-related oxidation/antioxidation disequilibrium is strongly involved in IAH-induced damage to intestinal barriers. MICU1-targeted treatment may hold promise for preventing the progression of IAH to gut-derived sepsis. Earlier in 2014, an animal study led by the same author found that acute exposure to slightly elevated IAP may result in adverse effects on intestinal permeability and the pro-oxidant-antioxidant balance and so monitoring IAP is very important in critical patients [38]. In another experiment in rats by Liu et al. [39], Melanocortin 4 (MC4 receptor) agonist counteracts the intestinal inflammatory response, ameliorating intestinal injury in experimental secondary IAH by MC4 receptor-triggered activation of the cholinergic anti-inflammatory pathway. This may represent a promising strategy for the treatment of IAH in the future.

A systematic review and individual patient data meta-analysis on intra-abdominal hypertension in critically ill patients: the wake-up project (World initiative on Abdominal Hypertension Epidemiology, a Unifying Project) [40] in 2014 looking at the outcome and mortality in IAH/ACS found that the only independent predictors for IAH were SOFA score and fluid balance on the day of admission. 513 patients out of 2707 patients (30.8%) died in ICU. The independent predictors for intensive care mortality were SAPS II score, IAH, SOFA score and admission category. This review showed that IAH is an independent predictor for mortality and is frequently present in critically ill patients more than anticipated.

New medical treatment options that are still experimental include tissue plasminogen activator (tPa), theophylline and octreotide. tPa was evaluated for retroperitoneal hematoma by Horer et al. [41]. They analysed 13 patients who developed ACS with multiple organ failure in the ICU. The mean IAP was 23.5 mmHg before decompression (range 12–35), and when tPA was given, IAP dropped to a mean of 16 mmHg (range 10–28.5) after 24 h of administration. Drainage of hematoma after tPa increased to 1520 mL (range 170–2900) from 370 mL (range 5–1000). This also coincided with improvement in urinary output and haemodynamics.

Bodnar et al. [42] found a positive correlation between IAH and increased levels of serum adenosine and interleukin10 concentrations in 45 surgical patients with IAP >12 mmHg. Based on these findings, they conducted another study [43] comparing standard medical treatment in patients with IAH versus standard medical treatment and theophylline infusions twice daily. Mortality in theophylline group was 0% when compared to standard group (55%). Theophylline improved renal function, splanchnic perfusion, and cardiac contractility possibly by counteracting adenosine binding to adenosine receptors. The authors postulated that by decreasing circulating adenosine concentrations, theophylline infusion improves IAH-related mortality in surgical patients

Octreotide, a synthetic somatostatin analogue, by decreasing myeloperoxidase (MPO) activity and malondialdehyde levels and thereby increasing levels of glutathione if given before decompression of IAP has been shown to improve the reperfusion-induced oxidative damage in rats with ACS [44]. This translates to that octreotide might have a therapeutic role as an agent limiting reperfusion injury among patients with IAH and ACS.

Free radical scavengers such as melatonin and vitamin C (ascorbic acid) were also tried in the medical management of IAH/ACS and found useful in animal studies [45]. Vitamin C was found to reduce resuscitation fluid requirements significantly thereby preventing secondary ACS and IAH in burns [46].

Another nonsurgical technique being investigated is continuous negative extra-abdominal pressure (CNAP). Bloomfield et al. [47] demonstrated a significant reduction in IAP when continuous negative pressure was applied by vacuum via a large poncho into which the entire animal was placed. There was a mean reduction in IAP from 30.7 ± 1.3 to 18.2 ± 1.3 mmHg. Apart from IAP, central venous pressure (CVP), inferior venae caval (IVC) pressure, intra cranial pressure (ICP), pulmonary artery occlusion pressure (PAOP) and peak airway pressure were also reduced. This was also evaluated in a human study by Sugerman et al. [48], which proved the above benefits although some patients expressed discomfort in lower chest and pelvic area. All the novel medical options for management of IAH/ACS apart from standard medical management-like evacuation of intra and extra luminal contents, improvement of abdominal wall compliance, are still in experimental stage and not recommended for routine use.

7. Conclusion

IAH/ACS is not a problem limited to the abdomen but rather a systemic problem affecting various body systems adversely with deleterious consequences. Addressing this important pathology in a timely manner is crucial for the better outcome of critically ill patients. Mainstay of the management in IAH/ACS is still surgical decompression but medical options are equally important interventions. Novel therapies in medical options are being explored and needs further validation to be recommended in routine management of patients with intra-abdominal hypertension and abdominal compartment syndrome.

Author details

Abdulgafoor M. Tharayil*, Adel Ganaw, Syed Abdulrahman, Zia M. Awan and Sujith M. Prabhakaran

*Address all correspondence to: atharayil@hamad.qa

Department of Anaesthesia, Hamad Medical Corporation, Doha, Qatar

References

[1] Hong JJ, Cohn SM, Perez JM, Dolich MO, Brown M, McKenney MG. Prospective study of the incidence and outcome of intra-abdominal hypertension and the abdominal compartment syndrome. British Journal of Surgery. 2002;**89**(5):591

[2] Balogh Z, McKinley BA, Holcomb JB, Miller CC, Cocanour CS, Kozar RA, Valdivia A, Ware DN, Moore FA. Both primary and secondary abdominal compartment syndrome can be predicted early and are harbingers of multiple organ failure. Journal of Trauma. 2003;**54**(5):848

[3] Balogh Z, McKinley BA, Cocanour CS, Kozar RA, Holcomb JB, Ware DN, Moore FA. Secondary abdominal compartment syndrome is an elusive early complication of traumatic shock resuscitation. American Journal of Surgery. 2002;**184**(6):538

[4] Malbrain ML, Cheatham ML, Kirkpatrick A, Sugrue M, Parr M, De Waele J, Balogh Z, Leppäniemi A, Olvera C, Ivatury R, D'Amours S, Wendon J, Hillman K, Johansson K, Kolkman K, Wilmer A. Results from the International Conference of experts on intra-abdominal hypertension and abdominal compartment syndrome. I. Definitions. Intensive Care Medicine. 2006;**32**(11):1722

[5] Sanchez NC, Tenofsky PL, Dort JM, Shen LY, Helmer SD, Smith RS. What is normal intra-abdominal pressure? American Surgeon. 2001;**67**(3):243

[6] Schein M, Ivatury R. Intra-abdominal hypertension and the abdominal compartment syndrome. British Journal of Surgery. 1998;**85**(8):1027.

[7] Vidal MG, Ruiz Weisser J, Gonzalez F, Toro MA, Loudet C, Balasini C, Canales H, Reina R, Estenssoro E. Incidence and clinical effects of intra-abdominal hypertension in critically ill patients. Critical Care Medicine. 2008;**36**(6):1823

[8] http://www.wsacs.org/consensus_summary.php [Accessed on October 11, 2011].

[9] Van Mook WN, Huslewe-Evers RP, Ramsay G. Abdominal compartment syndrome. Lancet. 2002;**360**(9344):1502

[10] Cullen DJ, Coyle JP, Teplick R, Long MC. Cardiovascular, pulmonary, and renal effects of massively increased intra-abdominal pressure in critically ill patients. Critical Care Medicine. 1989;**17**(2):118.

[11] Barnes GE, Laine GA, Giam PY, Smith EE, Granger HJ. Cardiovascular responses to elevation of intra-abdominal hydrostatic pressure. American Journal of Physiology. 1985;**248**(2 Pt 2):R208.

[12] Aprahamian C, Wittmann DH, Bergstein JM, Quebbeman EJ. Temporary abdominal closure (TAC) for planned relaparotomy (etappenlavage) in trauma. Journal of Trauma. 1990;**30**(6):719

[13] Quintel M, Pelosi P, Caironi P, Meinhardt JP, Luecke T, Herrmann P, Taccone P, Rylander C, Valenza F, Carlesso E, Gattinoni L. An increase of abdominal pressure increases

pulmonary edema in oleic acid-induced lung injury. American Journal of Respiratory Critical Care Medicine. 2004;**169**(4):534

[14] Papavramidis TS, Marinis AD, Pliakos I, Kesisoglou I, Papavramidou N. Abdominal compartment syndrome – Intra-abdominal hypertension: Defining, diagnosing, and managing. Journal of Emergencies, Trauma and Shock. 2011;**4**(2):279-291

[15] Richards WO, Scovill W, Shin B, Reed W. Acute renal failure associated with increased intra-abdominal pressure. Annals of Surgery. 1983;**197**(2):183-187.

[16] Le Roith D, Bark H, Nyska M, Glick SM. The effect of abdominal pressure on plasma antidiuretic hormone levels in the dog. Journal of Surgical Research. 1982;**32**(1):65

[17] Friedlander MH, Simon RJ, Ivatury R, DiRaimo R, Machiedo GW. Effect of hemorrhage on superior mesenteric artery flow during increased intra-abdominal pressures. Journal of Trauma. 1998;**45**(3):433

[18] Chang MC, Cheatham ML, Nelson LD, Rutherford EJ, Morris JA Jr. Gastric tonometry supplements information provided by systemic indicators of oxygen transport. Journal of Trauma. 1994;**37**(3):488

[19] Caldwell CB, Ricotta JJ. Changes in visceral blood flow with elevated intraabdominal pressure. Journal of Surgical Research. 1987;**43**(1):14

[20] Mark G. Abdominal compartment syndrome in adults. In: Hilary S, Eileen MB, editors. Up to Date. Waltham, MA. [Accessed on March 4, 2017]

[21] Diebel LN, Wilson RF, Dulchavsky SA, Saxe J. Effect of increased intra-abdominal pressure on hepatic arterial, portal venous, and hepatic microcirculatory blood flow. Journal of Trauma. 1992;**33**(2):279

[22] Gargiulo NJ 3rd, Simon RJ, Leon W, Machiedo GW. Hemorrhage exacerbates bacterial translocation at low levels of intra-abdominal pressure. Archives of Surgery. 1998; **133**(12):1351

[23] Luca A, Cirera I, García-Pagán JC, Feu F, Pizcueta P, Bosch J, Rodés J. Hemodynamic effects of acute changes in intra-abdominal pressure in patients with cirrhosis. Gastroenterology. 1993;**104**(1):222

[24] Citerio G, Vascotto E, Villa F, Celotti S, Pesenti A. Induced abdominal compartment syndrome increases intracranial pressure in neurotrauma patients: A prospective study. Critical Care Medicine. 2001;**29**(7):1466.

[25] Bloomfield GL, Dalton JM, Sugerman HJ, Ridings PC, DeMaria EJ, Bullock R. Treatment of increasing intracranial pressure secondary to the acute abdominal compartment syndrome in a patient with combined abdominal and head trauma. Journal of Trauma. 1995;**39**(6):1168

[26] Kirkpatrick AW, Brenneman FD, McLean RF, Rapanos T, Boulanger BR. Is clinical examination an accurate indicator of raised intra-abdominal pressure in critically injured patients? Canadian Journal of Surgery. 2000;**43**(3):207

[27] Pickhardt PJ, Shimony JS, Heiken JP, Buchman TG, Fisher AJ. The abdominal compartment syndrome: CT findings. American Journal of Roentgenology. 1999;**173**(3):575

[28] Kirkpatrick AW, Roberts DJ, De Waele J, Jaeschke R, Malbrain ML, De Keulenaer B, Duchesne J, Bjorck M, Leppaniemi A, Ejike JC, Sugrue M, Cheatham M, Ivatury R, Ball CG, Reintam Blaser A, Regli A, Balogh ZJ, D'Amours S, Debergh D, Kaplan M, Kimball E, Olvera C. Pediatric guidelines sub-committee for the world society of the abdominal compartment syndrome. Intra-abdominal hypertension and the abdominal compartment syndrome: Updated consensus definitions and clinical practice guidelines from the World Society of the Abdominal Compartment Syndrome. Intensive Care Medicine. 2013;**39**(7):1190-1206. Epub 2013 May 15.

[29] Malbrain ML. Different techniques to measure intra-abdominal pressure (IAP): Time for a critical re-appraisal. Intensive Care Medicine. 2004;**30**(3):357

[30] Hobson KG, Young KM, Ciraulo A, Palmieri TL, Greenhalgh DG. Release of abdominal compartment syndrome improves survival in patients with burn injury. Journal of Trauma. 2002;**53**(6):1129

[31] Cheatham ML, Safcsak K. Percutaneous catheter decompression in the treatment of elevated intraabdominal pressure. Chest. 2011;**140**(6):1428

[32] Cheatham ML. Nonoperative management of intraabdominal hypertension and abdominal compartment syndrome. World Journal of Surgery. 2009;**33**(6):1116-1122

[33] Cheatham ML, White MW, Sagraves SG, Johnson JL, Block EF. Abdominal perfusion pressure: A superior parameter in the assessment of intra-abdominal hypertension. Journal of Trauma. 2000;**49**(4):621

[34] Neils M, Babak S. In: Eileen M, Katthryn AC, editor. Up to Date. Waltham, MA. [Accessed on March 4, 2017]

[35] Chiara O, Cimbanassi S, Biffl W, Leppaniemi A, Henry S, Scalea, Thomas M, et al. Journal of Trauma and Acute Care Surgery. 2016;**80**(1):173-183

[36] Sugrue M. Abdominal compartment syndrome and the open abdomen: any unresolved issues? Current Opinion in Critical Care. 2017;**23**(1):73-78

[37] Leng Y, Ge Q, Zhao Z, Wang K, Yao G. MICU1 may be a promising intervention target for gut-derived sepsis induced by intra-abdominal hypertension. Cell Death Discovery. 2016;**2**:16080.

[38] Yuxin L,Kuo Z, Jie F, Min Y, Qinggang G, Li C, Lu Z, Gaiqi Y. Effect of acute, slightly increased intra-abdominal pressure on intestinal permeability and oxidative stress in a rat model. PLoS One. 2014;9(10) e109350.

[39] Liu D, Zhang HG, Chang MT, Li Y, Zhang LY. Melanocortin-4 receptor agonists alleviate intestinal dysfunction in secondary intra-abdominal hypertension rat model. Journal of Surgical Research. 2015;**195**(1):263-270

[40] Malbrain ML, Chiumello D, Cesana BM, Reintam Blaser A, Starkopf J, Sugrue M, Pelosi P. A systematic review and individual patient data meta-analysis on intra-abdominal hypertension in critically ill patients: The wake-up project. World initiative on Abdominal Hypertension Epidemiology, a Unifying Project (WAKE-Up!). Minerva Anaesthesiology. 2014;**80**(3):293-306.

[41] Horer T, Skoog P, Pirouzram A, Larzon T. Tissue plasminogen activator-assisted hematoma evacuation to relieve abdominal compartment syndrome after endovascular repair of ruptured abdominal aortic aneurysm. Journal of Endovascular Therapy. 2012;**19**:144–148

[42] Bodnar Z, Keresztes T, Kovacs I, Hajdu Z, Boissonneault GA, Sipka S. Increased serum adenosine and interleukin 10 levels as new laboratory markers of increased intra-abdominal pressure. Langenbecks Archives of Surgery. 2010;**395**:969–972

[43] Bodnar Z, Szentkereszty Z, Hajdu Z, Boissonneault GA, Sipka S. Beneficial effects of theophylline infusions in surgical patients with intra-abdominal hypertension. Langenbecks Archives of Surgery. 2011;**396**:793–800

[44] De Keulenaer B, Regli A, De laet I, Roberts DJ, Malbrain MLNG. What's new in medical management strategies for raised intra-abdominal pressure: Evacuating intra-abdominal contents, improving abdominal wall compliance, pharmacotherapy, and continuous negative extra-abdominal pressure. Anaesthesiology Intensive Therapy. 2015;**47**(1):54-62.

[45] Sener G, Kacmaz A, User Y, Ozkan S, Tilki M, Yegen BC. Melatonin ameliorates oxidative organ damage induced by acute intra-abdominal compartment syndrome in rats. Journal of Pineal Research. 2003;**35**:163–168

[46] Kremer T, Harenberg P, Hernekamp F et al. High-dose vitamin C treatment reduces capillary leakage after burn plasma transfer in rats. Journal of Burn Care Research. 2010;**31**:470–479

[47] Bloomfield G, Saggi B, Blocher C, Sugerman H. Physiologic effects of externally applied continuous negative abdominal pressure for intra-abdominal hypertension. Journal of Trauma. 1999;**46**:1009–1014

[48] Sugerman HJ, Felton IW, 3rd, Sismanis A, et al. Continuous negative abdominal pressure device to treat pseudotumor cerebri. International Journal of Obesity and Related Metabolic Disorders. 2001;**25**: 486

[49] Nissar Shaikh, et al. A rare and unsuspected complication of Clostridium difficile infection. Intensive Care Medicine. 2008:**34**:963-966

[50] Roberto, et al. Procedures for monitoring intra-abdominal pressure. Review of Medical Sciences. 2007 Jan-Mar;**11(**1) Pinar del Río

[51] Huang Q, Li J, Lau W-Y. Techniques for abdominal wall closure after damage control laparotomy: From temporary abdominal closure to early/delayed fascial closure—A review. Gastroenterology Research and Practice. 2016;2016:15. Article ID 2073260. DOI: http://dx.doi.org/10.1155/2016/2073260

6

Acute Kidney Injury in the Intensive Care Unit

Jose J. Zaragoza and Faustino J. Renteria

Abstract

Acute kidney injury (AKI) is defined as an abrupt decrease in glomerular filtration rate (GFR). Incidence varies from 20% to as high as 70% in critically ill patients. Classically, AKI has been divided into three broad pathophysiologic categories: prerenal AKI, intrinsic AKI, and postrenal (obstructive) AKI. The clinical manifestations of AKI vary among a wide range of symptoms and metabolic abnormalities. A sudden decrease in GFR will result in rising concentrations of solutes in the blood, which are normally excreted by the kidneys. Recently, new urinary and serum biomarkers have gained a place in the diagnosis, classification, and prognosis prediction of AKI. The best treatment for AKI is prevention. Patients with prerenal azotemia should have intravascular volume deficits corrected and cardiac function optimized. Obstructive (postrenal) kidney disease is treated by mechanical relief of the block. The primary management of acute interstitial nephritis is discontinuation of the inciting agent. Renal replacement therapy (RRT) has emerged as a supportive mechanism rather than just as a lifesaving measure. Continuous techniques are preferable in treating critically ill patients, although every modality has its benefits, indications, and contraindications.

Keywords: acute kidney injury, acute renal failure, intensive care unit, glomerular filtration rate, renal replacement therapy

1. Introduction

Acute kidney injury (AKI) is now recognized as a major health problem that affects millions of patients worldwide and leads to decreased survival and increased risk of progression to chronic kidney disease (CKD). It is often diagnosed along with other acute illnesses and is common in critically ill patients. AKI has also an important role since it is strongly associated with augmented costs of care, worse outcomes, and diminished quality of life after discharge. The impact and prognosis of AKI vary considerably depending on the severity, clinical setting, comorbid factors, and geographical location [1].

AKI in the ICU is common, and it is increasing in incidence. Reported mortality in ICU patients with AKI varies between studies depending on AKI definition and the patient population studied. In most studies, mortality increases proportionately with increasing severity of AKI. In patients with severe AKI requiring renal replacement therapy (RRT), mortality is approximately 50–70%. Although AKI requiring RRT in the ICU is a well-recognized independent risk factor for in-hospital mortality, even small changes in serum creatinine (SCr) are associated with increased mortality.

The definition of AKI has many perceptions, the simplest way to describe it is as a sudden decrease in glomerular filtration rate (GFR) resulting in the retention of metabolic waste products and the dysregulation of fluid, electrolyte and acid-base homeostasis. AKI is a heterogeneous syndrome that includes hemodynamic disarrangements that disturb normal renal perfusion and decrease GFR without overt parenchymal injury; partial or complete obstruction to urine flow; and acute parenchymal injury resulting in glomerular, interstitial, tubular, or vascular dysfunction. The most common causes of AKI in critically ill patients include hemodynamically mediated prerenal dysfunction and acute tubular necrosis (ATN) due to ischemia-reperfusion injury, nephrotoxic exposure, or sepsis [2].

The cardinal manifestation of AKI is the retention of metabolic waste products, most commonly represented by creatinine and urea, and/or fluid accumulation. More than 35 clinical definitions of AKI currently exist in the literature. The Acute Dialysis Quality Initiative convened in 2002 and proposed the RIFLE classification (risk, injury, failure, loss, end-stage kidney disease) specifically for AKI in critically ill patients. Using SCr and urine output, the RIFLE criteria define three grades of severity and two outcome classes. Later, the Acute Kidney Injury Network (AKIN) proposed another clinical and practical definition. Even small changes in serum creatinine concentrations are associated with a substantial increase in the risk of death. For this reason, in 2012, the Kidney Disease Improving Global Outcomes (KDIGO) classification defined AKI as a raise of serum creatinine of at least 0.3 mg/dl or as a urine output of less than 0.3 ml/kg/h for at least 6 h (**Table 1**) [3].

2. Epidemiology

The epidemiology of AKI varies depending on the type and characteristics of the population described. Using the current 0.3-mg/dl change in serum creatinine threshold, published data ranges the incidence of AKI in hospitalized patients from 3 to 50% and from 10 to 70% in the intensive care unit (ICU). A 2013 meta-analysis of AKI incidence per the kidney improving global outcomes staging system with a total number of patients included of 3,585,911, reported incidence in 23% overall hospitalized patients [4].

Stage	RIFLE	AKIN	KDIGO	Urine output
RIFLE–Risk AKIN/ KDIGO Stage 1	Increase in serum creatinine × 1.5 (within 7 days)	Increase in serum creatinine of 0.3 mg/dl or > × 1.5 (within 48 h)	Increase in serum creatinine of 0.3 mg/dl (within 48 h) or × 1.5 (within 7 days)	Urine output of < 0.5 mg/kg/h for > 6 h
RIFLE–Injury AKIN/ KDIGO Stage 2	Increase in serum creatinine × 2	Increase in serum creatinine × 2	Increase in serum creatinine × 2	Urine output of < 0.5 mg/kg/h for > 12 h
RIFLE–Failure AKIN/ KDIGO Stage 3	Increase in serum creatinine × 3 or above 4.0 mg/dl	Increase in serum creatinine × 3 or above 4.0 mg/dl	Increase in serum creatinine × 3 or above 4.0 mg/dl	Urine output of < 0.3 mg/kg/h for > 24 h or anuria for > 12 h
RIFLE–Loss	Need for RRT for >4 weeks			
RIFLE–End stage	Need for RRT for >3 months			

Table 1. AKI definition by clinical parameters per RIFLE, AKIN, and KDIGO.

Among critically ill patients, numerous cohort studies have been issued to define the incidence of AKI in ICU. Final reports suggest that it goes as high as 70% in some populations. Patients with ICU-associated AKI are younger, more likely to be male and prone to have AKI associated with multisystem organ failure as opposed to isolated AKI. The most important recognized risk factor for AKI in the ICU environment is sepsis. Other important risk factors include previous diagnosis of Diabetes, Hypertension or CKD, concomitant use of vasopressors and use of mechanical ventilation. Renal replacement therapy (RRT) rates and mortality associated to AKI are significantly higher among ICU population opposed to hospitalized patients [5].

Two distinct patterns of ICU-associated AKI have been described: community-acquired AKI, present at ICU admission, and hospital-acquired AKI. Patients with hospital-acquired AKI have more severe outcomes, showing higher in-hospital mortality rates, longer lengths of stay both in the ICU and hospital, and higher needs of RRT [6, 7].

3. Pathophysiology

AKI can be divided into three broad etiologic categories: prerenal AKI, intrinsic AKI, and postrenal (**Figure 1**). Prerenal refers to states of hypoperfusion of the kidneys without a parenchymal damage, this kind of AKI occurs often in ICU patients. Postrenal or obstructive AKI is characterized by acute block of the urinary tract. Regarding intrinsic dysfunction, acute damage to the renal parenchyma exists, as in acute tubular necrosis, acute interstitial nephritis and/or acute glomerular nephritis. The terms "prerenal," "intrinsic," and "postrenal" are used to group common pathophysiologic features and not diagnosis. It was a long-held view that "prerenal AKI" or "transient" AKI were synonymous with "hypovolemic AKI" and "fluid responsiveness," this is no longer the case and must not be used in this manner. Approach to the diagnosis and treatment is described below [8, 9].

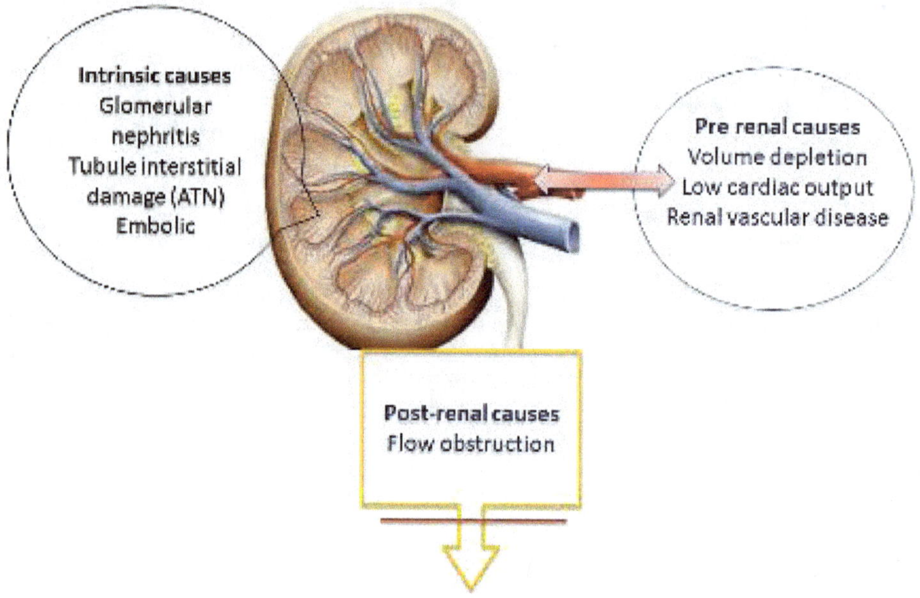

Figure 1. Traditional etiologic categories for AKI.

3.1. Prerenal AKI

Prerenal AKI is the most common pathophysiologic cause of AKI, contributing to the development 30–60% of all cases of AKI in ICU. Prerenal AKI develops when the capacity of the normal physiologic responses to hypovolemia is exceeded. This response initiates with a decrease in mean arterial pressure, triggering baroreceptors that lead the activation of the sympathetic nervous system, activation of the renin-angiotensin-aldosterone system (RAAS), and secretion of the antidiuretic hormone vasopressin. The activation of the renal sympathetic nerves constricts the afferent (preglomerular) arterioles and stimulates release of renin from the juxtaglomerular apparatus. Renin secretion is also directly stimulated in response to hypovolemia by changes in intrarenal hemodynamic. Secretion of renin activates a cascade with the final production of angiotensin II. Angiotensin II stimulates both afferent and efferent (postglomerular) arteriolar vasoconstriction; however, the effect on the afferent vessel is opposed by vasodilatory prostaglandins, kallikrein, kinins, and nitric oxide. The net effect is vasoconstriction of both afferent and efferent arterioles and decrease of GFR to maintain circulating volume at near normal levels by the production of concentrated urine with low sodium content (i.e., fractional excretion of sodium) [10–12].

In classic forms of prerenal AKI, reduced renal perfusion pressure (or increased renal venous pressure) and afferent arteriolar constriction combined lower the glomerular capillary hydrostatic pressure below the autoregulation capacity and consequently the net ultrafiltration pressure, hence diminishing GFR. Prerenal AKI may be caused by extracellular fluid volume loss or shifts, reduced cardiac output, systemic vasodilation, intrarenal vasoconstriction, or increased renal venous pressure.

3.2. Renal AKI

Intrinsic AKI is commonly divided into tubular, interstitial, glomerular, and vascular processes depending on the nephron region that is the most affected. The most common intrinsic cause of AKI is ATN, accounting for 85–90% of intrinsic ICU-associated AKI. The causes of ATN can be broken down into three major categories: ischemia-reperfusion injury, nephrotoxic, and septic. Sepsis-associated ATN has unique features and may develop in the absence of overt renal ischemia [13].

3.2.1. Sepsis-associated ATN

Sepsis has long been recognized as a foremost precipitant of AKI and deserves a distinction. Sepsis-associated AKI (SA-AKI) portends a high burden of morbidity and mortality in both children and adults with critical illness. Observational data suggest that injury during SA-AKI occurs early of the critical illness and after ICU admission. In a large recent cohort, 68% of 5443 patients with septic shock had evidence of AKI within 6 h after presentation. The development of AKI later during an episode of sepsis has been associated with worse clinical outcome and increased mortality rates (76.5 vs. 61.5% in early AKI) [14].

Sepsis-mediated hypo perfusion leading to tubular necrosis has been traditionally cited as the main pathophysiology for SA-AKI; however, mounting evidence has challenged this paradigm. Numerous drivers for injury now are recognized as playing a role in SA-AKI, including ischemia-reperfusion injury, nephron inflammation, hypoxic and/or oxidant stress, cytokine and chemokine-driven direct tubular injury, and tubular and mesenchymal apoptosis. For instance, renal vein thermodilution measurement of RBF in eight septic critically ill patients did not show hypoperfusion to the glomerulus consistently. Tubular cellular injury contributes to the propagation of AKI during sepsis. Several causal mechanisms appear to be involved, but tubular necrosis, traditionally cited as the major cellular switch for injury, is not supported by the available experimental evidence. Renal tubular apoptosis in response to the stress of systemic sepsis now is cited as a potential contributing mechanism of injury in SA-AKI [14–16].

Similarly, cellular hypoxia is a molecular driver of injury during SA-AKI. Tissue hypoxia in the kidney during sepsis may be defined by inflammation, changes in intrarenal nitric oxide, nitrosative stress or oxygen radical homeostasis, and dysregulation. Downregulation of mediators of oxidative phosphorylation occurs during sepsis and protection of mitochondrial respiration may mitigate renal injury during sepsis [14, 17, 18].

3.3. Postrenal AKI

AKI resulting from obstruction usually causes fewer than 5% of ICU-associated AKI. Obstruction above the level of the bladder is referred to as upper tract obstruction. The development of AKI from upper tract obstruction requires the presence of bilateral obstruction or unilateral obstruction in the setting of a single functioning kidney or dysfunction of the contralateral kidney.

Patients with obstructive disease may present with anuria if obstruction is complete, with normal or increased urine volume in a partial obstruction, or with fluctuating urine output with periods of anuria alternating with rapid passage of urine as the pressure in the collecting system rises and overcomes the block. In the acute phase of obstruction, intratubular pressure rises over venous renal pressure replacing the latter in the net filtration pressure equation. When intratubular pressure reaches close to mean arterial pressure, net filtration pressure falls below the autoregulation range, sometimes almost to zero [19].

4. Clinical findings

The clinical manifestations of AKI vary from a wide range of signs and symptoms. The syndrome encompasses from laboratory abnormalities without symptoms to organ failure exhibiting fluid overload and severe electrolyte and/or acid-base disturbances [20].

A sudden decrease in GFR results in rising concentrations of waste products, commonly represented by urea end creatinine in the blood. The relationship between the GFR and the concentration of urea and creatinine in blood stream is nonlinear and may be affected by a variety of other factors. The level of blood urea nitrogen (BUN) generally correlates with the symptoms, with uremic manifestations usually absent until the BUN is above 100 mg/dl. Creatinine is derived from the nonenzymatic hydrolysis of creatine, which is usually released at a constant rate from skeletal muscle and is excreted primarily by filtration at the glomerulus. There is essentially no tubular reabsorption of creatinine. That is why, in the absence of glomerular filtration, serum creatinine typically increases by 1–2 mg/dl/day. The role of creatinine as a marker of renal function is limited by the fact that the serum concentration may take 24–36 h to rise after a renal insult. Additionally, ICU patients commonly accumulate fluid due to intravenous administration and concomitant AKI. Fluid overload decreases creatinine concentration since it dilutes the total amount of creatinine in the extracellular fluid. A true change in GFR may not be adequately reflected by serum creatinine in patients with sepsis, liver disease, fluid overload, and/or muscle wasting [20].

Urine output of less than 400–500 ml/day or a sustained urine output of less than 20 ml/h in a high-risk patient in the absence of volume depletion almost always indicates the presence of AKI. By KDIGO definition, a urine output of less than 0.5 ml/kg/h for 6 h indicates the occurrence of AKI [3].

4.1. Biomarkers

Cystatin C is a cysteine protease inhibitor that is released into the bloodstream at a constant rate from all nucleated cells. It is filtered at the glomerulus and reabsorbed and catabolized by renal proximal tubular epithelial cells such that virtually no cystatin C appears in the urine. The interindividual variability in cystatin C production appears to be less than that for creatinine. Cystatin C may be a more reliable marker of GFR [21].

Several relatively new biomarkers of tubular injury have been proposed as novel diagnostic tests for the early diagnosis of AKI. These markers include kidney injury molecule-1 (KIM-1), neutrophil gelatinase-associated lipocalin (NGAL), interleukin 18 (IL-18), liver fatty acid binding protein (L-FABP), and α- and π-glutathione-S-transferase (GST), among others. They have been tested particularly amid cardiac surgery patients, with good predicting values. Even though these markers seem promising, these are not suitable for indiscriminate use in every ICU patient, and their exact specific role at the bedside remains uncertain [22, 23].

A novel test method measures two small tubular cell–derived molecules, Insulin-like Growth Factor Binding Protein 7 (IGFBP7) and Tissue Inhibitor of Metalloproteinase 2 (TIMP-2). IGFBP7 and TIMP-2 are markers of cell cycle arrest and possibly apoptosis, inflammation, and tubular cell repair. The above-stated conditions appear to be the most relevant in the development of tubular cell injury, when the loss of cell polarity, brush border derangement, and cell sloughing might occur. Such injury may deflect the organism from normal repair toward maladaptive and lead to CKD, which further predisposes the individual to recurrent AKI [24].

According to recently published data, this test possesses the highest sensitivity for detecting AKI at an early stage. The Astute140™ meter is a device based on a fluorescence labeling technique, which detects fluorescent signals from the immunoassay and calculates concentrations of IGFBP7 and TIMP-2 from the inserted cartridge. The device converts the measured signals into a single number, defining the relative risk of the patient developing AKI. The result, known as the AKIRisk score, is obtained within 20 min [25].

5. Approach

The first step in evaluating a patient with AKI in the ICU is to determine whether kidney hypo perfusion plays a role in the current state. Physical examination should focus on assessing for evidence of volume depletion, such as dry mucous membranes, decreased skin turgor, and absence of sweat in the axilla and inguinal regions. If necessary, a more complete assessment should be done before or at the ICU. Advance hemodynamic monitoring is reasonable in high-risk patients, particularly using dynamic measurements of cardiac function, or even a complete ultrasound and echocardiographic evaluation at the bedside [26].

Placement of a bladder catheter should be performed to exclude urethra obstruction as a cause of AKI, but primarily, to initiate real-time urinary flow monitoring. Urinary output express information of whether our actions and treatment result in the patients' improvement. Urinary sediment should be examined under the microscope to discard other causes of AKI, especially intrinsic causes. In the presence of proteinuria, a urinary sediment containing abundant cells or casts suggests an intrinsic cause of AKI rather than hypoperfusion as the primary mechanism. Precisely, the presence of renal tubular epithelial cells, epithelial cell casts, or pigmented (muddy brown) granular casts suggests the diagnosis of ATN and is associated with the increased risk for bad outcomes. A normal urine sediment suggests the presence of either a prerenal or postrenal pathophysiology of AKI, although obstructive uropathy may be associated with haematuria, pyuria, or crystalluria. The electrolyte composition of the urine may be helpful in differentiating between prerenal and ATN (i.e., fractional excretion of sodium), but not to guide the treatment [27, 28].

Imaging of the kidneys and bladder is required for the diagnosis of obstructive kidney disease and might provide information about the prehospital kidney function. Enlarged kidneys in a diabetic patient suggest that a previous damage was present, and GFR was diminished at baseline. This is especially helpful in a community-acquired AKI patient in whose previous renal function is unknown.

5.1. Clinical vs. subclinical AKI

The pitfalls of currently recommended diagnosis of AKI (i.e. creatinine and urinary flow) and the discovery of the above-mentioned new biomarkers have created new insights in AKI approach. The alteration of tubular and cellular arrest biomarkers, without creatinine elevation or a diminish of urinary flow, has led to the theory that at least some of the nephrons in the kidneys have suffered damage despite lack of azotemia (i.e. subclinical AKI). New classification for AKI has been proposed based on this. This new classification encompasses both clinical (i.e., with elevation in creatinine) and subclinical (i.e., alteration in biomarkers without creatinine elevation) AKI (**Figure 2**) [3, 23].

6. Treatment

The best treatment for AKI is acknowledging the existing risk factors and prevention. Diminish the time of hypo perfusion in every patient with AKI by a rapid recognition of cardiac output deficits, keeping an adequate intravascular effective volume and avoid nephrotoxic are keystones of prevention.

There is no specific management that accommodates the clear majority of patients with established AKI. Patients with prerenal AKI, as mentioned, should have intravascular volume deficits corrected and cardiac function optimized. Obstructive (postrenal) kidney disease is treated by mechanical relief of the obstruction. The primary management of acute interstitial

Type of AKI	Creatinine BUN	Urine Output	Biomarkers
Clinical AKI	↑	↓	↓
Subclinical AKI	↓	↑	↑

Figure 2. Clinical vs. subclinical AKI.

nephritis is discontinuation of the inciting agent; in patients with persistent AKI, there may be a role for treatment with glucocorticoids.

Once volume status and cardiac output have been optimized, if the patient remains oliguric, the use of a unique trial of diuretics to establish urine output can be considered. Although nonoliguric forms of ATN are associated with significantly lower risk of morbidity and mortality than oliguric forms, the primary rationale for a trial of diuretic therapy is to facilitate volume management not to improve AKI. None of the most common diuretics used in ICU worldwide increase the GFR. Positive fluid balance after development of AKI is associated with increased mortality rate, and avoiding fluid accumulation has a protective effect over mortality. The use of renal vasodilators, including dopamine, fenoldopam, and atrial natriuretic peptide, has not been shown to be beneficial in AKI, and its use should be discouraged [3].

AKI is associated with the development of sometimes serious electrolyte and acid-base disturbances, including hyperkalemia, hyponatremia, hyperphosphatemia, hypo- and (less commonly) hypercalcemia, hypermagnesemia, hyperuricemia, and metabolic acidosis. In addition, AKI is associated with anemia, bleeding diatheses, increased risk of infections, and dysfunction of other organ systems, including cardiovascular dysfunction, respiratory failure, gastrointestinal complications, and neurologic disturbances. These complications should be in mind of the treating physician in the ICU at every time [29, 30].

6.1. Renal replacement therapy

In patients with severe AKI, RRT is the cornerstone of supportive management. One objective of RRT includes allowing the removal of fluid and solutes that accumulate during renal failure. The available modalities of RRT comprise intermittent hemodialysis (IHD), the various forms of continuous renal replacement therapy (CRRT), and the hybrid modalities of prolonged intermittent RRT (PIRRT; also, extended duration dialysis [EDD] or sustained low-efficiency dialysis [SLED]) [31, 32].

Solute removal during RRT may occur by diffusion down a concentration gradient from the blood across a semipermeable membrane into dialysate or by convective transport of solute across the membrane during filtration. Fluid removal occurs by filtration, driven by either a hydrostatic or osmotic pressure gradient across the semipermeable membrane. In conventional IHD, the patient's blood passes through a semipermeable hemodialyzer counter current to the flow of dialysate on the other side of the membrane. The dialysis solution has a composition that approximates the normal electrolyte conformation of extracellular fluids and creates equilibrium to the blood, normalizing solutes. CRRT utilizes either diffusive hemodialysis, convective hemofiltration, or a combination of both. In addition to the duration of therapy, the major difference between intermittent and continuous hemodialysis is the dialysate flow rate. In intermittent hemodialysis, dialysate flow rates (typically 500–800 ml/min) are equal to or greater than blood flow rates, allowing rapid solute clearance. In continuous hemodialysis, the dialysate flow rate (typically 15–30 ml/min) is slow compared to that of the blood, permitting virtual equilibration of low-molecular-weight solutes such as urea between the blood and dialysate. Thus, solute clearance for low-molecular-weight solutes approximates the dialysate flow rate. Nonetheless, the total daily or weekly clearance is greater with continuous treatment, due to the extended time of therapy.

In continuous hemofiltration, a high filtration rate is generated, and physiologic replacement fluid is administered at an equal rate. Negative fluid balance (ultrafiltration) is accomplished by administering less milliliter per hour (usually 50–400 ml/h). Solute removal occurs exclusively by convection, and clearance is approximately equal to the ultrafiltration rate. The convective transport is limited primarily by the pore size of the membrane, so hemofiltration provides more efficient clearance of higher molecular weight (>500–15,000 KDa) solutes. Although it has been proposed that removal of higher molecular weight solutes with hemofiltration as compared to hemodialysis would be of clinical benefit, this has not been borne out in clinical trials. Because of their prolonged duration, the net ultrafiltration rate required to attain the same daily fluid removal is lower with CRRT than with IHD. Thus, CRRT is generally considered to cause less hemodynamic instability than conventional IHD [33].

Finally, PIRRT is a modification of conventional IHD, utilizing lower blood and dialysate flow rates while prolonging the treatment duration to 8–16 h.

There has been considerable debate regarding which modality is most appropriate for use in critically ill patients with AKI. Current data suggest that no individual modality of RRT provides either better patient survival or recovery of kidney function. These modalities should be complementary and must not be considered as mutually exclusive. According to the KDIGO guidelines, CRRT must be considered the first-line treatment in hemodynamically unstable patients and those with neurological illness whom require RRT and might be prone to develop cerebral edema [3].

Conventional indications for initiation of RRT include volume overload unresponsive to diuretic therapy, electrolyte and acid-base disturbances refractory to medical management, severe hyperkalemia, metabolic acidosis, overt uremia, characterized pericarditis, or encephalopathy. Most of the AKI patients in the ICU do not spent enough time in the hospital to express most of these indications. Initiating RRT in a patient with some of the conventional indications is unquestionable, although the use in other cases when the alterations do not endanger life immediately is uncertain. Studies have shown conflictive results when comparing the so-called early and late initiation strategies, with no clear benefit from one over the other. Even, there is no definition of either of them. Benefits of connecting a specific patient should be opposed to the risks of the same action, and each case should be individualized. Keep in mind, the potential harms of connecting too early include unnecessary exposure to the risks related to the catheter insertion, diminishing intravascular effective volume (especially in IHD), and resources utilization that increase costs. The unwanted adverse effect of taking too long in initiating might be death [34].

7. Outcomes

The mortality rate increases with AKI, independently associated to the underlying disease and baseline characteristics. Much higher mortality rates are associated with intrinsic forms of AKI over prerenal or postrenal disease. In severe septic-related AKI, short-term mortality rates approach 50–70% and have changed little over the past three decades. Factors associated to increased mortality risk include sepsis, male gender, advanced age, the use of RRT, degree of creatinine increase and coexistent nonrenal organ failure. For those patients who survive, AKI is associated with prolonged length of hospitalization and substantial health resource utilization [35].

More than half of patients who recover their renal function can be demonstrated to have subclinical kidney disease including modest decrements in GFR, diminished renal functional reserve, defects in tubular function and urinary concentration, and tubule-interstitial scarring on kidney biopsy [36].

8. Conclusions

AKI in hospitalized patients is a contributing factor for poor prognosis and outcomes. In critically ill patients, AKI etiologies differ, but the core one is the occurrence of renal hypo perfusion during shock states. Therefore, the best treatment of AKI is prevention. Additionally, hemodynamic optimization and diminishing offending factors are also crucial. Several modalities for RRT are available, and they should be considered complimentary. The ideal initiation timing depends on every patient's needs and benefits should be opposed to risk continuously during each patient's evolution.

Author details

Jose J. Zaragoza[1,2]* and Faustino J. Renteria[1]

*Address all correspondence to: zaragozagalvan@hotmail.com

1 Intensive Care Unit, Hospital Español, Mexico City, Mexico

2 Mexican College of Critical Care Medicine, Mexico City, Mexico

References

[1] Ostermann M, Joannidis M. Acute kidney injury 2016: Diagnosis and diagnostic workup. Critical Care 2016;**20**:299. DOI: 10.1186/s13054-016-1478-z

[2] Lameire N, Van Biesen W, Vanholder R. Acute renal failure. Lancet 2005;**365**:417-430. DOI: 10.1016/S0140-6736(05)17831-3

[3] Khwaja A. KDIGO clinical practice guidelines for acute kidney injury. Nephron Clinical Practice 2012;**120**:c179–c184. DOI: 10.1159/000339789

[4] Susantitaphong P, Cruz DN, Cerda J, Abulfaraj M, Alqahtani F, Koulouridis I, et al. World incidence of AKI: A meta-analysis. Clinical Journal of the American Society of Nephrology 2013;**8**:1482-1493. DOI: 10.2215/CJN.00710113.

[5] Hoste EAJ, Bagshaw SM, Bellomo R, Cely CM, Colman R, Cruz DN, et al. Epidemiology of acute kidney injury in critically ill patients: The multinational AKI-EPI study. Intensive Care Medicine 2015;**41**:1411-1423. DOI: 10.1007/s00134-015-3934-7

[6] Hsu C-N, Lee C-T, Su C-H, Wang Y-CL, Chen H-L, Chuang J-H, et al. Incidence, outcomes, and risk factors of community-acquired and hospital-acquired acute kidney injury. Medicine (Baltimore) 2016;**95**:e3674. DOI: 10.1097/MD.0000000000003674

[7] Nash K, Hafeez A, Hou S. Hospital-acquired renal insufficiency. American Journal of Kidney Diseases 2002;**39**:930-936. DOI: 10.1053/ajkd.2002.32766

[8] Doi K, Katagiri D, Negishi K, Hasegawa S, Hamasaki Y, Fujita T, et al. Mild elevation of urinary biomarkers in prerenal acute kidney injury. Kidney International 2012;**82**:1114-1120. DOI: 10.1038/ki.2012.266

[9] Endre ZH, Kellum JA, Di Somma S, Doi K, Goldstein SL, Koyner JL, et al. Differential diagnosis of AKI in clinical practice by functional and damage biomarkers: Workgroup Statements from the Tenth Acute Dialysis Quality Initiative Consensus Conference. Contributions to Nephrology 2013;**182**:30-44. DOI: 10.1159/000349964

[10] Thadhani R, Pascual M, Bonventre JV. Acute renal failure. The New England Journal of Medicine 1996;**334**:1448-1460. DOI: 10.1056/NEJM199605303342207

[11] Yared A, Kon V, Ichikawa I. Mechanism of preservation of glomerular perfusion and filtration during acute extracellular fluid volume depletion: Importance of intrarenal vasopressin-prostaglandin interaction for protecting kidneys from constrictor action of vasopressin. Journal of Clinical Investigation 1985;**75**:1477-1487. DOI: 10.1172/JCI111851

[12] Oliver JA, Sciacca RR, Cannon PJ. Renal vasodilation by converting enzyme inhibition: Role of renal prostaglandins. Hypertension 1983;**5**:166-171. DOI: 10.1161/01.HYP.5.2.166

[13] Uchino S, Kellum JA, Bellomo R, Doig GS, Morimatsu H, Morgera S, et al. Acute renal failure in critically ill patients: A multinational, multicenter study. Journal of the American Medical Association 2005;**294**:813-818. DOI: 10.1001/jama.294.7.813

[14] Alobaidi R, Basu RK, Goldstein SL, Bagshaw SM. Sepsis-associated acute kidney injury. Seminars in Nephrology 2015;**35**:2-11. DOI: 10.1016/j.semnephrol.2015.01.002

[15] Bellomo R, Wan L, Langenberg C, Ishikawa K, May CN. Septic acute kidney injury: The glomerular arterioles. Contributions to Nephrology., 2011;**174**:98-107. DOI: 10.1159/000329246

[16] Brenner M, Schaer GL, Mallory DL, Suffredini AF, Parrillo JE. Detection of renal blood flow abnormalities in septic and critically ill patients using a newly designed indwelling thermodilution renal vein catheter. Chest 1990;**98**:170-179

[17] Gomez H, Ince C, De Backer D, Pickkers P, Payen D, Hotchkiss J, et al. A unified theory of sepsis-induced acute kidney injury: Inflammation, microcirculatory dysfunction, bioenergetics, and the tubular cell adaptation to injury. Shock 2014;**41**:3-11. DOI: 10.1097/SHK.0000000000000052

[18] Heyman SN, Evans RG, Rosen S, Rosenberger C. Cellular adaptive changes in AKI: Mitigating renal hypoxic injury. Nephrology Dialysis Transplantation 2012;**27**:1721-1728. DOI: 10.1093/ndt/gfs100

[19] Liaño F, Junco E, Pascual J, Madero R, Verde E. The spectrum of acute renal failure in the intensive care unit compared with that seen in other settings. The Madrid Acute Renal Failure Study Group. Kidney International. 1998;**66**:S16-S24

[20] Thomas ME, Blaine C, Dawnay A, Devonald MAJ, Ftouh S, Laing C, et al. The definition of acute kidney injury and its use in practice. Kidney International. 2015;**87**:62-73. DOI: 10.1038/ki.2014.328

[21] Inker LA, Schmid CH, Tighiouart H, Eckfeldt JH, Feldman HI, Greene T, et al. Estimating glomerular filtration rate from serum creatinine and cystatin C. The New England Journal of Medicine 2012;**367**:20-29. DOI: 10.1056/NEJMoa1114248

[22] Han WK, Bailly V, Abichandani R, Thadhani R, Bonventre J V. Kidney Injury Molecule-1 (KIM-1): A novel biomarker for human renal proximal tubule injury. Kidney International. 2002;**62**:237-244. DOI: 10.1046/j.1523-1755.2002.00433.x

[23] Koyner JL, Vaidya VS, Bennett MR, Ma Q, Worcester E, Akhter SA, et al. Urinary biomarkers in the clinical prognosis and early detection of acute kidney injury. Clinical Journal of the American Society of Nephrology 2010;**5**:2154-2165. DOI: 10.2215/CJN.00740110

[24] Aregger F, Uehlinger DE, Witowski J, Brunisholz RA, Hunziker P, Frey FJ, et al. Identification of IGFBP-7 by urinary proteomics as a novel prognostic marker in early acute kidney injury. Kidney International. 2014;**85**:909-919. DOI: 10.1038/ki.2013.363

[25] Pajenda S, Ilhan-Mutlu A, Preusser M, Roka S, Druml W, Wagner L. NephroCheck data compared to serum creatinine in various clinical settings. BMC Nephrology 2015;**16**:206. DOI: 10.1186/s12882-015-0203-5

[26] McGee S, Abernethy WB, Simel DL. The rational clinical examination: Is this patient hypovolemic? Journal of the American Medical Association. 1999;**281**:1022-1029.

[27] Chawla LS, Dommu A, Berger A, Shih S, Patel SS. Urinary sediment cast scoring index for acute kidney injury: A pilot study. Nephron Clinical Practice. 2008;**110**:c145-c150. DOI: 10.1159/000166605

[28] Singer E, Elger A, Elitok S, Kettritz R, Nickolas TL, Barasch J, et al. Urinary neutrophil gelatinase-associated lipocalin distinguishes pre-renal from intrinsic renal failure and predicts outcomes. Kidney International. 2011;**80**:405-414. DOI: 10.1038/ki.2011.41

[29] Zaragoza JJ, Villa G, Garzotto F, Sharma A, Lorenzin A, Ribeiro L, et al. Initiation of renal replacement therapy in the intensive care unit in Vicenza (IRRIV) score. Blood Purification. 2015;**39**:246-257. DOI: 10.1159/000381009

[30] Wald R, Bagshaw SM. The timing of renal replacement therapy initiation in acute kidney injury: Is earlier truly better?. Critical Care Medicine. 2014;**42**:1933-1934. DOI: 10.1097/CCM.0000000000000432

[31] Ronco C, Cruz D, Bellomo R. Continuous renal replacement in critical illness. Contributions to Nephrology. 2007;**156**:309-319. DOI: 10.1159/0000102121

[32] Marshall MR, Golper TA, Shaver MJ, Alam MG, Chatoth DK. Sustained low-efficiency dialysis for critically ill patients requiring renal replacement therapy. Kidney International. 2001;**60**:777-785. DOI: 10.1046/j.1523-1755.2001.060002777.x

[33] Ronco C, Ricci Z, De Backer D, Kellum JA, Taccone FS, Joannidis M, et al. Renal replacement therapy in acute kidney injury: Controversy and consensus. Critical Care. 2015;**19**:146. DOI: 10.1186/s13054-015-0850-8

[34] Joannidis M, Forni LG. Clinical review: Timing of renal replacement therapy. Critical Care 2011;**15**:223. DOI: 10.1186/cc10109

[35] Manns B, Doig CJ, Lee H, Dean S, Tonelli M, Johnson D, et al. Cost of acute renal failure requiring dialysis in the intensive care unit: Clinical and resource implications of renal recovery. Critical Care Medicine 2003;**31**:449-455. DOI: 10.1097/01.CCM.0000045182.90302.B3

[36] Lewers DT, Mathew TH, Maher JF, Schreiner GE. Long-term follow-up of renal function and histology after acute tubular necrosis. Annals of Internal Medicine. 1970;**73**:523. DOI: 10.7326/0003-4819-73-4-523

7

Sepsis in Children

Selim Öncel

Abstract

Sepsis is systemic inflammatory response syndrome due to a documented or suspected infection. Causative agents of sepsis include group B streptococcus, *Escherichia coli*, and *Listeria monocytogenes* in infants younger than 2 months, and community-acquired organisms. Bacteremia may ensue in patients whose defense mechanisms have become vulnerable due to many factors. Sepsis and septic shock can be viewed as clinical pictures, which develop as consequences of proinflammatory processes/cytokines leading to a state that cannot be restrained by anti-inflammatory processes/cytokines. As yet, a cytokine, which is uniquely associated with severe sepsis and septic shock and can be used as a biomarker, has not been discovered. Sepsis is a cytokine storm, which may adversely affect almost any organ system. Whether there is an association between the severity of sepsis or septic shock and cytokine gene polymorphisms is an important field of study. Mottled skin and prolongation of capillary refill time may help the physician recognize septic shock before hypotension emerges. The management of severe sepsis and septic shock involves (1) the hemodynamic support, (2) inotropes, vasopressors, and vasodilators, (3) antimicrobial therapy, (4) transfusions, and (5) corticosteroids as indicated. Hospital mortality of pediatric sepsis is 2–10%.

Keywords: sepsis, pediatrics, cytokines, sepsis-associated encephalopathy, systemic inflammatory response syndrome, neonatal sepsis

1. Introduction

Although sepsis can affect any individual at any time during her/his lifetime, it is more apt to occur and be destructive at the extremes of life, the very old and the very young.

It is sometimes referred to as "blood poisoning" in anglophone countries and in various manners elsewhere (e.g., "microbe in blood" in Turkey). The sepsis is the body's deadly response to infection. Once sets in, sepsis can progress to septic shock and death if left untreated. One-third of people who develop sepsis die worldwide. These deaths occur more frequently in economically developing countries [1].

This chapter deals with pediatric sepsis with much greater emphasis on beyond neonatal period.

2. Definitions

Systemic inflammatory response syndrome (SIRS) is defined as two or more of the following items, one of which has to be the one marked with an asterisk (*) [2]:

1. Body core temperature of higher than 38.5°C or lower than 36°C*.
2. Except leukopenia caused by chemotherapy, a leukocyte count exceeding or lower than normal limit for age or immature leukocyte count above 10% of total leukocyte count*.
3. Abnormal heart rate:
   (a) In children 1 year of age and over
   - Average heart rate in excess of two standard deviations from the age normal in the absence of external stimuli, long-term drug use, or painful stimuli
   - Persistent elevation in heart rate in 24 h without any other explanation

   (b) In children less than 1 year of age
   - Average heart rate below 10th percentile for age in the absence of external vagal stimulus, beta-blocker, or congenital heart disease
   - Persistent depression in heart rate in half an hour without any other explanation
4. Average respiratory rate of more than two standard deviations above normal for mechanical ventilation that is being carried out for an acute process irrelevant of general anesthesia or an underlying neuromuscular disease.

Sepsis is SIRS due to a documented or suspected infection [2–5].

Organ dysfunction definitions are explained below:

1. If at least one of the following items is present despite isotonic intravenous fluid bolus (≥40 mL/kg in 1 h), this is called **cardiovascular dysfunction** [2]:
   (a) Criteria for drop in blood pressure:

- Blood pressure is below fifth percentile for age OR.
- Systolic blood pressure below two standard deviations of normal for age.

(b) Vasoactive drugs required for maintaining normal blood pressure (5 μg/kg/min dopamine or dobutamine of any dosage, epinephrine, or norepinephrine).

(c) Presence of more than two of the following items:

- Unexplained metabolic acidosis with a base deficit of more than 5 mmol/L.
- Arterial lactate concentration of more than two times the upper limit.
- Urine output of less than 0.5 mL/kg/h.
- Capillary refill time of more than 5 s.
- The difference between core and peripheral temperature of more than 3°C.

2. If at least one of the following items is present, this is called **respiratory dysfunction** [2]:

   (a) Arterial oxygen partial pressure (PaO_2)/inspired oxygen fraction (FiO_2) ratio of less than 300 in the absence of pulmonary disease or cyanotic heart disease.

   (b) Initial measurement of arterial carbon dioxide partial pressure ($PaCO_2$) above 65 Torr or 20 mmHg.

   (c) Proven requirement for maintaining the saturation at or above 92% or FiO_2 of more than 50%.

   (d) Nonelective invasive or noninvasive mechanical ventilation requirement.

3. If at least one of the following items is present, this is called **neurological dysfunction** [2]:

   (a) Glasgow Coma Score of 11 or less.

   (b) Acute change in mental status together with a drop of Glasgow Coma Score of three or more points from abnormal baseline value.

4. If at least one of the following items is present, the situation is called **hematological dysfunction** [2]:

   (a) International normalized ratio (INR) above 2.

   (b) Platelet count below 80,000/μL or has decreased 50% from the highest value recorded in the last 3 days (for chronic hematology-oncology patients).

5. **Renal dysfunction** is serum creatinine concentration of two times the upper limit for normal or more or twofold increase in baseline serum creatinine [2].

6. The presence of at least two of the following items is called **liver dysfunction** [2]:

   (a) Alanine transaminase (ALT) concentration of two times the upper limit for age.

   (b) Total bilirubin concentration of 4 mg/dL or more (not applicable for newborns).

For establishing the diagnosis of **acute respiratory distress syndrome (ARDS)**, the following criteria should be met [2]:

- PaO_2/FiO_2 ratio <200 mmHg.
- Bilateral infiltrates on chest X-ray.
- Acute onset.
- No sign of left heart failure present.

If, in addition to sepsis, there is cardiovascular organ dysfunction, ARDS, or two or more other organ dysfunctions, this situation is called **severe sepsis** [2].

3. Causative agents

Sepsis may be a consequence of infections due to bacteria, viruses, fungi, or parasites. Causative agents of sepsis include group B streptococcus, *Escherichia coli, Listeria monocytogenes* in infants younger than 2 months of age, and community-acquired organisms like *S. pneumoniae* and *Neisseria meningitidis* in children of 1–2 years. In a Canadian study of 6-year duration, the most common pathogens in bloodstream infections of childhood were *S. pneumoniae, Staphylococcus aureus,* and *E. coli* [6].

4. Pathophysiology

The site of infection, as the cause of sepsis, varies according to age. In infants, it is usually primary bacteremia. There is respiratory tract infection in nearly half of older children with sepsis [7].

Since sepsis is defined as SIRS, or in other words, pathological changes in body temperature, heart, or respiratory rates, and leukocyte count in the presence of proven or suspected infection, it would be prudent that we review the pathogeneses of the components of SIRS and infection that form sepsis and changes due to organ dysfunction in severe sepsis separately [2, 8].

4.1. Formation of infection

One of the most important clinical situations causing sepsis and septic shock is bacteremia. Bacteria must pass through the dermal or mucosal barrier in order that bacteremia takes place.

The pathogenesis of bacteremia is closely associated with the self-defense of the host and the characteristics of the bacteria. Organisms like *S. pneumoniae*, *N. meningitidis* and *Haemophilus influenzae* type b, which form a part of nasopharyngeal flora, cause bacteremia by overcoming mucosal defense systems with the aid of facilitating factors like upper respiratory infections. *N. meningitidis* is taken into the cylindrical epithelial cell with phagocytosis. After traversing the cytoplasm in the phagosome, it passes into subepithelial tissues. *H. influenzae* type b passes into subepithelial tissues by clinging to the epithelial cell and loosing the intercellular tight junctions making its way toward pharyngeal capillaries. *S. pneumoniae* attaches to specific receptors by means of which it enters the cell. The number of platelet-activating factor receptors located on surfaces of respiratory epithelial cells increases during viral infections. These receptors serve as attachment sites for pneumococci. Gram-negative organisms that are a part of gut flora also attach to specific receptors. Pili and adhesins on the microorganism surface play a pivotal role in this attachment. Pili were also shown to be important in the pathogenesis of sepsis caused by *Streptococcus pyogenes*, Group B streptococcus, and *S. pneumoniae* [9].

Bacteremia may ensue in patients whose defense mechanisms have become vulnerable due to many factors. The examples are as follows:

- With the intubation of an intensive care patient, protease activity increases whereas cell-bound fibronectin diminishes rendering cell surface receptors "sheathless," which make them ideal binding sites for predominantly Gram-negative bacteria of gut flora [9].
- Viridans streptococci, elements of oral flora, may cause bacteremia in neutropenic children who have severe oral mucositis and receiving antineoplastic chemotherapy.
- Gram-negative gut bacteria cause bacteremia by traversing the gut mucosa (translocation), whose integrity has been disrupted by antineoplastic drugs.
- Staphylococci, thanks to their ability to adhere to hard surfaces, cause catheter-related bacteremia by colonizing in catheter lumina.

4.2. The process of cytokine synthesis

The word "cytokine" is made up of two Greek words, "cyto-" (cell) and kinos (movement). The cytokine concept was introduced to scientific world by Barry Bloom and John David, who, being unaware of each other's similar research, discovered a cytokine, known as macrophage migration inhibitor factor today. Although cytokines were once classified as lymphokines, interleukins, and chemokines, according to their functions, and target and release sites, such a classification is avoided due to the abundance and substitution characteristics of cytokines [10].

Every cytokine has a corresponding cell surface receptor, with the stimulation of which begin signaling cascades, as a consequence of which some genes are upregulated or downregulated. In the end, either other cytokines or cell receptors for various molecules are synthesized, or the rate of synthesis of these substances decreases [10].

Sepsis and septic shock can be viewed as clinical pictures, which develop as consequences of pro-inflammatory processes/cytokines leading to a state that cannot be restrained by anti-inflammatory processes/cytokines (**Table 1**). The human body responds in a pathological manner to infection, which is a pathological situation itself. The occurrence of sepsis or immune compromise depends on whether systemic inflammatory response or its opposite end, compensatory anti-inflammatory response syndrome, predominates the inner environment as a response to infection. Compensatory anti-inflammatory response syndrome is a clinical entity, which progresses primarily with T-helper depression due to catecholamine discharge and apoptosis of splenic B-lymphocytes [11].

When the causative organism enters the body, nonspecific (innate) immune system is stimulated. Mammals perceive the pathogen by means of pattern-recognition receptors, the most important and evolutionally the oldest of which are Toll-like receptors (TLRs), found in insects, plants, and mammals. TLRs are transmembrane proteins, so-called because of their similarity to a product protein of the gene Toll, which is named after the remark ("Das ist ja toll!" ("That's really cool!")) by Nobel Prize in Physiology or Medicine winner (1995) Christina Nüsslein-Volhard, who has reportedly shouted out as so in surprise when she realized a *Drosophila melanogaster* (common fruit fly) had assumed an amazing appearance as a result of

Proinflammatory	Anti-inflammatory
TNF-α	IL-1Ra
IL1b, IL-2, IL-6, IL-8, IL-15	IL-4
Neutrophil elastase	IL-10
IFN-γ	IL-13
Thromboxane	Type II IL-1 receptor
Platelet-activating factor	Transforming growth factor-b
Vasoactive neuropeptides	Adrenaline
Phospholipase A_2	Soluble TNF-α receptors
Plasminogen activator inhibitor-1	Leukotriene B4-receptor antagonist
Prostaglandins	
Prostacyclin	
Free radicals	
Soluble adhesion molecules	
Tyrosine kinase	
Protein kinase	
H_2S	
NO	
High mobility group box 1 protein	

TNF: tumor necrosis factor, IL: interleukin, IFN: interferon.

Table 1. Major proinflammatory and anti-inflammatory mediators [12].

polymorphism of one of its proteins [13]. Transmembrane proteins have their extracellular, transmembrane, and intracellular parts. Humans have at least 10 different TLRs [14]. TLRs are found in abundance on leukocytes, macrophages, and some kinds of endothelial cells [11]. It is noteworthy that some TLRs are found on cytoplasmic membrane and some on the membrane of endocytic vesicules. These receptors recognize many organisms, from bacteria to fungi, and from protozoa to viruses. Although a part of nonspecific immune system, TLRs vary with respect to the patterns concerning the component of the organism they recognize. For instance, whereas TLR4 is unique in recognizing lipopolysaccharide of Gram-negative bacteria, mannan of *Candida albicans*, and glucuronoxylomannan of *Cryptococcus neoformans*, glycosylphosphatidylinositol moieties of *Plasmodium falciparum* are recognized by either TLR4 or TLR2. Hemozoin of *P. falciparum* is exclusively recognized by TLR9 [15].

Stimulated TLRs cause many protein kinases to be phosphorilized, in other words, become active. Reactions of these highly complex biochemical pathways take place in cytosol or endosome. Some of the biochemical pathways are dependent on a mediator molecule named MyD88, and some are not. For example, proinflammatory cytokines in sepsis and septic shock are released in a MyD88-dependent pathway. The end products of these pathways (nuclear factor kappa B ($NF_{\kappa}B$), interferon regulatory factor 3 (IRF3)) traverse the nuclear membrane and induce related genes by adhering to promotor regions of deoxyribonucleic acid (DNA). $Nf_{\kappa}B$ activity is inhibited by the most-studied heat-shock protein HSP70, which, thus, diminishes the inflammatory response. HSP70 reduces the damage caused by excessive inflammation by decreasing apoptosis and preserving cell proteins [16].

Significant information has been obtained with the study of inflammatory processes, especially those induced by Gram-negative bacteria. Septic shock occurs via similar mechanisms with Gram-positive organisms. Here, instead of lipopolysaccharide, which is found in abundance in Gram-negative organisms, less potent cell wall molecules, such as peptidoglycan and teicoic acid, cause similar inflammatory responses.

Gram-negative bacteria have a thin cell wall made up of a single layer of peptidoglycan, out of which there is a cell membrane consisting of lipopolysaccharide, which is a strong stimulator of immune response. The lipopolysaccharide molecule has three main components [17]:

1. **Lipid A** is responsible for the biological activity of endotoxin. Its structure is almost the same in different strains.
2. **Core polysaccharide** is made up of oligosaccharides, but its structure is highly diverse among species, even within strains.
3. **Oligosaccharide side chains** vary among strains. It consists of repeating units (e.g., 40 repetitions in O antigen) and is the moiety which provides the O antigen its antigenic specificity.

Lipopolysaccharide first binds to lipopolysaccharide-binding protein (LBP) in plasma. LBP-lipopolysaccharide complex binds to CD14 molecule on the plasma membrane. This new complex binds to TRL4/MD ("myeloid differentiating factor")-2, which is also on the plasma membrane [18]. This structure, activating various protein kinases, as outlined above, causes cytokine release when the end products bind to promotor regions on DNA [19].

There are countless cytokines playing roles in sepsis and septic shock. These mediators, causing release of each other, create an enormous mediator cascade. The mediator cascade is initiated by the stimulation of tumor necrosis factor (TNF) (cachectin) production by stimulators like lipopolysaccharide, C5a, viruses, and enterotoxins. TNF appears to be the main cytokine initiating and playing a pivotal role in the progression of the mediator cascade. TNF, released from many cells, such as monocytes, macrophages, natural killer cells, microglial cells, and hepatic Kupfer cells, causes countless mediators (e.g., interleukin(IL)-1β, IL-6, eicosanoids, platelet activation factor) to spill into blood in an uncontrolled manner resulting in a very severe inflammatory response and endothelial damage. However, there are many cytokines, the productions of which do not necessitate the presence of TNF [20]. As a consequence of this process, typical signs of endotoxic shock will show up. Some of the cytokines released (e.g., TNF-α, IL-1, and IL-6) cause free oxygen radical and protease release from other immune system cells, such as neutrophils, prostanoids leukotrienes, thromboxanes, nitric oxide, and endothelin from endothelial cells. Some of these substances are useful in killing bacteria but some (e.g., nitric oxide) are known to cause mitochondrial dysfunction by deactivating the catecholamines in the circulation. Mediators, whose release is induced by lipopolysaccharide, increase nitric oxide synthase II production and thus nitric oxide (endothelial-origin relaxation factor) production. Nitric oxide is a potent vasodilator and is the primary substance responsible for the hypotension in septic shock. Besides, nitric oxide causes vasodilation, which in turn causes diminished perfusion pressure in capillary network and blood flow by opening collateral channels. Decreased capillary flow results in organ hypoxia despite high blood flow because of vasodilation.

We have enough knowledge on how sepsis and septic shock develop, but it is surprising that only a few histopathologic changes concerning cell death are present in patients who have died of severe sepsis. Apart from cellular apoptosis in spleen and intestines, myopathic changes in skeletal muscle, and changes in vascular morphology in meningococcal sepsis, there is no serious sign of necrosis in main organs.

Then, studies have concentrated on microcirculation and mitochondrial dysfunction, and theories on how adenosine triphosphate (ATP) production can decrease under normal, even supranormal oxygen partial pressures, have been put forward. These theories include diminished pyruvate entry into tricarboxylic acid cycle, activation of poly-(ADP-ribose) polymerase, and uncoupling of oxidation from phosphorylation. Another cause of tissue hypoxia is nitric oxide's combining with free oxygen radicals (O_2^-) to form peroxynitrite ($ONOO^-$) resulting in reversible or irreversible binding of these three substances to proteins in the electron transport chain, such as succinate dehydrogenase and cytochrome c oxidase. As a result, ATP production decreases, being unable to meet the needs of the energy-consuming cell, and cell death takes place. This process accounts for the unexpectedly few histopathologic changes in autopsies. Complement system is activated through contact with bacterial molecules or binding of proteins, such as antibody or mannose-binding lectin, to these molecules. Complements like C3b and C5a cause migration of leukocytes and increase inflammation [11].

The balance between thrombogenesis and thrombolysis has been disrupted in sepsis. There is endothelial damage due to direct effect of microorganisms, cytokines, and fibrin deposition triggered by endothelial dysfunction. As a result of this, a process of simultaneous thromboses and bleedings, which is known as consumption coagulopathy or disseminated intravascular coagulation (DIC), develops. DIC is more frequently encountered in Gram-negative sepsis (e.g., meningococcal sepsis) than in Gram-positive sepsis. The most common complications of DIC are thromboses of great vessels, liver infarction, acute renal failure, cerebral hemorrhage, and cerebral infarction [21].

4.3. Cytokines as sepsis biomarkers

TNF, IL-1b, and IL-6 are the first cytokines to regulate the initial response of the innate immune system. TNF and IL-1b activate endothelial cells and attract the granulocytes in circulation to inflammation site. TNF and IL-1b cause fever and other systemic signs by entering the circulation. IL-6 increases the production of what is known as acute phase proteins (e.g., C-reactive protein) in liver and more granulocytes in bone marrow. As can easily be seen, TNF, IL-1b, and IL-6 are responsible for the formation of SIRS and could be thought of being used as sepsis biomarkers [22].

TNF and IL-1b concentrations increase in endotoxin-associated Gram-negative sepsis. TNF or IL-1b administration to laboratory animals is as effective in the formation of septic shock as the endotoxin itself, but in clinical studies, TNF and IL-1b could not be used as sepsis biomarkers because

- TNF concentrations before anti-TNF antibody treatment do not affect the outcome.
- IL-1b does not rise as TNF does.

Of the three cytokines mentioned above, IL-6 has attracted the most attention. The causes of this include

- The role of IL-1b, IL-1a, and the receptor antagonist of IL-1 in the development of sepsis is debated [22].
- The relatively higher reliability of measurement of the plasma concentration of IL-6.
- The usability of IL-6 in the diagnosis and treatment of autoimmune rheumatologic diseases.
- The availability of commercial immunoassay kits, contrary to TNF and IL-1b.

Nevertheless exactly as in TNF and IL-1b, IL-6 is not specific to sepsis and its role as sepsis biomarker is prognostic, rather than diagnostic. In many studies, rise in IL-6 concentration is associated with higher mortality. This characteristic can be used to detect patients who may benefit from therapy [22].

Since the clinical signs of sepsis in neonates are very subtle and nonspecific, predictive biomarkers are needed, particularly in economically developing countries, where the incidence, morbidity, and mortality of early neonatal sepsis (ENS) (sepsis diagnosed less than 72 h after birth) are particularly high. Evidence published to date is still far from convincing the physician to use procalcitonin as a biomarker for routine use in clinical practice as a risk stratifier and a prognostic predictor or even to guide the duration of antibiotic treatment and bedside decision making [23]. The results of a new study by He et al. indicate that elevated IL-27 strongly correlates with ENS and may provide additional diagnostic value along with procalcitonin [24].

The usage of IL-6 and LBP in pediatrics is also promising. In newborns with late sepsis risk, IL-6 rises 48 h before bacterial sepsis becomes clinically manifest [25]. Initial high IL-6 concentrations predict future septic shock in hospitalized children [26]. Initial high IL-6 concentrations foretell high risk of septic shock and mortality in pediatric burn patients [27]. LBP points to invasive bacterial infections and bacterial infections in children and newborns over 28 weeks of gestational age, respectively [28–30]. LBP can differentiate between SIRS and ENS in newborns within the first 48 h of their lives [30].

While homing chemokines serve to regulate adaptive immune system, especially in secondary lymphoid tissue, proinflammatory chemokines attract granulocytes and monocytes to the site of inflammation and promote their extravasation. Chemokines, thanks to these properties, can be used as biomarkers in sepsis, and some of them have been shown to be superior to IL-6 in that aspect. Examples are IL-8 (in the diagnosis of sepsis) and monocyte chemoattractant protein (MCP)-1 (in the determination of sepsis mortality) [31]. According to the results of a study, among 17 cytokines (IL-1β, IL-2, IL-4, IL-5, IL-6, IL-7, IL-8, IL-10, IL-12, IL-13, IL-17, interferon-γ, granulocyte colony-stimulating factor, granulocyte-macrophage colony-stimulating factor, MCP-1, macrophage inflammatory protein-1, and TNF-α), the cytokines most closely associated with organ dysfunction within 24 h are IL-8 and MCP-1 [31]. As yet, a cytokine which is uniquely associated with severe sepsis and septic shock and can be used as a biomarker has not been discovered [32].

4.4. Effect of cytokine storm on tissues and organs

- Cardiovascular system

  Myocardium is depressed in septic shock. The reason for this depression is not hypoperfusion, but depressing cytokines like TNF and IL-1β in the circulation. Ventricules dilate and ejection fraction drops. As a result, hypoperfusion ensues in peripheral tissues. Peripheral hypoperfusion and hypoxia lead to overproduction of lactic acid, which is another myocardial depressor. This chain of events persists as a vicious cycle [21].

- Respiratory system

  Alveoli are diffusely damaged because of circulating endotoxins. In the exudative phase of this damage, proteinaceous edema fluid accumulates in alveoli, and type I epithelial cells are injured. In this clinical picture, which is also known as shock lung, alveolar collapse, hemorrhage, edema, hyaline membrane formation, which is made up of fibrin and necrotic epithelial cells on epithelial surfaces of respiratory bronchioles and alveolar ducti, and neutrophil accumulation in alveolar capillaries occur. Unless treated, severe pulmonary edema develops despite low central venous pressure, and as a result, ventilation-perfusion mismatch ensues. This clinical picture is called ARDS. In the regeneration phase, healing occurs via return to normal structure or pulmonary fibrosis. Lost type 1 cells are replaced by proliferating type 2 cells. Superimposing infections and barotrauma due to mechanical ventilation worsen respiratory system functions [21].

- Kidneys

  Nitric oxide disrupts blood distribution in renal medulla and cortex. With the effect of nitric oxide and cytokines, renal tubule function, which requires high energy input, deteriorates due to decreasing ATP production. As a consequence of hypotension, increase in the release of endothelin, which is a vasopressor hormone, and activation of renin-angiotensin-aldosterone system pave the way to sodium and water retention, which makes a ground for renal failure. Neutrophil adhesion and microthrombi further diminish the glomerular filtration rate. The question of why renal failure in sepsis, despite anuria and despite its presence even in patients who die of sepsis, can develop without acute tubular necrosis and why it takes renal function so long (months) to return to normal while systemic inflammation has already disappeared and circulatory function has returned to normal still stands as an enigma and awaits to be elucidated [11, 21].

- Central and peripheral nervous system

  The most important one among the effects of sepsis on central nervous system is sepsis-related encephalopathy and critical illness polyneuropathy. The causes of encephalopathy include disruption of blood-brain barrier, coagulopathy-related cerebral hemorrhage, microinfarctions, hypoxic-ischemic encephalopathy, metastatic brain abscesses, meningitis, and cytokine storm. While this clinical entity, which manifest itself with delirium and confusion, is often reversible, it may lead to self-mutilism of the patient in intensive care and development of cognitive and behavioral dysfunction in the long term.

  The diagnosis of this clinical picture, which manifests itself also with flaccid paralysis and loss of deep tendon reflexes, is usually made only during or after separation of the patient from ventilator due to encephalopathy, administration of neuromuscular drugs, and the unfavorable general situation of the patient. Prognosis varies according to the severity of illness and patient's age. Muscle weakness may last for months [21].

- Gastrointestinal system

  Gastrointestinal system is negatively affected by sepsis due to hypoperfusion. Gastrointestinal bleeding may ensue as a consequence of splanchnic hypoperfusion, increase in intestinal permeability, bacterial translocation, stress ulcers, and coagulopathy.

  Although liver is relatively resistant to sepsis, transaminase elevation, peribiliary infarctions, and cholestatic jaundice may ensue as a result of hypotension [21].

- Immune system

  Although an immunologic hyperreaction itself, sepsis further disrupts the integrity of the immune system. In survivors of sepsis, mortality rate is higher in the following several years than that in normal population, which can be attributed to a vague immune disorder with cytokines and chemokines [21, 33]. Overproduction of anti-inflammatory cytokines may be a cause of immune deficiency in sepsis, but there is no evidence that the abundance of anti-inflammatory cytokines (such as IL-1 receptor antagonist and soluble TNF receptors) in the environment is sufficient for putting away the effects of proinflammatory cytokines [20].

- Extremities

  A clinical picture of skin bleeding and necrosis due to microvascular thrombi and subsequent perivascular hemorrhage may develop, especially in the presence of disseminated intravascular coagulation. This is called purpura fulminans (PF). Although most frequently encountered in *N. meningitidis* bacteremia, PF may ensue in bloodstream infections due to *S. pneumoniae* and capsulated microorganisms of any kind. In addition to necroses in PF, vasoconstriction in sepsis may be severe enough to cause infarctions of fingers and autoamputation. Vasopressor drugs, if administered without fluid resuscitation, increase the risk for this complication [21, 33].

- Mental status

  Psychological disorders, such as posttraumatic stress disorder (in 20% of ARDS patients), depression, panic attack, public isolation, inability to stay alone or in crowded areas, and decrease in sexual activity, are seen frequently in survivors of sepsis [21].

4.5. The role of gene polymorphisms in predisposition to sepsis

Whether there is an association between the severity of sepsis and septic shock and cytokine gene polymorphisms is an important field of study. Such a connection could not be shown with IL-1, IL-1 receptor antagonist, and IL-10 genes. It has been postulated that TNF2, being a rare TNF gene (adenine at −308 position), may be associated with high promoter activity, but no elevation in the prevalence of TNF2 allele in patients having frequent attacks of severe sepsis and infections due to Gram-negative organisms has been noted. There is a publication stating that rare Arg753Gln mutation of TLR2 renders individuals prone to staphylococcal sepsis [33]. Single-nucleotide polymorphism in IL-1β gene was found associated with higher mortality [34].

5. Medical history

In sepsis, complaints leading to the child being brought to the physician vary according to the source of infection or SIRS. Fever, hypothermia tachypnea, stomach ache, vomiting, diarrhea, clouding of consciousness, or several of these may be present in the child. Features in the history such as the child's immunization status, past infections, and attending daycare should be taken into notice [35].

6. Physical examination

Fever or hypothermia (core body temperature <36°C) may be observed [5]. Abnormalities in other vital signs may also be detected. Normal limits of vital signs according to age are depicted in **Table 2** [36].

Shock may not be present in sepsis. Hypotension is not a prerequisite for shock. Mottled skin and prolongation of capillary refill time may help the physician recognize septic shock before hypotension emerges [2, 5].

Age group	Bradycardia (pulse/min)	Tachycardia (pulse/min)	Respiratory rate (respirations/min)	Systolic blood pressure (mmHg)
0 day to 1 week	<100	<180	>50	<65
1 week to 1 month	<100	<180	>40	<75
1 month to 1 year	<90	<180	>34	<100
2–5 years	<80	<140	>22	<94
6–12 years	<70	<130	>18	<105
13–18 years	<60	<110	>14	<117

Table 2. Normal of vital signs according to age [36].

7. Laboratory tests

In a child suspected of having sepsis, the following tests may be ordered: complete blood count (always with differentials), a reasonable metabolic panel (electrolytes, glucose, liver function tests, and albumin), serum lactate, arterial blood gases, coagulation studies, amylase, lipase, urinalysis, sputum culture, and Gram stain [35]. Leukocytosis or leukopenia may be present in children with sepsis (**Table 3**) [2].

Antibiotics should be started after blood and other cultures being drawn unless a delay of longer than 45 min is expected because of this process. According to the results of a recent study, the diagnosis of pediatric septicemia through BACTEC 9240 is quicker with high yield and great sensitivity compared to the conventional technique [37]. Blood cultures are recommended to be taken from a peripheral vein and a catheter, which has been in place for more than 48 h into a set of aerobic and anaerobic bottles and as at least two sets. In case the volume of the blood is insufficient, the sensitivity of the blood culture will decrease, and vice versa [38, 39]. The author suggests that anaerobic blood cultures not be taken from children routinely, since

- The volume of blood that can be taken from children is limited.
- True anaerobic blood stream infections are rare (<5%) in children.
- Instead of sets consisting of one aerobic and one anaerobic bottle, selective culture for anaerobic organisms with two aerobic bottles yields better results (6% more positives).

- Since sensitivity patterns of anaerobes are well known, they can be covered effectively with empirical therapy.

Age group	Leukocyte count (×10³/μL)
0–7 days	>34
1 week to 1 month	>19.5 or <5
1 month to 1 year	>17.5 or <5
2–5 years	>15.5 or <6
6–12 years	>13.5 or <4.5
12–18 years	>11 or <4.5

Table 3. Leukocyte counts according to age [2].

Even if anaerobic blood cultures are to be drawn, the indications should be limited to risky situations as below [40–42]:

- Children displaying abnormal abdominal symptoms and signs.
- Children with sacral decubitus ulcers or cellulitis.
- Patients with poor oral hygiene, severe oral mucositis, or chronic sinusitis.
- Neutropenic children receiving high-dose corticosteroid therapy, which may mask abdominal symptoms.
- Children with sickle cell disease.
- Infants of mothers with prolonged rupture of membranes or chorioamnionitis.
- Children thought to have bacteremia due to a human bite or crushing trauma.

When clinically indicated, cultures may be taken from urine, cerebrospinal fluid, wounds, respiratory secretions, and other body fluids. Most accurate results will probably be obtained with double quantitative blood cultures in case of an intravascular device-related bloodstream infection. Mannan, antimannan, and 1,3 beta-D-glucan tests may be used if invasive candidiasis is suspected. Imaging techniques are very useful to delineate the foci of infection and to decide whether the patient's condition is suitable for transport [5].

8. Diagnosis and differential diagnosis

Risk-scoring systems may guide the physician in deciding the presence of a serious bacterial infection [43]. As mentioned above, if a probable or proven infection is present with SIRS, the child is in sepsis. Sepsis should be differentiated from other causes of SIRS (e.g., trauma, burn, acute pancreatitis, drug reaction (acetaminophen, cytarabine, IL-2)) and hypotension (e.g., hypovolemic shock, cardiogenic shock, neurogenic shock, and adrenocortical insufficiency) [4, 44–46]. The value of procalcitonin and other biomarkers in the differential diagnosis of sepsis is under investigation [5].

9. Management

The management of severe sepsis and septic shock involves the following phases:

9.1. Hemodynamic support

Hemodynamic support should be started promptly without waiting for the intensive care admission. A protocol on recognizing septic shock in emergency ward may shorten the time that is passed for the initiation of appropriate therapy [47]. Although central venous line is preferred, fluids may be given through peripheral veins or via intraosseous route if a central venous catheter is not present or cannot be placed [5, 48]. Initial recommended fluid is crystalloid (e.g., normal saline) in boli of 20 mL/kg, each administered in 5–10 min. It should be kept in mind that mortality in children may be reduced if albumin is used in the initial fluid [49]. These crystalloids or colloid boli are continued until the perfusion returns to normal and the total given fluid volume reaches 60 mL/kg or more unless hepatomegaly or rales develop [48]. It is imperative that fluid resuscitation be given as rapidly as possible and not sparingly. The mortality in children who were given a total of more than 40 mL/kg is about 40% lower than those given a total of less than 20 mL/kg. The duration of intensive care and hospital stay become shorter (2–3 days) in patients given 60 mL/kg of fluid in the first 60 min than those who are not [50–52]. Inotropic support is recommended instead of fluid replacement if hepatomegaly or crackles are present. If the child has severe hemolytic anemia and blood pressure is normal, blood transfusion should be preferred to crystalloid or albumin boli [5].

For children in respiratory distress or hypoxia, oxygen should be administered with a mask; thereafter, if needed and if possible, high-flow oxygen through nasal cannula or nasopharyngeal continuous positive air pressure (CPAP) may be carried out [5, 48]. An adequate cardiovascular resuscitation reduces the likelihood of cardiovascular instability if mechanical ventilation is needed [5].

In the early management (in the first hour and in emergency ward), clinical goals for the septic shock patient are the following:

- Bring the capillary refill time back to 2 s or less.
- Provide blood pressure normal for age.
- Obtain a normal pulse and heart rate by removing the difference between central and peripheral pulses.
- Warm the extremities.
- Raise the urine output above 1 mL/kg/h.

- Restore hypoglycemia and hypocalcemia back to normal.
- Restore mental status.

Antibiotics should have been started meanwhile [5, 48, 53].

Goals to be realized by invasive monitorization of the patient are as follows:

- Central venous oxygen saturation of 70% or above and
- Cardiac index of 3.3–6 L/min/m^2 [5, 54]

9.2. Inotropes, vasopressors, and vasodilators

The patients whose initial fluid therapy has been completed in 10–15 min and who are unresponsive to this therapy (twice crystalloid or colloid boli) should have been started inotrope support at about 15th min of management through a peripheral vein if necessary until central venous route is assured [5, 55]. The goals at this stage of the management are as follows [5]:

- Normal perfusion pressure (mean arterial pressure, central venous pressure): 55 mmHg for term newborns, 60 mmHg for children 1 month to 1 year of age, 65 mmHg for children aged 1–15 years.
- Central venous oxygen saturation ($ScvO_2$) = 70%.
- Cardiac index = 3.3–6 L/min/m^2.

In cold shock with normal blood pressure but abnormal capillary refill time (>2 s), the dosage of dopamine given through central vein can be increased to 10 μg/kg/min. If shock is refractory to dopamine, epinephrine (0.05–3 μg/kg/min) should be given; $ScvO_2$ and hemoglobin (Hb) should be kept above 70% and 10 g/dL, respectively. If $ScvO_2$ persists below 70%, a vasodilator, such as milrinone and imrinone, should be added to therapy; levosimendan should be considered to be started [5, 48].

In cold shock with low blood pressure, $ScvO_2$ and Hb should be kept above 70% and 10 g/dL, respectively. If shock is refractory to dopamine, epinephrine (0.05–3 μg/kg/min) should be given; if hypotension persists, norepinephrine should be started. If $ScvO_2$ is still below 70%, dobutamine, milrinone, enoksimone, or levosimendan should be considered [5, 48].

In warm shock with low blood pressure, the rate of norepinephrine should be adjusted such that $ScvO_2$ stays above 70%. If hypotension persists, vasopressin, terlipressin, or angiotensin should be considered. If $ScvO_2$ is still below 70%, low-dose epinephrine should be considered [5, 48].

In some patients, in whom systemic vascular resistance is very low despite norepinephrine administration, vasopressin, and terlipressin were used, but no benefit from these drugs has been shown in randomized studies [56–60]. In patients with low cardiac output, but high systemic vascular resistance, vasodilators such as

- Calcium sensitizer (levosimendan).
- Type III phosphodiesterase inhibitors (amrinone, enoximone, or milrinone).

- Nitrovasodilators.
- Prostacyclin.
- Fenoldopam.
- Pentoxifylline.

have been proposed in addition to inotropes [5].

If no response is taken with this therapy, the case is accepted as catecholamine-resistant shock, and the patient should be started hydrocortisone if at risk for absolute adrenal insufficiency [5, 48].

If catecholamine-resistant shock persists, pneumothorax, pericardial effusion, and high intraabdominal pressure should be excluded or corrected if present; pulmonary artery catheter, pulse contour cardiac output catheter, and femoral artery thermodilution catheter should be used or Doppler ultrasonography should be considered to receive some guidance on therapy [48].

If, despite all these measures, shock cannot be taken under control, extracorporeal membrane oxygenation (ECMO) should be considered [5, 61, 62].

9.3. Antimicrobial therapy

After severe sepsis is recognized, antibiotics should be started in the first hour, even in the first 15 min if possible. Cultures should be taken before initializing therapy if feasible, but therapy should not be delayed for this reason. The choice of antibiotic should be in accordance with endemic or epidemic data. Intramuscular or oral route may be used until intravenous access is made. In toxic shock syndromes with refractory hypotension, clindamycin and antitoxin are recommended. The management of *Clostridium difficile* colitis is preferentially carried out with enteral antibiotics; vancomycin should be used for severe colitis. Antimicrobial therapy should continually be reevaluated with regard to deescalation [5].

Combination empirical therapy is recommended for neutropenic patients with severe sepsis and in places where difficult-to-treat organisms, such as Acinetobacter and Pseudomonas, are prevalent. This therapy should be in the form of a wide-spectrum beta-lactam antibiotic + an aminoglycoside/quinolone in places where the risk of infection due to Pseudomonas is high. If the prevalence of *S. pneumoniae* is high, a beta-lactam + macrolide combination is recommended. Combination therapy should be of short duration (3–5 days or less) according to antibiotic-sensitivity results [5].

The duration of antimicrobial therapy should be limited to 7–10 days unless

- The response is slow,
- The infection focus is undrainable,
- *S. aureus* bacteremia is present,
- Some fungus or virus infections are present,

- An immunologic disorder with neutropenia is present, or
- Pneumonia due to *Pseudomonas spp.* or other Gram-negative rods is present [5, 63].

Narrowing the antimicrobial spectrum and shortening the duration of antimicrobial therapy would prevent superinfections due to other agents, such as *Candida* spp., *C. difficile*, and vancomycin-resistant *Enterococcus faecium* [5].

Antiviral therapy should be started in sepsis or septic shock due to viruses. Antimicrobial therapy should be stopped in case that the cause of sepsis was detected as something other than infection. The removal of infected intravascular devices, especially central venous catheters, if possible and if preferred to antibiotic lock methods, will reduce mortality and increase the chances that the infection will be cured [5, 64].

9.4. Transfusions

If superior vena cava oxygen saturation is low (<70%), Hb concentration should be maintained at 10 g/dL. After hypoxemia and shock subside, the goal for Hb should be over 7 g/dL. Higher concentrations may be needed if acute bleeding, severe hypoxemia, or ischemic heart disease is present [5, 65, 66].

Platelet transfusion is indicated if the platelet count is

- Below 10,000/μL without a detectable bleeding.
- Below 20,000/μL if the patient has significant bleeding risk.
- Below 50,000/μL in the presence of active bleeding or in situations requiring either surgical or invasive procedures.

Plasma therapy should be brought to the agenda in case of thrombotic purpura situations, such as progressive disseminated intravascular coagulation due to sepsis, secondary thrombotic microangiopathy, and thrombotic thrombocytopenic purpura. In the absence of planned invasive intervention or bleeding, antithrombin therapy, erythropoietin administration for sepsis-associated anemia, and fresh-frozen plasma therapy should be avoided.

9.5. Corticosteroids

Hydrocortisone should be given to children with severe sepsis only in the presence of suspected or proven adrenal insufficiency, because there are publications both favoring (for reduction in mortality) and discouraging (for increasing mortality) its use [5, 67, 68]. Risk factors for adrenal insufficiency include severe septic shock with purpura, steroid use for chronic illness, and hypophysis or adrenal gland abnormalities. Hydrocortisone infusion is started with the dosage of 50 mg/m^2/24, which may be needed to be increased up to 50 mg/kg/day in a short time. The measurement of baseline serum cortisol concentration may be useful at the onset of therapy [5].

9.6. Miscellaneous recommendations

In ARDS, tidal volumes exceeding 10 mL/kg should be avoided. Plateau pressure, arterial pH, and arterial partial oxygen pressure should be maintained at 30 cmH_2O or below, between 7.3–7.45 and 60–80 Torr (8–10.7 kPa), respectively. The Hb goal of 10 g/dL in unstable patients should be taken as 7 g/dL after recovery from shock and deep hypoxia [69].

Water retention in patients recovering from shock should be treated with diuretics. If this fails, continuous venovenous hemofiltration or intermittent dialysis should be carried out in order to prevent water retention of more than 10% of the body weight [5].

In children with septic shock, glucose concentration should be maintained below 180 mg/dL since concentrations of 178 mg/dL and over are associated with higher mortality. In newborns and children, insulin therapy should be given along with glucose infusion, the rate of which should be 4–6 mg/kg/min (6–8 mg/kg/min in newborns). The alternative is giving maintenance fluids prepared with 10% dextrose in water [5, 70].

Although no sedative or sedation protocol is recommended for patients with sepsis and mechanical ventilation support, long-term propofol should be avoided in children below 3 years for its association with fatal metabolic acidosis. Etodomidate and dexmedetomidine should also be avoided due to its inhibitory effect on adrenal axis and sympathetic nervous system, the integrity of which is essential for hemodynamic stability in septic shock [5].

Enteral route should be preferred to parenteral route in nutrition. Glucose requirements of newborns and children can be met with sodium-containing fluids prepared with 10% dextrose in water and administered at maintenance rate.

10. Prognosis

Hospital mortality of pediatric sepsis is 2–10% [5]. In United States, hospital mortality in severe sepsis has declined from 10% in 1995 to 4% in 2003 [71, 72]; this is probably because septic shock is increasingly recognized more readily and earlier in the course and treated more aggressively [73].

Seven and six percent of children who are discharged from hospital after surviving postneonatal sepsis die within 28 days and afterward, respectively (early and late mortality). About half of those who survive these 28 days are rehospitalized at least once. Comorbidity is important in the development and late mortality of and rehospitalization in pediatric sepsis [74, 75].

11. Conclusion

As sepsis in children continues to take lives of children, especially in economically developing countries, it will continue to be the focus of attention for physicians, scientists, and the public. Although there are a few newer antibiotics in the pipeline, other novel therapies hold promise for overcoming this "cytokine storm disease" in near future.

Author details

Selim Öncel

Address all correspondence to: selimOncel@doctor.com

Division of Pediatric Infectious Diseases, Department of Pediatrics and Child Health, Section of Internal Medical Sciences, Kocaeli University Faculty of Medicine, Kocaeli, Turkey

References

[1] Sepsis Alliance. Sepsis and Children [Internet]. 2017. Available from: http://www.sepsis.org/sepsis-and/children/[Accessed: 2017-02-05].

[2] Goldstein B, Giroir B, Randolph A, International Consensus Conference on Pediatric Sepsis. International pediatric sepsis consensus conference: definitions for sepsis and organ dysfunction in pediatrics. Pediatr Crit Care Med. 2005;**6**:2-8. DOI: 10.1097/01.PCC.0000149131.72248.E6

[3] Lever A, Mackenzie I. Sepsis: definition, epidemiology, and diagnosis. BMJ. 2007;**335**:879-883. DOI: 10.1136/bmj.39346.495880.AE

[4] Martin GS. Sepsis, severe sepsis and septic shock: changes in incidence, pathogens and outcomes. Expert Rev Anti Infect Ther. 2012;**10**:701-6. DOI: 10.1586/eri.12.50

[5] Dellinger RP, Levy MM, Rhodes A, Annane D, Gerlach H, Opal SM, et al. Surviving Sepsis Campaign: international guidelines for management of severe sepsis and septic shock, 2012. Intensive Care Med. 2013;**39**:165-228. DOI: 10.1007/s00134-012-2769-8

[6] Laupland KB, Gregson DB, Vanderkooi OG, Ross T, Kellner JD. The changing burden of pediatric bloodstream infections in Calgary, Canada, 2000-2006. Pediatr Infect Dis J. 2009;**28**:114-117. DOI: 10.1097/INF.0b013e318187ad5a

[7] Watson RS, Carcillo J. Scope and epidemiology of pediatric sepsis. Pediatr Crit Care Med. 2005;6(3 Suppl):S3-5. DOI: 0.1097/01.PCC.0000161289.22464.C3

[8] Tibby S, Nadel S, Paolo, Arenas-Lopez S, Ewald U, Härtel C, et al. Report on the expert meeting on neonatal and paediatric sepsis. European Medicines Agency [Internet]. 2010.

Available from: http://www.ema.europa.eu/docs/en_GB/document_library/Report/2010/12/WC500100199.pdf [Accessed: 2017-02-05]

[9] Kaplan SL, Vallejo JG. Bacteremia and septic shock. In: Feigin RD, Cherry JD, Demmler-Harrison GJ, Kaplan SL, editors. Feigin & Cherry's Textbook of Pediatric Infectious Diseases. 6th ed. Philadelphia: Saunders Elsevier; 2009. p. 837-851.

[10] Wikipedia contributors. Cytokine. Wikipedia, The Free Encyclopedia [Internet]. 2013. Available from: http://en.wikipedia.org/wiki/Cytokine [Accessed: 2017-02-05]

[11] Mitchell E, Whitehouse T. The pathophysiology of sepsis. In: Daniels R, Nutbeam T, editors. ABC of Sepsis. 1st ed. West Sussex: Blackwell Publishing Ltd; 2010. p. 20-24.

[12] Ramnath RD, Weing S, He M, Sun J, Zhang H, Manmish Singh B, et al. Inflammatory mediators in sepsis: Cytokines, chemokines, adhesion molecules and gases. J Org Dysfunct. 2006;**2**:80-92. DOI: 10.1080/17471060500435662

[13] O'Neill LAJ, Brint E, editors. Toll-like Receptors in Inflammation. 1st ed. Basel: Birkhäuser Verlag; 2005.

[14] Takeda K, Yamamoto M, Honda K. Assessing the response of cells to TLR stimulation. In: Konat GW, editor. Signaling by Toll-like Receptors. 1st ed. Boca Raton: CRC Press; 2008. p. 1-22.

[15] Uematsu S, Akira S. Toll-like receptors (TLRs) and their ligands. In: Bauer S, Hartmann G, editörler. Toll-Like Receptors (TLRs) and Innate Immunity. 1st ed. Heidelberg: Springer-Verlag; 2008. p. 1-20.

[16] Bromberg Z, Weiss YG, Deutschman CS. Heat shock proteins in inflammation. In: Abraham E, Singer M, editors. Mechanisms of Sepsis-Induced Organ Dysfunction and Recovery. 1st ed. Heidelberg: Springer-Verlag Berlin Heidelberg; 2007. p. 113-121.

[17] Silipo A, Molinaro A. The diversity of the core oligosaccharide in lipopolysaccharides. In: Wang X, Quinn PJ, editörler. Endotoxins: Structure, Function and Recognition. 1st ed. Dordrecht: Springer; 2010. p. 69-99.

[18] Gangloff M, Gay NJ. MD-2: the Toll "gatekeeper" in endotoxin signalling. Trends Biochem. Sci. 2004;**29**:294-300. DOI: 10.1016/j.tibs.2004.04.008

[19] Hoebe K, Beutler B. TLRs as bacterial sensors. In: O'Neill LAJ, Brint E, editors. Toll-like Receptors in Inflammation. 1st ed. Basel: Birkhäuser Verlag; 2005. p. 1-17.

[20] Cavaillon J-M, Adib-Conquy M, Fitting C, Adrie C, Payen D. Cytokine cascade in sepsis. Scand J Infect Dis. 2003;**35**:535-544. DOI: 10.1080/00365540310015935

[21] Cilliers H, Whitehouse T, Tunnicliffe B. Serious complications of sepsis. In: Daniels R, Nutbeam T, editors. ABC of Sepsis. 1st ed. West Sussex: Blackwell Publishing Ltd; 2010. p. 15-19.

[22] Faix JD. Biomarkers of sepsis. Crit Rev Clin Lab Sci. 2013;**50**:23-36. DOI: 10.3109/10408363.2013.764490

[23] Lanziotti VS, Póvoa P, Soares M, Silva JR, Barbosa AP, Salluh JI. Use of biomarkers in pediatric sepsis: literature review. Rev Bras Ter Intensiva. 2016;**28**:472-482. DOI: 10.5935/0103-507X.20160080

[24] He Y, Du WX, Jiang HY, Ai Q, Feng J, Liu Z, Yu JL. Multiplex cytokine profiling identifies interleukin-27 as a novel biomarker for neonatal early onset sepsis. Shock. 2017;**47**:140-147. DOI: 10.1097/SHK.0000000000000753

[25] Küster H, Weiss M, Willeitner AE, Detlefsen S, Jeremias I, Zbojan J, et al. Interleukin-1 receptor antagonist and interleukin-6 for early diagnosis of neonatal sepsis 2 days before clinical manifestation. Lancet. 1998;**352**:1271-1277. DOI: 10.1016/S0140-6736(98)08148-3

[26] Fioretto JR, Martin JG, Kurokawa CS, Carpi MF, Bonatto RC, Ricchetti SMQ, et al. Interleukin-6 and procalcitonin in children with sepsis and septic shock. Cytokine. 2008;**43**:160-164. DOI: 10.1016/j.cyto.2008.05.005

[27] Finnerty CC, Herndon DN, Chinkes DL, Jeschke MG. Serum cytokine differences in severely burned children with and without sepsis. Shock. 2007;**27**:4-9. DOI: 10.1097/01.shk.0000235138.20775.36

[28] Behrendt D, Dembinski J, Heep A, Bartmann P. Lipopolysaccharide binding protein in preterm infants. Arch Dis Child Fetal Neonatal Ed. 2004;**89**:F551-554. DOI: 10.1136/adc.2003.030049

[29] Ubenauf KM, Krueger M, Henneke P, Berner R. Lipopolysaccharide binding protein is a potential marker for invasive bacterial infections in children. Pediatr Infect Dis J. 2007;**26**:159-162. DOI: 10.1097/01.inf.0000253064.88722.6d

[30] Pavcnik-Arnol M, Hojker S, Derganc M. Lipopolysaccharide-binding protein in critically ill neonates and children with suspected infection: comparison with procalcitonin, interleukin-6, and C-reactive protein. Intensive Care Med. 2004;**30**:1454-1460. DOI: 10.1007/s00134-004-2307-4

[31] Bozza FA, Salluh JI, Japiassu AM, Soares M, Assis EF, Gomes RN, et al. Cytokine profiles as markers of disease severity in sepsis: a multiplex analysis. Crit Care. 2007;**11**:R49. DOI: 10.1186/cc5783

[32] Lvovschi V, Arnaud L, Parizot C, Freund Y, Juillien G, Ghillani-Dalbin P, et al. Cytokine profiles in sepsis have limited relevance for stratifying patients in the emergency department: a prospective observational study. PLoS One. 2011;**6**:e28870. DOI: 10.1371/journal.pone.0028870

[33] Munford RS, Suffredini AF. Sepsis, severe sepsis, and septic shock. In: Mandell GL, Bennett JE, Dolin R, editors. Mandell, Douglas, and Bennett's Principles and Practice of Infectious Diseases. Philadelphia: Churchill Livingstone Elsevier; 2010. p. 987-1010.

[34] Stüber F. Cytokine gene polymorphism and host susceptibility to infection. In: Kotb M, Calandra T, editors. Cytokines and Chemokines in Infectious Diseases Handbook. 1st ed. Totowa: Humana Press Inc.; 2003. p. 23-30.

[35] DynaMed Editorial Team. Sepsis in children [Internet]. DynaMed [database online]. 2017 [updated: 2013 Jan 26; cited: 2017 Feb 05]. Available from: http://www.ebscohost.com/dynamed

[36] Fleming S, Thompson M, Stevens R, Heneghan C, Plüddemann A, Maconochie I, et al. Normal ranges of heart rate and respiratory rate in children from birth to 18 years of age: a systematic review of observational studies. Lancet. 2011;**377**:1011-1018. DOI: 10.1016/S0140-6736(10)62226-X

[37] Ahmad A, Iram S, Hussain S, Yusuf NW. Diagnosis of paediatric sepsis by automated blood culture system and conventional blood culture. J Pak Med Assoc. 2017;**67**:192-195. PMID: 28138169

[38] Connell TG, Rele M, Cowley D, Buttery JP, Curtis N. How reliable is a negative blood culture result? Volume of blood submitted for culture in routine practice in a children's hospital. Pediatrics. 2007;**119**:891-896. DOI: 10.1542/peds.2006-0440

[39] Isaacman DJ, Karasic RB, Reynolds EA, Kost SI. Effect of number of blood cultures and volume of blood on detection of bacteremia in children. J Pediatr. 1996;**128**:190-195. PMID: 8636810

[40] Morris AJ, ilson ML, Mirrett S, Reller LB. Rationale for selective use of anaerobic blood cultures. J Clin Microbiol. 1993;**31**:2110-2113. PMCID: PMC265706

[41] Zaidi AK, Knaut AL, Mirrett S, Reller LB. Value of routine anaerobic blood cultures for pediatric patients. J Pediatr. 1995;**127**:263-268. PMID: 7636652

[42] Shoji K, Komuro H, Watanabe Y, Miyairi I. The utility of anaerobic blood culture in detecting facultative anaerobic bacteremia in children. Diagn Microbiol Infect Dis. 2013;**76**:409-412. DOI: 10.1016/j.diagmicrobio.2013.05.003

[43] Brent AJ, Lakhanpaul M, Thompson M, Collier J, Ray S, Ninis N, et al. Risk score to stratify children with suspected serious bacterial infection: observational cohort study. Arch Dis Child. 2011;**96**:361-367. DOI: 10.1136/adc.2010.183111

[44] Craig DGN, Reid TWDJ, Martin KG, Davidson JS, Hayes PC, Simpson KJ. The systemic inflammatory response syndrome and sequential organ failure assessment scores are effective triage markers following paracetamol (acetaminophen) overdose. Aliment Pharmacol Ther. 2011;**34**:219-228. DOI: 10.1111/j.1365-2036.2011.04687.x

[45] Ek T, Jarfelt M, Mellander L, Abrahamsson J. Proinflammatory cytokines mediate the systemic inflammatory response associated with high-dose cytarabine treatment in children. Med Pediatr Oncol. 2001;**37**:459-464. PMID: 11745875

[46] Schwartzentruber DJ. Guidelines for the safe administration of high-dose interleukin-2. J. Immunother. 2001;**24**:287-293. PMID: 11565830

[47] Cruz AT, Perry AM, Williams EA, Graf JM, Wuestner ER, Patel B. Implementation of goal-directed therapy for children with suspected sepsis in the emergency department. Pediatrics. 2011;**127**:e758-766. DOI: 10.1542/peds.2010-2895

[48] Brierley J, Carcillo JA, Choong K, Cornell T, Decaen A, Deymann A, et al. Clinical practice parameters for hemodynamic support of pediatric and neonatal septic shock: 2007 update from the American College of Critical Care Medicine. Crit Care Med. 2009;**37**:666-688. DOI: 10.1097/CCM.0b013e31819323c6

[49] Delaney AP, Dan A, McCaffrey J, Finfer S. The role of albumin as a resuscitation fluid for patients with sepsis: a systematic review and meta-analysis. Crit Care Med. 2011;**39**:386-391. DOI: 10.1097/CCM.0b013e3181ffe217

[50] Oliveira CF, Nogueira de Sá FR, Oliveira DSF, Gottschald AFC, Moura JDG, Shibata ARO, et al. Time- and fluid-sensitive resuscitation for hemodynamic support of children in septic shock: barriers to the implementation of the American College of Critical Care Medicine/Pediatric Advanced Life Support Guidelines in a pediatric intensive care unit in a developing world. Pediatr Emerg Care. 2008;**24**:810-815. DOI: 10.1097/PEC.0b013e31818e9f3a

[51] Paul R, Neuman MI, Monuteaux MC, Melendez E. Adherence to PALS sepsis guidelines and hospital length of stay. Pediatrics. 2012;**130**:e273-280. DOI: 10.1542/peds.2012-0094

[52] Carcillo JA, Davis AL, Zaritsky A. Role of early fluid resuscitation in pediatric septic shock. JAMA. 1991;**266**:1242-1245. PMID: 1870250

[53] Raimer PL, Han YY, Weber MS, Annich GM, Custer JR. A normal capillary refill time of ≤ 2 seconds is associated with superior vena cava oxygen saturations of ≥70%. J Pediatr. 2011;**158**:968-972. DOI: 10.1016/j.jpeds.2010.11.062

[54] De Oliveira CF, de Oliveira DSF, Gottschald AFC, Moura JDG, Costa GA, Ventura AC, et al. ACCM/PALS haemodynamic support guidelines for paediatric septic shock: an outcomes comparison with and without monitoring central venous oxygen saturation. Intensive Care Med. 2008;**34**:1065-1075. DOI: 10.1007/s00134-008-1085-9

[55] Ceneviva G, Paschall JA, Maffei F, Carcillo JA. Hemodynamic support in fluid-refractory pediatric septic shock. Pediatrics. 1998;**102**:e19. PMID: 9685464

[56] Polito A, Parisini E, Ricci Z, Picardo S, Annane D. Vasopressin for treatment of vasodilatory shock: an ESICM systematic review and meta-analysis. Intensive Care Med. 2012;**38**:9-19. DOI: 10.1007/s00134-011-2407-x

[57] Choong K, Bohn D, Fraser DD, Gaboury I, Hutchison JS, Joffe AR, et al. Vasopressin in pediatric vasodilatory shock: a multicenter randomized controlled trial. Am J Respir Crit Care Med. 2009;**180**:632-639. DOI: 10.1164/rccm.200902-0221OC

[58] Rodríguez-Núñez A, López-Herce J, Gil-Antón J, Hernández A, Rey C, RETSPED Working Group of the Spanish Society of Pediatric Intensive Care. Rescue treatment with terlipressin in children with refractory septic shock: a clinical study. Crit Care. 2006;**10**:R20. DOI: 10.1186/cc3984

[59] Lindsay CA, Barton P, Lawless S, Kitchen L, Zorka A, Garcia J, et al. Pharmacokinetics and pharmacodynamics of milrinone lactate in pediatric patients with septic shock. J Pediatr. 1998;**132**:329-334. PMID: 9506650

[60] Irazuzta JE, Pretzlaff RK, Rowin ME. Amrinone in pediatric refractory septic shock: an open-label pharmacodynamic study. Pediatr Crit Care Med. 2001;**2**:24-28. PMID: 12797884

[61] MacLaren G, Butt W, Best D, Donath S. Central extracorporeal membrane oxygenation for refractory pediatric septic shock. Pediatr Crit Care Med. 2011;**12**:133-136. DOI: 10.1097/PCC.0b013e3181e2a4a1

[62] Skinner SC, Iocono JA, Ballard HO, Turner MD, Ward AN, Davenport DL, et al. Improved survival in venovenous vs venoarterial extracorporeal membrane oxygenation for pediatric noncardiac sepsis patients: a study of the Extracorporeal Life Support Organization registry. J Pediatr Surg. 2012;**47**:63-67. DOI: 10.1016/j.jpedsurg.2011.10.018

[63] Chastre J, Wolff M, Fagon J-Y, Chevret S, Thomas F, Wermert D, et al. Comparison of 8 vs 15 days of antibiotic therapy for ventilator-associated pneumonia in adults: a randomized trial. JAMA. 2003;**290**:2588-2598. DOI: 10.1001/jama.290.19.2588

[64] Millar M, Zhou W, Skinner R, Pizer B, Hennessy E, Wilks M, et al. Accuracy of bacterial DNA testing for central venous catheter-associated bloodstream infection in children with cancer. Health Technol Assess. 2011;**15**:1-114. DOI: 10.3310/hta15070

[65] Lacroix J, Hébert PC, Hutchison JS, Hume HA, Tucci M, Ducruet T, et al. Transfusion strategies for patients in pediatric intensive care units. N Engl J Med. 2007;**356**:1609-1619. DOI: 10.1056/NEJMoa066240

[66] Karam O, Tucci M, Ducruet T, Hume HA, Lacroix J, Gauvin F, et al. Red blood cell transfusion thresholds in pediatric patients with sepsis. Pediatr Crit Care Med. 2011;**12**:512-518. DOI: 10.1097/PCC.0b013e3181fe344b

[67] Zimmerman JJ, Williams MD. Adjunctive corticosteroid therapy in pediatric severe sepsis: observations from the RESOLVE study. Pediatr Crit Care Med. 2011;**12**:2-8. DOI: 10.1097/PCC.0b013e3181d903f6

[68] Markovitz BP, Goodman DM, Watson RS, Bertoch D, Zimmerman J. A retrospective cohort study of prognostic factors associated with outcome in pediatric severe sepsis: what is the role of steroids? Pediatr Crit Care Med. 2005;**6**:270-274. DOI: 10.1097/01.PCC.0000160596.31238.72

[69] Randolph AG. Management of acute lung injury and acute respiratory distress syndrome in children. Crit Care Med. 2009;**37**:2448-2454. DOI: 10.1097/CCM.0b013e3181aee5dd

[70] Branco RG, Garcia PCR, Piva JP, Casartelli CH, Seibel V, Tasker RC. Glucose level and risk of mortality in pediatric septic shock. Pediatr Crit Care Med. 2005;**6**:470-472. DOI: 10.1097/01.PCC.0000161284.96739.3A

[71] Odetola FO, Gebremariam A, Freed GL. Patient and hospital correlates of clinical outcomes and resource utilization in severe pediatric sepsis. Pediatrics. 2007;**119**:487-494. DOI: 10.1542/peds.2006-2353

[72] Watson RS, Carcillo JA, Linde-Zwirble WT, Clermont G, Lidicker J, Angus DC. The epidemiology of severe sepsis in children in the United States. Am J Respir Crit Care Med. 2003;**167**:695-701. DOI: 10.1164/rccm.200207-682OC

[73] Han YY, Carcillo JA, Dragotta MA, Bills DM, Watson RS, Westerman ME, et al. Early reversal of pediatric-neonatal septic shock by community physicians is associated with improved outcome. Pediatrics. 2003;**112**:793-799. PMID: 14523168

[74] Czaja AS, Zimmerman JJ, Nathens AB. Readmission and late mortality after pediatric severe sepsis. Pediatrics. 2009;**123**:849-857. DOI: 10.1542/peds.2008-0856

[75] Van de Voorde P, Emerson B, Gomez B, Willems J, Yildizdas D, Iglowstein I, et al. Paediatric community-acquired septic shock: results from the REPEM network study. Eur J Pediatr. 2013;**172**:667-674. DOI: 10.1007/s00431-013-1930-x

8

Airway Management in ICU Settings

Nabil Abdelhamid Shallik, Mamdouh Almustafa,

Ahmed Zaghw and Abbas Moustafa

Abstract

Maintenance of patent airway, adequate ventilation, and pulmonary gas exchange is very important in critically ill patients. Airway management in intensive care patients differs significantly from routine surgical procedures in the operating room. The airway competence in intensive care unit (ICU) should be coping with the rapidly evolving advances in airway management. Therefore, efforts should be focused on the three pillars of airway master: airway providers as intensivists or critical care physicians, equipment, and operational plans. Not all institutions can afford all airway equipment in the market; however, they should make sure that critical care providers have a full access to the available tools and they are comfortable using it. Educational sessions and refresher courses should be tailored to meet the competence level of the ICU providers and equipment availability. Operational plan includes developing institutional airway protocols and implementing difficult airway guidelines. The protocols should consider different staffing models of ICU and make sure all the time at least one member of the team with the highest experience in airway should be always available. The aim of writing this chapter is to enable the intensivist to optimize their use of airway equipment and managing high-risk patients in ICU.

Keywords: tracheal intubation, videolaryngoscopy (VL), flexible fiberoptic intubation, bronchoscopy, percutaneous tracheostomy, extubation in ICU, high-flow nasal cannula (HFNC), virtual endoscopy (VE), airway ultrasound, supra-glottic airway devices, tube exchange

1. Tracheal intubation in ICU

1.1. Introduction

Tracheal intubation (TI) is one of daily practiced procedures in the intensive care unit (ICU), especially when the patient has respiratory failure or cardiovascular collapse. It involves highly skilled techniques that require much of training, practice, and expertise. The excellence in airway management in ICU is necessary for intensivist's every day practice, which when it is lacking does not only compromise the quality of care but also has a potential impact on patient safety.

The optimal intubation condition prevailing in surgical theaters differs a lot in nature than harsh and chaotic scenarios in ICU. The nature of those situations has three factors: the highly skilled anesthesiologists versus the intensivists; the compensated, well-controlled surgical patient versus the decompensated sick ICU patients; and equipment availability. That is why in ICU settings, the airway instrumentation-related complications have higher incidence than anesthesia settings. Among the contributory factors for high failure rates are the highly stressful environment, limited expertise level of the providers with different techniques of airway management, the physiological baseline for the patients, inadequate pre-oxygenation, unfamiliarity with new airway equipment, and the critical time factor in distressed situations in addition to the negative hemodynamic effects for the intubation medications.

2. Challenges in airway management in the critically ill patients

2.1. Response to pre-oxygenation

Effective pre-oxygenation is the first step for airway management. If it is done optimally by reaching PEO_2 of >90%, it extends the apnea safety time margin for critical ICU patients with already limited oxygen transport and when the intubation for airway control would be time consuming. The apnea time for oxy-hemoglobin to desaturate below 85% in postoperative period is 23 s in critically ill patients compared to 502 s in healthy adults [1].

The standard pre-oxygenation used in optimized surgical patients would fail to sustain adequate PaO_2 in critically ill patients with hyper-metabolic profile during apneic period for intubation.

The airway management encountered in a rapidly deteriorating patient with hypoxia from a life-threatening cardiopulmonary failure is not an uncommon daily ICU scenario. Lack of airway expertise is a high risk for multiple intubation attempts, airway trauma, esophageal intubation, and intubation failure, and consequences were adverse with high percentage of cardiac arrest or brain damage. Moreover, multiple traumatic trials by inexperienced provider could easily convert a simple airway to a difficult one due to airway edema.

2.2. Assessment and evaluation of the airway

Airway evaluation prior to tracheal intubation (TI) is the standard of care in anesthesia settings and should be routinely practiced in ICU before any TI. Many studies about airway evaluation in controlled anesthesia settings showed that combined airway tests are better than each test alone in terms of sensitivity and reliability.

Airway tests include Mallampati classification, thyromental distance, neck mobility, inter-incisor distance, and body mass index (BMI), which are all reliable predictors for difficult airway. Other scores include El Ganzouri test and LEMON test. El Ganzouri test is a numerical score, involves all the abovementioned tests: Mallampati classification, thyromental distance, neck mobility, inter-incisor distance, and BMI plus under-bite and previous difficult intubation history. LEMON test involves **L**ook **E**xternally, **M**allampati class, **O**bstruction, and **N**eck mobility.

2.3. Drugs used for tracheal intubation, rapid sequence intubation

Hemodynamic changes during TI are predictable physiological consequences after airway management, which are attributed to three main factors: sympathetic system, cardiac contractility, and mechanical ventilation. Vaso-dilatory and cardio-depressive effects of medications, preexisting hypovolemia, and positive-pressure ventilation are major contributors to any predictable hemodynamic changes. Ketamine and Etomidate are anesthetic agents with a fast onset, short half-life, and tolerable hemodynamic changes. They are widely used in emergency settings to improve intubation conditions. Etomidate is an anesthetic agent with adrenal inhibition effect. A cardio-stable agent as Ketamine is preferable in ICU. The critical illness of ICU patients compromises the gastric emptying, making a rapid sequence intubation (RSI) a wise decision. Succinylcholine is a fast acting muscle relaxant with ultra short duration that is commonly used in emergency setting when there are no contraindications to its use. Muscle relaxants have its role in facilitating intubation; however, encountering cannot-ventilate-cannot-intubate (CVCI) scenario after giving muscle relaxants could lead to a fatal airway emergency. Studies found that physicians other than anesthesiologists are reluctant to use muscle relaxants before intubation in the ICU. A large data set found fewer complications, including in patients with difficult airways when muscle relaxants were used. In a prospective multicenter study, Jaber showed that tracheal intubation by muscle relaxants has less complications by 22 versus 37% when muscle relaxants were not used [2]. In another study in emergency department, Li et al. found a significant decrease in esophageal intubation with the use of muscle relaxants (3 vs. 18%) [3]. Succinylcholine should not be used in patients with hyperkalemia, congenital muscle disorders, and burn patients with difficult airway as it could lead to hyperkalemic cardiac arrest. As alternative to Succinylcholine, Rocuronium Bromide (1 mg/kg) can be used for rapid sequence intubation in critical care patients and can be reversed by Sugammadex Sodium.

2.4. Pre-oxygenation and tracheal tube confirmation

Pre-oxygenation before intubation is the standard of care. The standard pre-oxygenation used in optimized surgical patients could fail to sustain adequate PaO_2 in patients with respiratory failure. Randomized control trial (RCT) by Baillard et al. confirmed that pre-oxygenation done by noninvasive positive-pressure ventilation (NIPPV) prior to TI is superior to that done classically by a bag-valve mask device for a 3-min duration [2]. The patients who have been pre-oxygenated by NIPPV have higher pulse oximetric saturation (98 ± 2 vs. 93 ± 6%) and higher PaO_2 values during TI (203 vs. 97 mmHg) and up to 5 min into the post-intubation period compared with the bag-valve mask method. In acute respiratory failure,

NIPPV improves oxygenation by delivering high oxygen concentration, by unloading respiratory muscle, recruiting alveoli, and thereby increasing the functional residual capacity in such hypoxemic patients. To confirm the endotracheal tube placement after TI, classically chest inspection for bilateral equal expansion and chest auscultation for equal air entry on both sides have been routinely used. Recently, the American Society for Anesthesiology (ASA) has adopted end tidal CO_2 monitor as the standard of care inside the operating room. Confirmation of endotracheal intubation by capnography has 100% sensitivity and specificity. Continuous capnography waveform is recommended as well during chest compression for cardiac arrest victims [4]. Esophageal detector device is an alternative carbon dioxide-monitoring device. The endobronchial intubation must be ruled out by chest radiograph, as a part of post-intubation care.

2.5. Intubation "care bundle" management

Care bundles are the best evidence-based therapies that could guarantee the best outcomes when applied together than each therapy alone in the bundle. Intubation bundle has been developed to enhance the quality of intubation procedure by setting a package tool to be followed by any provider in any intubation scenario with every patient. This bundle focuses on standardization of the stepwise process and eliminating the individual preferences and technical variability. The bundle involves maintaining cardiovascular stability, gas exchange, and the neurological status while securing the airway. The proposed ICU intubation management protocol includes 10 elements bundle [2].

2.5.1. Pre-intubation

1. Presence of two persons.
2. (Normal saline 500 ml or colloid 250 ml) as fluid loading in the absence of cardiogenic causes of pulmonary edema.
3. Long-term sedation ready to start.
4. Pre-oxygenation for 3 min by NIPPV with the following parameters:

(FiO_2 100%, pressure support ventilation level of 5–15 cm H_2O, tidal volume of 6–8 ml/kg, and PEEP of 5 cm H_2O).

2.5.2. During intubation

5. Rapid sequence induction: Anesthetic medications include Etomidate 0.2–0.3 mg/kg or ketamine 1.5–3 mg/kg or Propofol-Ketamine mixture. Muscle relaxants include Succinylcholine 1–1.5 mg/kg or Rocuronium Bromide 1 mg/kg. Succinylcholine is contraindicated in the following condition, hyperkalemia, severe acidosis, acute or chronic neuromuscular disease, burn patient for more than 48 h and spinal cord trauma, otherwise Rocuronium Bromide is preferred.
6. Cricoid pressure or Sellick maneuver should be applied.

2.5.3. Post-intubation

7. Immediate confirmation of tube placement by capnography.

8. Nor-adrenaline infusion if diastolic blood pressure still low.

9. Start long-term sedation.

10. Initial "protective ventilation": Tidal volume 6–8 ml/kg of ideal body weight, PEEP 5 cm H_2O and respiratory rate between 10 and 20 cycles/min, FiO_2 100%, plateau pressure <30 cm H_2O.

Studies showed that the bundle lowered the life-threatening complications as severe desaturation, hypotension, or cardiac arrest by 21 versus 34%. Other moderate complications have lowered as well (9 vs. 21%) compared with the non-bundle group [2].

TI in emergency settings in unstable patients could lead to an acute airway emergency. The airway morbidity and mortality increase with unstable hemodynamics and failing oxygenation during emergency intubations. That is why tracheal intubation in the ICU may be life-saving or life threatening. Airway management in a deteriorating sick patient is a real ICU emergency which cannot be delayed. Rescue airway equipment as THRIVE, NIPPV, and tracheostomy should be ready as a backup when difficult airway is encountered. Fewer complications have been noticed when the TI was done by experienced providers. Familiarity with rescue airway techniques is helpful. The rhythm of ICU environment necessitates precise guidelines that are tailored to ICU settings. Hence, implementation of an intubation care bundle along with a pre-planned approach to difficult airway is essential for safe TI in the ICU.

2.6. Tracheal re-intubation

Particular issues as the need to re-intubate following a trial of extubation or accidental extubation are common in ICU. Re-intubation may be unexpectedly difficult in hypoxic, distressed, or uncooperative patients with multiple risk factors and in patients who have been extubated after prolonged intubation as airway edema is common sequela.

3. Videolaryngoscopy in ICU

3.1. Introduction

Videolaryngoscopy (VL) is an indirect visualization technique for the larynx mainly for the purpose of airway assessment or airway management especially in ICU area. The images from the video can be displayed, magnified, and recorded on a monitor. Video-assisted visualization has been evolved in airway practice after the pressing clinical need of difficult airway scenario and lack of new tools other than Macintosh/Miller blades. That was invented in 1940. After many years of clinical practice, the VL techniques have been approved by the American Society of Anesthesia (ASA) and incorporated in their difficult airway algorithms. VL is promoted as a first step to go in anticipated difficult airway scenario.

3.2. Indication or advantage over ordinary laryngoscopy

1. The first choice of elective oral or nasal intubation in adults, pediatrics, or neonates, in case of anticipated and unanticipated difficult laryngoscopy.
2. Reduces strain and stress of operator during intubation.
3. Diagnostic and recording of airway lesions, abnormal anatomy, and pathology.
4. Can be used for TEE probes [5], naso-gastric tube [6], double lumen bronchial tube [7], and throat-pack insertion.
5. VAFI techniques (video-assisted fiberoptic intubation).
6. Good teaching tool for junior staff.
7. Guide the assistant where to apply external laryngeal manipulation: BURP (Backward Upward Rightward Pressure).
8. Help presbyopic doctors especially in neonatal intubation.
9. Awake tracheal intubation [8] and in abnormal intubating position as lateral decubitus [9].
10. Less traumatic over ordinary laryngoscopy.
11. Reduce the cervical spine mobility in patients with unstable cervical spine or reduced spinal mobility [10].

3.3. Types of videolaryngoscopy (VL)

Many types have been introduced into the market, which has created many dilemmas for the practitioners which one to choose (**Table 1**). Each VL device is unique in its size, shape, and profile, which gives specific strength and weakness to each. As a dozen devices are being continuously added to the market, it would be challenging and impractical for the anesthesiologists to obtain and train on all of them. Ideal VL should be intuitive, lightweight, low profile, inexpensive, easily maneuverable, easy to learn and master, remote view screen, with memory storage capacity, and long-lasting rechargeable batteries. Special features are being added as antifog capabilities by heating of the lens. The device should be easily adaptable to different intubation techniques, for example, nasal and oral.

3.3.1. Video stylets

The rigid stylets were in practice for the last 25 years to facilitate retromolar intubation. The bending angle is 40° at the distal end with a view angle of 110°. The video RIFL has a rigid rod with a flexible tip to articulate till 135° by closing the lever by a handgrip.

The stylets are advocated when the mouth opening is limited; however, its applicability is restricted to oral intubation. The video stylets are bulky, requiring space in the room,

Rigid blades		Guided channels-Automatically shaped		Video stylets	
Standard blade	**Angled blade**	**Channeled blade**	**Channeled airway**	**Rigid stylet**	**Rigid stylet + Flexing tip**
Storz C-Mac	Coopdech VLP100	AirTraq	Total track (VLM) Video Laryngeal Mask	Bonfils	RIFL
	Storz DCI	Pentax AWS			Shikani optical stylet
	McGrath "AIRCRAFT"	Res-Q-Scope II			
	GlideScope				
Storz V-Mac	Storz D-Blade				
	King Vision				
	Venner A.P. Advance				
	MedAn				

Table 1. Summary of different types of VL devices.

with no antifogging mechanism. It has the longest intubation time among other video techniques and higher learning curve but is very useful in restricted mouth opening using retromolar space. The Shikani optical stylet is a malleable, stainless steel, J-shaped endoscope with illumination fibers and a fiberoptic bundle that can be used with a separate camera and monitor system, or on its own with an optical eyepiece. **Figure 1** shows Bonfils retromolar videolaryngoscope.

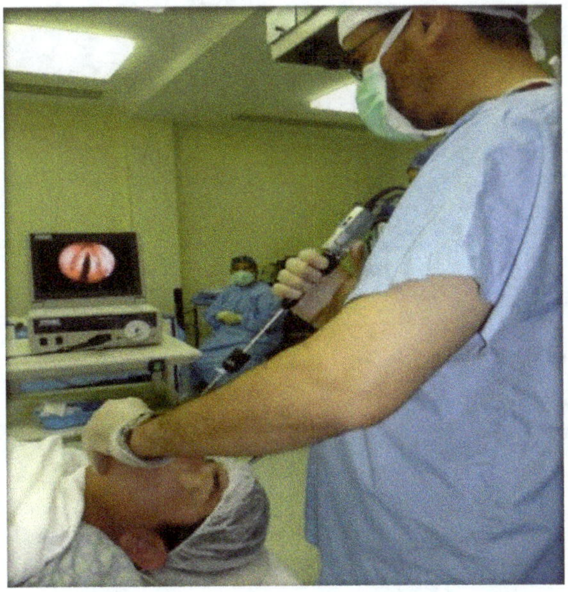

Figure 1. Bonfils retromolar videolaryngoscope (Storz-Company).

3.3.2. *Channeled videolaryngoscopy*

The representatives of the family are Pentax and AirTraq. All channeled devices have been designed mainly for oral intubation; however, the recent version of AirTraq has been studied and used in nasal intubation. The AirTraq is a single-use optical device with optional video camera attachment. It is available in different sizes and could be used for nasal intubation and double lumen tube insertion; however, it is single use and it requires 30–40 s to reduce fogging. Pentax is similar to AirTraq, with the advantage of the only plastic guide blades which are disposable. The tip is angled by 135° and it cannot be used with an endotracheal tube (ETT) less than 6.5, making it impractical for pediatric population. Both Pentax and AirTraq have been proved to reduce the cervical spine mobility in patients with unstable cervical spine or reduced spinal mobility. Res-Q-Scope is a similar device, but the clinical studies are so limited.

3.3.3. *Rigid blades*

Rigid blades are classified into standard blade or angled blade. In general, the standard blades use the various modifications of typical Macintosh blades as C-Mac (**Figure 2**). However, the angled blades offer more angulations near the distal tip to widen the view angle. In some equipment, as in Coopdech D-scope, sizes of 0,1 and Miller's blades are available, etc. C-scope sizes (sizes 0 and 1) Miller blades are available, but in most of the others Macintosh blades sizes 2, 3, and 4 are the standard.

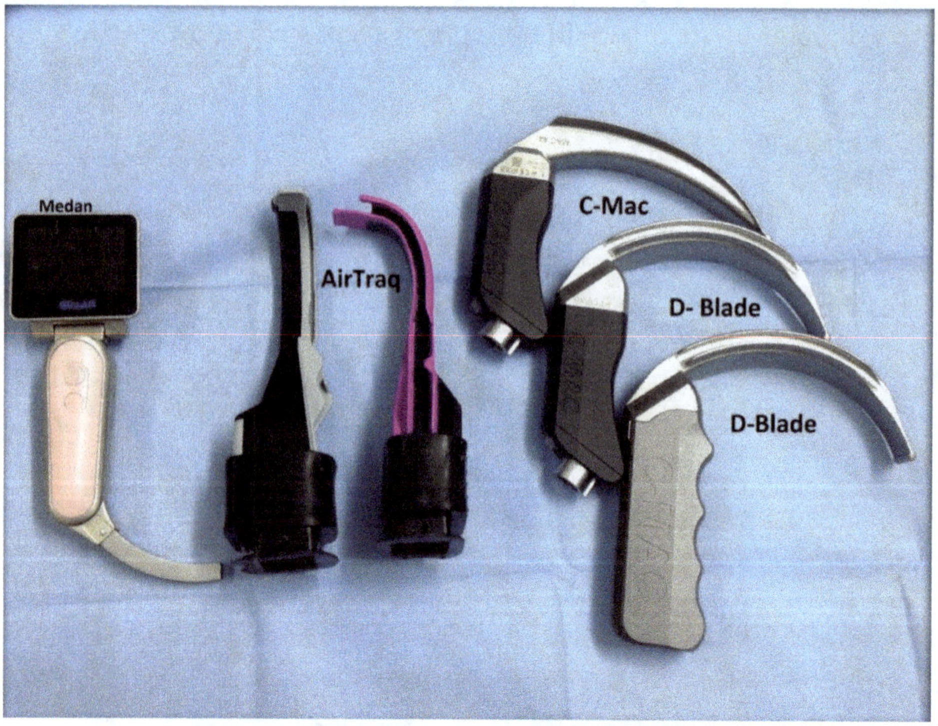

Figure 2. Videolaryngoscopes.

It was shown that the design familiarity with standard Macintosh blades, side screen, and enhanced view has reduced the learning curve for the inexperienced providers.

The main difference among rigid blades is the blade angulation and the position of the side view screen. In Coopdech VLP100, it has a build-in screen on top of the device with the view angle of 39-52°, with the option of sizes 2, 3, and 4 Macintosh or size 0, 1 Miller blade. The McGrath "AIRCRAFT" is similar to Coopdech VLP100 in having a build-in side screen over the handle, but different in having adjustable variable length blades that snaps in place once the length is adjusted. The GlideScope (**Figure 3**) has an angulation of 60°, with antifogging camera, plastic disposable blades, and separate view screen. GlideScope appeared to be the most intuitive, easy to learn with the steepest learning curve [11] but a little bit bulky in relation to C-Mac blade; that is why most of clinicians prefer C-Mac over GlideScope. Venner A.P. Advance and MedAn videolaryngoscopes are also available in the market from these VL types but the clinical studies are so limited.

In general, not one device has shown to have a 100% success rate and none has shown to be superior to another. All studies concluded that VL offers better laryngoscopic view if not the same as direct laryngoscopy. Most of the studies have concluded that the intubation time is more with videolaryngoscopy than with the direct laryngoscopy. Relative devices were faster than others by few seconds, DCI Storz Videolaryngoscope is relatively faster by 10 s than GlideScope (34 s) and McGarth (38 s); other study showed that the time for intubation for GlideScope was 33 s, CMAC was 17 s, and McGarth was 41 s [12]. Intubation with the GlideScope has been found to be 99% successful after initial failure of direct laryngoscopy, helping to reduce the incidence of failed intubation. It should be noted that the relative learning curves could affect the performance of GlideScope in some studies, as in

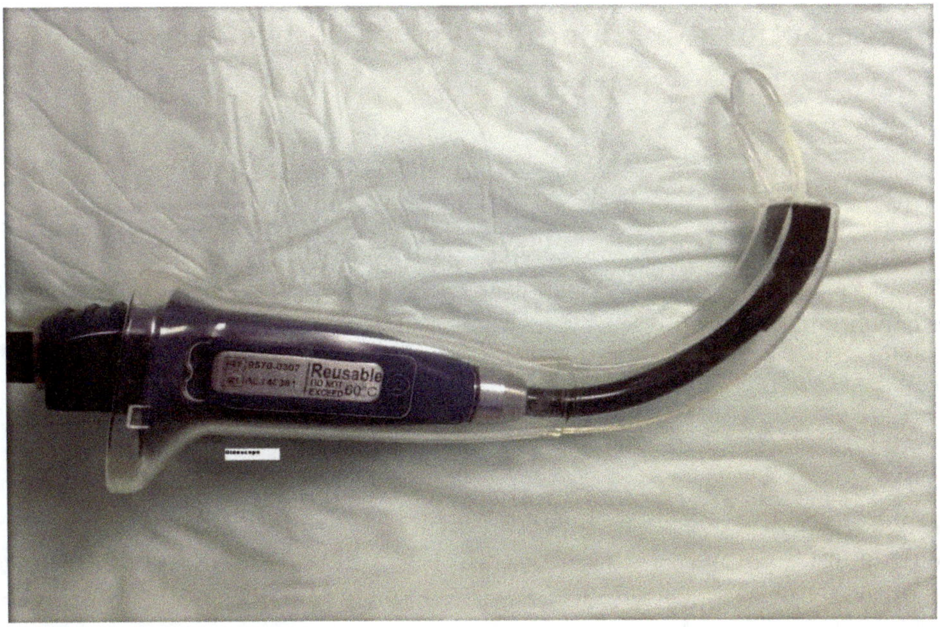

Figure 3. GlideScope (Verathon Inc., US).

the study of Platts-Mills in emergency department, which showed no difference in intubation failure between GlideScope and Macintosh, and intubation time in GlideScope was longer (12 s) [13] (**Figure 3**).

The main advantage for the videolaryngoscopy is minimal cervical spine mobility during intubation as the pharyngeal and laryngeal axis should not align together, offering least mobility for cervical instability. Moreover, it is helpful in case of limited accessibility, for example, magnetic resonance imaging (MRI) scanning, beach chair position, or prone position. It also allows sharing the airway view with beyond the operator for teaching or assistance purposes (**Figure 2**).

The devices of VL have been evaluated and adopted for practice outside the operative room.

3.4. Disadvantages of VL

The most common disadvantages of VL could be variable learning curve that depends on the level of training and experience, difficult passage of tube despite satisfactory laryngeal view, and loss of the depth perception. The fogging and secretion that could obstruct the camera are among other technical issues. Other disadvantage is the cost that could range from 5000 to 10,000$, which could be a burden in some part of the world; however, the cost could be justifiable in the industrialized part of the world if it could prevent such fatal airway events with its subsequent million dollar lawsuits. One study for VL adoption in Massachusetts emergency departments in 2012 has showed that adoption rate for VL was 43%, a relatively fast rate. The 69% of non-adopters have attributed that to the cost of the device [14].

4. Flexible fiberoptic intubation in ICU

4.1. Introduction

It is an airway device used for indirect visualization of the airway either for airway management or for other diagnostic and therapeutic purposes. Traditionally, all old scopes have used the fiberoptic fiber technology; however, the newer scopes, out of reliability issues, do not use the fiberoptic technology anymore and that's why the nomenclature changed to flexible intubation scope.

4.2. Types

Flexible intubation scope is a flexible cord that has fiberoptic fibers (old scopes) or optical fibers with a small camera on the tip of the scope using complementary metal oxide semiconductor (CMOS) technology and the so-called flexible intubation video endoscope (FIVE) from Storz Company. The proximal handle has a working channel port for oxygen and suction, lever to flex or extend the tip and light source. The diameter of adult scope is of 3.8 and 4.2 mm which can hold ETT of 6.5 mm or more. The diameter of children scope is of 2.2 and 3.1 mm which can hold 3 and 4 mm EET, respectively. Both adult and pediatric scopes have working channel of 1.2 mm. Most of flexible intubation scopes are reusable; however, recently a single-use flexible intubation scope started to be in the market from Ambu Company.

4.3. Indications

The main indication of flexible scope intubation (FSI) in anesthesia care and ICU settings is to secure the placement of endotracheal tube when there is anticipated airway difficulty and confirmation of tube position after intubation if necessary. It can be used as well in the management of abnormal airway anatomy, obstructive upper airway lesion, and unstable cervical spine to limit the cervical mobility, and the evaluation of airway obstruction is another anesthetic indication as a preoperative assessment (preoperative naso-endoscopy in pre-assessment anesthesia clinic) or directly prior to intubation for the patients with known anatomical abnormalities in the upper airway. The choice of the route has its indications as well, as nasal route is used in a case of limited mouth opening or a strong gag reflex, or if the surgery needs nasal intubation. Other indications other than primary anesthetic care involve diagnostic and therapeutic purposes, see **Table 2**.

4.4. Contraindications

There are no absolute contraindications for the FSI, but in the following situations difficult to impossible scenarios could be encountered. Large airway bleeding and secretions could make the view impossible. The limited clinical experience of the operator, the necessities for rapid airway control, the need to insert the tube under vision to minimize further trauma to the upper airway, and uncooperative patient are other contraindications. However, it is not absolute, as uncooperative patient can be intubated as sleep FSI and the visualization for ETT

Diagnostic indications	Therapeutic indications
• Evaluation of pneumonia, atelectasis, infiltrate of unclear etiology.	• Mucus impaction.
• Evaluation of hemoptysis.	• Foreign body removal.
• Evaluation of toxic burn inhalation.	• Laser coagulation for lesions.
• Evaluation of chest trauma.	• Photodynamic therapy.
• Evaluation of chronic cough.	• Electrocoagulation.
• Placement of artificial airways.	• Cryotherapy.
• Evaluate complications of tracheostomy.	• Dilation by balloon.
• Evaluation of precancerous lesions.	• Brachytherapy.
• Evaluation of tracheoesophageal fistula.	• Tracheobronchial stents.
• Evaluation of bronchopleural fistula.	• Bronchopleural fistula.
• Confocal microbronchoscopy.	• Needle aspiration of mediastinal cysts.

Table 2. Indications of flexible scope intubation (FSI).

insertion could be achieved by adjuvant airway as in fiberoptic-assisted videoscopic intubation (FAVI), a technique, when other indirect visualization technique, as C-Mac VL (**Figure 2**), is used to facilitate the insertion of ETT under vision. Nasal route is contraindicated in case of severe craniofacial deformity and skull base fracture.

4.5. Preparation for flexible scope intubation (FSI)

The preparation step for FSI is the most important step for a successful procedure. It involves patient selection and preparation, airway anesthesia and equipment preparation. The patient selection will determine whether the FSI will be through the oral or nasal route and whether it will be awake or sleep FSI. Generally, the awake has better visualization than the deep, due to loss of muscle tone and pharyngeal collapse after induction of anesthesia.

4.5.1. Patient preparation

It starts by good communication with the patient and proper assessment of the underlying condition. Anti-sialagogues should be applied for all patients whether it is oral or nasal, as secretions do not only affect the view but also limit the action of the local anesthetics. Commonly, it is recommended to use intravenous 0.2 mg glycopyrrolate, 15 min before the procedure. For patients with high risk for aspiration, risk and benefit should be analyzed as airway anesthesia and long intubation time could compromise the airway reflexes and increase aspiration risk. Certain measures have been recommended to minimize that risk: as intubation in head-up position, administration of 0.3 M sodium citrate 30 ml and Metoclopramide 10 mg or Ranitidine 50 mg within 1 h before the start of the procedure. Patient positioning depends on the technique and patient and operator's preference as well. Positions could be sitting (beach-chair), lateral decubitus for awake FSI or supine positions for sleep FSI and prone position as a rescue technique.

Airway anesthesia is a critical step in the procedure. It can be done by applying the local anesthetic solutions, gel, or ointment by atomizer, nebulizer, or "spray as you go technique." Airway anesthesia equipment includes atomizing devices, nebulizers, syringes and needles, and cotton swabs.

Combined techniques are always recommended to optimize the outcome. Combination of 4% lidocaine nebulization, atomization spray to tongue, and oropharynx followed by "spray as you go" through the working channel of the scope using epidural catheter are commonly applied together.

Cautions should be taken not to exceed with the lidocaine dosage above 6 mg/kg to avoid systemic toxicity. Trans-tracheal local anesthetic infiltration and nerve blocks could be used with a skilled operator but it is not commonly done. Glossopharyngeal nerve block, superior laryngeal nerve block, sphenopalatine nerve block, and anterior ethmoidal nerve block are among the nerves that could be blocked; however, the discussion of each nerve technique will be beyond the scope of this chapter. For nasal anesthesia, vasoconstrictors as 1% phenylephrine or 0.05% oxymetazoline are added to the local anesthetics to minimize nasal bleeding.

Airway equipment includes flexible intubating scope, face mask, specialized oral airway, and endotracheal tube, antifogging agent, lubricating agent, nasopharyngeal airway, oral or nasal mucosal atomization device (MAD) and video monitor. All equipment should be checked for functionality before any operation.

4.6. Technique

Oral intubation is the most common route. Stepwise approach should be followed: as ETT is loaded first to the scope, then oropharyngeal suction before insertion of scope, then applying of bite blocker or fiberoptic plastic airway (e.g., Ovassapian, Williams, or Berman). FSI should always be in the midline till satisfactory view is achieved. The working channel offers a source for suction, oxygen insufflation, or channel for epidural catheter during the procedure.

Nasal intubation has its advantage in avoiding the gag reflex; however, the chance of epistaxis is high. Topical nasal decongestant such as 0.05% oxymetazoline and 1% phenylephrine should be used to decrease the nasal mucosal irritation and bleeding.

Awake intubation necessitates patient cooperation, adequate airway anesthesia; however, sedation may be required. The patient is asked to swallow or breathe deeply and smoothly. Sedation could be titrated on individual basis, based on the underlying comorbidities. Commonly used sedation is Remifentanil infusion starting with 0.05 μg/kg/min or Remifentanil target-controlled infusion (TCI) mode with or without 1–2 mg Midazolam or Dexmedetomidine 0.3 μg/kg/h with or without Midazolam 1–2 mg or incremental doses of Midazolam 1 mg alone. Propofol TCI is another alternative to Midazolam as a sedative agent.

Sleep intubation could be done after induction of anesthesia in certain circumstances.

4.7. Strategies for success

It is important to keep in mind that FSI is a complex clinical procedure with requirements of special skills, which make even good preparation not enough to guarantee the success. Practicing certain adjuvant measures as strategies for enhancing the laryngoscopic view and facilitated ETT insertion could decrease the failure rate. Enhancing the view could be achieved by keeping airway patent by one or more of the following: jaw thrust, pulling tongue out by a gauze, fiberoptic oral airway placement, external laryngeal manipulation, insertion of laryngoscopic blade with lifting the epiglottis away from the pharyngeal wall (VAFI technique), and clearing the lens fogging by gentle touch of mucus membrane. Facilitated ETT insertion aims to minimize a possible trauma from the blind insertion of the tube after the FIS has reached the carina. The facilitation could be done by a 90° anticlockwise rotation of the tube to avoid getting caught at right arytenoid, warming the tube, flexible tube and combination of direct and indirect laryngoscopic technique or using video-assisted fiberoptic intubation (VAFI) technique.

4.8. Advantages

Flexible intubation scope is unique airway visualization equipment that offers great clinical help, not only in the management of difficult airway scenarios but also in the diagnosis and treatment as well. More details are described under bronchoscopy section.

4.9. Disadvantages

FSI is a complex procedure with no straightforward steps. To master the technique, it requires a lot of practice with high learning curve. Extra equipments are always necessary; moreover, it requires time for preparation and cannot help in emergency situation. Nasal epistaxis, minor airway trauma as erythema, and vocal cord injury could occur.

5. Bronchoscopy in ICU

5.1. Introduction

Flexible fiberoptic bronchoscopy is frequently used for diagnosis and therapy, performed in ventilated patients via an endo-tracheal tube or tracheostomy tube in ICU and other critical areas. Indication may be diagnostic or therapeutic (**Table 2**). *The most common indications* include clearance of retained secretion, mucous plug, lung collapse, endobronchial brush, removal of blood clot, diagnosis of ventilator-associated pneumonia by broncho-alveolar lavage (BAL), trans-bronchial biopsy, detection of airway lesions (e.g., neoplastic), endobronchial ultrasound (US), and visualization of instruments during percutaneous tracheostomy. Contraindications are relative so each patient should be carefully assessed for risk benefits. *Contraindications* include uncooperative patient, unstable patient as severe hypoxemia, hypercarbia, unstable asthma, recent myocardial infarction, or any situation of possible serious hemorrhage after biopsy as uremia, tracheal obstruction or stenosis and pulmonary hypertension.

5.2. Management of the airway for bronchoscopy

Separate operator should manage airway and ventilation. The bronchoscopist should be prepared to interrupt the procedure immediately if there is destabilization. Patients are preoxygenated, anesthetized, paralyzed, and ventilated on 100% O_2. Positive end expiratory pressure (PEEP) should be maintained. Impairment of gas exchange is common due to tube obstruction and when suction is applied through the scope.

Endotracheal tubes smaller than 8-mm internal diameter may be significantly occluded by flexible fiberoptic bronchoscopy and this could impair ventilation and oxygenation. A lubricated swivel (or elbow) connector with a fitted rubber cap prevents loss of ventilation. If pressure-controlled ventilation is used, peak pressure setting should be increased to compensate for the loss of tidal volume. Suction periods should be limited to 5 s or less. Thick secretions often require instillation of saline (10–20 ml) down the injection port to dissolve them. During broncho-alveolar lavage (BAL), a sputum trap should be used between bronchoscope and wall suction.

5.3. Special situation with flexible fiberoptic bronchoscopy

- *Bleeding dyscrasias:* Coagulation studies, platelet counts, and hemoglobin concentration are necessary before the procedure especially when there are clinical risk factors for abnormal coagulation. Bronchoscopy with lavage can be performed with platelet counts of >20,000 per/µl.

- *Pneumothorax:* A chest radiograph should be obtained if a patient is symptomatic or if there is a clinical suspicion of possible pneumothorax after trans-bronchial biopsy. Patients should be advised of the potential for delayed complications following trans-bronchial biopsy.
- *Fever and infection:* Antibiotic prophylaxis is not warranted before bronchoscopy for the prevention of endocarditis, fever, or pneumonia.
- *Ischemic heart disease:* flexible fiberoptic bronchoscopy should ideally be delayed for 4 weeks after MI.

6. Percutaneous tracheostomy

6.1. Introduction

Mechanical ventilation can be delivered to the patient who requires ventilatory support either initially through endotracheal tube (ETT) for short-term period or through tracheostomy tube, in cases where the respiratory support will be prolonged due to underlying medical reasons [15].

Tracheostomy versus intubation: The relative advantages and disadvantages of tracheostomy and endotracheal intubation are outlined in **Table 3** [16–20].

Tracheostomy techniques: Bedside percutaneous tracheostomy is an alternative to operative (open) tracheostomy, as it could be done either at the bedside or in the operating room. Successful performance of the bedside percutaneous procedure is related to the expertise of the operator and supportive personnel. Surgeons or well-trained critical care clinicians could do with fewer complications. Choosing between open or percutaneous tracheostomy depends upon the availability of each procedure and institutional expertise.

	Intubation	Tracheostomy
Advantage	• Highly skilled personnel are required. • Stoma complication is less. • Procedural complication is less.	• Ability to speech, swallowing. • Ability to mobile and discharged outside ICU. • Easy suction. • Better patient satisfaction and comfort.
Disadvantage	• Possible mouth, nasal or laryngeal injury. • Cuff pressure complication. • Requirement of tube exchange or possible ICU care.	• Cuff pressure complication. • Stoma and fistula complications. • Possible laryngeal injury, pulmonary and mediastinum complication. • Mortality complication due de-cannulation in improper time.

Table 3. Advantage and disadvantage tracheostomy versus intubation.

Percutaneous versus operative: Percutaneous tracheostomy offers numerous advantages compared to operative tracheostomy: it requires less time to perform, it is less expensive, and it is typically performed sooner (because an operating room doesn't have to be scheduled). In addition, overall complications may be less frequent with percutaneous tracheostomy than surgical tracheostomy, even though percutaneous tracheostomy has an increased risk of anterior tracheal injury and posterior tracheal wall perforation.

Data describing outcomes comparing both techniques are conflicting, which may reflect the different techniques used to perform percutaneous tracheostomy (e.g., ultrasound-guided, bronchoscopy-guided, dilatational, other).

6.2. Complication

Infection: In two meta-analyses of randomized controlled trials, percutaneous dilatational tracheostomy reduced wound infections (e.g., odds ratio: 0.28, 95% CI: 0.16–0.49) compared to both surgical tracheostomy performed in the ICU and surgical tracheostomy performed in the operating room. A separate meta-analysis of 29 randomized and non-randomized studies reported a similar reduction in the rate of wound infection with percutaneous tracheostomy [21].

Bleeding and mortality: When compared to surgical tracheostomy performed in the operating room, only percutaneous dilatational tracheostomy has also been associated with reduced bleeding (odds ratio: 0.29, 95% CI: 0.12–0.75) and mortality (odds ratio: 0.71, 95% CI: 0.50–1.0). A similar reduction in overall mortality was reported in another 10-year review of 616 trauma patients that compared those who underwent percutaneous tracheostomy with those who underwent open tracheostomy (10 vs. 15%) [17].

By contrast, another meta-analysis of 20 trials reported no difference in mortality or major bleeding [18]. In a separate meta-analysis, perioperative complications (including death, serious cardiorespiratory events, and minor complications) were rare, but more common with percutaneous tracheostomy than with surgical tracheostomy. In another meta-analysis of 29 studies, no significant difference in bleeding or tracheal stenosis was reported [20].

Scarring: While one meta-analysis reported no difference in the rate of tracheal stenosis or scarring, another reported significant reduction on the rate of scarring.

Taken together, the data suggest that percutaneous dilatational tracheostomy offers numerous advantages compared to surgical tracheostomy. However, the benefit of percutaneous tracheostomy may be substantially less dependent upon the technique employed.

6.3. Contraindications

Relative contraindications to percutaneous tracheostomy include age under 15 years of age; uncorrectable bleeding diathesis; gross distortion of the neck from hematoma, tumor, thyroid gland enlargement, or scarring from previous neck surgery; documented or clinically suspected tracheomalacia; evidence of infection in the soft tissues of the neck; obese and/or short neck which obscures landmarks; and inability to extend the neck because of cervical fusion, rheumatoid arthritis, or other causes of cervical spine instability.

It should be reiterated that these contraindications are relative. Percutaneous dilatational tracheostomy has been performed successfully by skilled operators in patients who were very old, were morbidly obese, had a history of previous tracheostomy, or had thrombocytopenia (the patients received pre-procedure platelet transfusions). It has also been performed successfully in patients receiving high-frequency oscillation ventilation or positive end expiratory pressure (PEEP) at a level of >10 cm H_2O.

A study that evaluated the rates of bleeding complications during percutaneous tracheostomy showed that bleeding complications could be predicted by a platelet count less than 50,000/μl, an activated partial thromboplastin time longer than 50 s, or the presence of two or more coagulation disorders. Administration of prophylactic subcutaneous heparin did not increase the risk of bleeding [18].

For patients undergoing a bronchoscopic-guided percutaneous tracheostomy, a bedside checklist, similar to that performed for open tracheostomy performed in the operating room, may be associated with reduced procedural complications.

6.4. Complications

Acute: The most common acute (e.g., first few days) complications include obstruction and pneumothorax as well as postoperative hemorrhage and infection.

Obstruction: Percutaneous tracheostomy tubes can become partially obstructed by the posterior membranous trachea following initial placement, although symptomatic obstruction is uncommon. This complication appears to be related to the experience of the clinician performing the procedure. However, the swelling of the posterior tracheal wall could cause symptomatic compression of the tube up to 1 week after placement.

Subcutaneous emphysema and pneumothorax: The incidence of subcutaneous emphysema and pneumothorax is 1.4 and 0.8%, respectively [19]. Cadaver models revealed that imperfect positioning of fenestrated cannula and posterior wall perforation are possible mechanisms for these complications [19].

Chronic complications of tracheostomy (i.e., weeks and months) that are specific to tracheostomy include the following:

- *Tracheal stenosis:* Granulation tissue is the main reason for tracheal obstruction in patients under long mechanical ventilation by tracheostomy, which differs from the stenosis that develops in endotracheal tube that will be appearing earlier and be web-like. Stenosis of the trachea is not only below the tracheostomy tube, but it may occur above the tracheal stoma but below the glottis. That could contribute to high-peak airway pressures and difficulty in weaning. Treatment includes the placement of a longer tracheostomy tube, surgical intervention, or the placement of a tracheal stent [20].
- *Tracheoarterial fistula:* Massive hemorrhage due to a tracheoarterial fistula is the most devastating complication. Tracheoarterial fistula (most often a tracheoinnominate artery fistula) was more common in the past from low-positioned tracheostomy tubes and is now rarely encountered

with several studies reporting an incidence of <1% in both short-term and long-term tracheostomies [21]. The development of a tracheoarterial fistula is a life-threatening complication with a reported survival of 14%. Tracheoarterial fistulas are due to erosion from the tube tip or cuff into the anterior wall of the trachea resulting in a fistulous communication with the innominate artery as it passes anteriorly across the trachea. Patients may develop a "sentinel" bleeding followed by massive hemoptysis. Diagnosis is dependent upon a high index of suspicion, and when suspected, immediate action should be undertaken to stop the bleeding since diagnostic modalities such as angiography or bronchoscopy may lead to delay and death.

The following temporizing maneuvers may be performed while waiting for definitive therapy, which is surgical repair [22].

- In an attempt to compress the innominate artery, the tracheostomy or endotracheal tube cuff may be overinflated.
- If the above fails, an ETT may be placed orally, the tracheostomy removed, and the cuff inflated distal to the tracheostomy site.
- If that fails, a finger can be placed through the tracheostomy stoma and positioned distally into the trachea ("The little Dutch boy maneuver"); the finger is then pulled anteriorly to compress the artery against the sternum (pressure should be sufficient to lift the torso anteriorly). Pressure should be maintained during transport to the operating room. Ventilation and oxygenation need to be preserved with a bag-valve mask or intubation with an ETT orally.

Reduced phonation: Following tracheostomy, many patients experience a reduction in or loss of phonation, the duration of which may be prolonged or indefinite, and the effect of which can be devastating to some patients. Traditionally, speech valves are used in tracheostomized patients (with the cuff deflated) who successfully wean from mechanical ventilation and are able to self-ventilate. Preliminary data suggest that early phonation is feasible and may be beneficial when instituted during mechanical ventilation in tracheostomized patients. As an example, one randomized trial of 30 ventilated tracheostomized patients reported that early intervention with cuff deflation plus an in-line speaking valve during mechanical ventilation shortened the time to phonation by 11 days, when compared with late intervention using the standard approach. Further research is needed before in-line speaking valves can become routine for this population [22].

Others: Tracheoesophageal fistula is more commonly encountered with prolonged endotracheal intubation and is discussed separately.

Although not studied in a randomized trial, the complication rate associated with tracheostomy may be increased in obese patients with a body mass index of ≥35 [22].

Changing a tracheostomy tube: There are no universally accepted indications for changing a tracheostomy tube. Therefore, the following indications are based on clinical experience rather than on empirical evidence:

Routine changes: Tracheostomy tubes are routinely changed from 7 to 14 days after initial insertion and then every 60 to 90 days. Observational data suggest that changing the tracheostomy tube before 7 days may be associated with earlier use of a speaking valve and earlier ability to tolerate oral intake. A consensus statement recommends changing the tracheostomy tube at 3–7 days if inserted operatively but 10–14 days if placed via the percutaneous dilatational method.

Patient discomfort: Patient discomfort may respond to a reduction in the size of the tracheostomy tube.

Malposition: Tracheostomy tube malposition may respond to a change in the length or size of the tracheostomy tube.

Patient-ventilator asynchrony: Patient-ventilator asynchrony that is related to the tracheostomy tube may respond to changing the tube.

Cuff leak: A cuff leak may be due to malposition of the tracheostomy tube (particularly in the setting of tracheomalacia) and may respond to changing the tube.

Fracture: Fracture of the tracheostomy tube or flange is an indication for a new tracheostomy tube.

Type change: Changing a tracheostomy tube from one type to another may be indicated by the clinical circumstances; as an example, changing from a balloon cuff to either a foam cuff or a cuff-less tracheostomy tube.

Bronchoscopy: Flexible bronchoscopy generally requires a tracheostomy tube with an inner diameter of at least 7.5 mm; thus, the tracheostomy tube may need to be changed to one with a larger inner diameter to facilitate bronchoscopy.

Decannulation: Appropriate candidates for tracheal decannulation after weaning from mechanical ventilation include patients who fulfill all the following criteria:

No upper airway obstruction, ability to clear secretions that are neither too copious nor too thick, and presence of an effective cough. In patients with neuromuscular disease, a peak cough flow greater than 160 ml/min generally predicts successful decannulation. The value of this measurement in patients without neuromuscular disease is unknown.

Failed decannulation has been associated with age, greater severity of illness, the presence of renal failure, and a shorter duration of spontaneous breathing prior to decannulation or the insertion of a tracheostomy plug.

7. Extubation in ICU

7.1. Introduction

The removal of endotracheal tube (ETT) termed as extubation is the last step of ventilatory weaning. Extubation step necessitates consideration of patient condition, experience with extubation techniques, and post-extubation management.

Before extubation: Successful weaning from mechanical support is not the only prerequisite for safe extubation. Extubation is carried on patent airway with adequate airway reflex after independence from ventilatory support.

Airway protection: Airway protection requires a conscious patient with a strong cough reflex and minimal secretions.

Typical criteria for successful weaning: Fully awake and cooperative, good muscle tone and function, intact bulbar function, stable hemodynamic, no dysrhythmias, Hb greater than 8.0 gm%, minimal inotropic requirements, optimal fluid balance, respiratory $FiO_2 < 0.4$, PEEP < 10 cm H_2O, no significant respiratory acidosis (PH > 7.3 or $PaCO_2$ <6.5 kPa), good cough, normal metabolic pH, normal electrolyte balance, non-distended abdomen, adequate nutritional status, normal CO_2 production, and normal oxygen demands [23].

Some patients will be extubated without difficulty and others will rapidly deteriorate as a result of inadequate respiratory effort or clearance of secretions. Those patients will require re-intubation, ventilation, and another period of optimization and consideration for tracheostomy. Some patients will benefit from weaning straight onto mask CPAP or NIV [23].

Difficult extubation: Extubation of a patient with a known difficult airway requires careful planning in anticipation for potential re-intubation. If there are doubts about airway patency prior to extubation, then direct laryngoscopy, fiberoptic bronchoscopy, and assessment of leak upon cuff deflation are useful checks. Patients who are considered likely to be difficult to re-intubate can be extubated with an airway exchange catheter in situ, to allow rapid re-intubation. Intravenous dexamethasone, nebulized adrenaline, and Heliox have been used with variable success in such circumstances.

Risk factors for extubation failure are peak expiratory flow rate (PEFR) of ≤ 60 L/min, sputum volume production of > 2.5 ml/h, and compromised neurological status. Combination of three risk factors reliably predicts extubation failure by 100% compared to 3% if no risk factor mentioned above is present [24].

Post-extubation management: Post-extubation care includes suctioning, bronchodilator therapy, diuresis, or noninvasive ventilation (NIV). Those measures could aid to prevent re-intubation by improving the oxygenation and airway clearance.

Oxygen (including high-flow nasal cannula (HFNC)): Every patient should be oxygenated post-extubation. We prefer using devices that provide adequate oxygenation and comfort for the patient. For most patients, this goal is achieved with low-flow devices (nasal prongs, simple, or venturi face masks). When higher flows of oxygen are required, high-flow nasal cannula (HFNC) may offer improved oxygenation, provide a small amount of positive end expiratory pressure (PEEP), and is better tolerated when compared with oxygen delivered through low- or high-flow face masks.

The efficacy of HFNC in the post-extubation setting was best illustrated in a trial of 527 patients who were mechanically ventilated for an average of only 1–2 days and considered to be at low risk for re-intubation following extubation. Compared to conventional low-flow oxygen therapy, HFNC reduced the rate of re-intubation at 72 h (5 vs. 12%) as well as the rate of respiratory failure (14 vs. 8%). However, methodologic flaws such as imperfect blinding and the high proportion of postsurgical and neurologic patients, where HFNC may have improved secretion clearance, may have biased results in favor of HFNC. Although encouraging, this trial does not support the routine use of HFNC following extubation [25].

In addition, while further studies are required to clarify who benefits the most from HFNC after extubation, its use in those who are severely hypoxemic is appropriate (e.g., partial arterial pressure of oxygen/fraction of inspired oxygen ratio <300). Further details regarding HNFC in other medical and postoperative populations and efficacy compared with NIV in post-extubation patients are discussed separately.

8. High-flow nasal cannula (HFNC)

8.1. Introduction

Different names and descriptions of this therapy:

HFNC: **H**igh-**F**low **N**asal **C**annula.

THRIVE: **T**ransnasal **H**umidified **R**apid **I**nsufflation **V**entilatory **E**xchange.

POINT: **P**erioperative **O**xygenation **I**nsufflatory **N**asal **T**herapy (**Figure 4**).

Or transnasal insufflation or nasal high-flow or nasal high-flow ventilation or high-flow therapy or high-flow nasal cannula oxygen therapy.

HFNC oxygen delivery system involves a mixture of oxygen/air, an active humidified, heated circuit, and nasal cannula. The active heater and humidifier are able to deliver heated and humidified high flow reaching 60 L/min than has many physiological advantages. High flow is able to reduce dead space by maintaining PEEP inside the airway and supplying constant fraction of oxygen. In spite of limited evidence in literature in ICU, it has gained popularity among physicians in various critical conditions. The existing evidence in neonates proves that HFNC decreases the work of breathing by reducing the respiratory rate and sufficiently supports the patient ventilation, reducing the escalation of ventilator support [26].

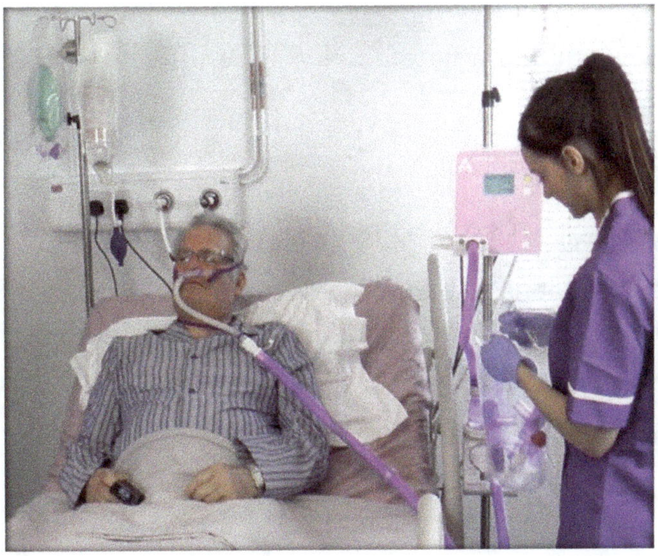

Figure 4. High-flow nasal cannula (HFNC) (Aqua VENT FD 140® from Armstrong Medical Company, Northern Ireland).

As the evidence is still evolving, still the indications and contraindications should be considered for each case individually.

8.2. Indications

- Hypercapnic respiratory failure.
- Hypoxemic respiratory failure.
- Post-extubation.
- Pre-intubation oxygenation.
- Sleep apnea.
- Acute heart failure.

8.3. Contraindication

- Bilateral nasal blockade as postnasal operations.
- Nasal bleeding.
- Nasal tumors.
- Nasal infection.
- It is also unlikely that HFNC can readily rescue those patients who have total airway obstruction and its use in the presence of a known or suspected cranial base fracture is also not advised.

8.4. Advantages

- Better tolerated in some patients than face masks.
- Fixed performance, permitting accurate delivery of up to 100% oxygen in most clinical situations.
- Gas is warmed and humidified.
- Low-level positive airways pressure is possible.
- An additional benefit is that nasal high-flow devices have been shown to produce positive airway pressures of over 5 cm H_2O, thus permitting their use in place of low-level CPAP [26].
- It is an open system and we do not have to care about the tight contact of interfaces, and HFNC can be applicable to patients with claustrophobia.

8.5. Disadvantages

- Results of large-scale clinical trials are still awaited.

- More expensive than standard oxygen delivery devices.
- Not yet available in all hospitals, and rarely outside of critical care.

9. Usage of supraglottic airway devices (SGAD) in ICU

9.1. Introduction

Airway management in the critical care is challenging and differs from the operating theatre. The supra-glottic airway devices (SGADs), especially the laryngeal mask airway (LMA), provide a fast and lifesaving way in the critical events.

9.2. Advantages

- Can solve "Cannot Intubate, Cannot Ventilate" (CICV) scenario.
- Passing a Bougie through it, then intubation over a Bougie or using an Aintree Intubating Catheter (Cook Critical Care, Bloomington, IN, USA).
- Bronchoscopy through LMA.
- Used as an airway while performing a tracheostomy.
- Ventilation during cardiac arrest instead of an ETT, if no skilled staffs are available.
- Minimal skills requirements to use an LMA.
- No muscle relaxant is required.
- No contact with vocal cords, less irritating than ETT.

9.3. Disadvantages

- No guarantee for a good airway, as the tip may fold on itself blocking the airway.
- No good seal with no protection from aspiration.
- Intubating through the LMA could be problematic. As it has shown that the LMA opening sits perfectly above the cords only in 45–60% of the time [27]. This means almost half of the time the LMA is directing the ETT away from the cords. The situation is worse in difficult airway as the provider was perfectly capable of shoving the tube the wrong way without any help.

9.4. Evidence for and against the use of LMAs in critical care

- Experts have recommended the use of LMA in a "Cannot Intubate, Cannot Ventilate" (CICV) scenario while waiting for a better airway. It has shown that LMAs have saved lives in such situations [28].

- The dilemma of LMAs not offering a good seal has no effect on clinical outcomes. Risk of aspiration has never been demonstrated, even with the old generations of LMA [29].
- No difference between the LMA and routine bag-mask and ETT anesthesia [29]
- Using the LMA as an airway while performing a tracheostomy has no sufficient evidence in the literature. There is no difference in the rate of complications, but the tracheostomies involving LMAs seemed to be quicker, may be due to less time to adjust the ETT cuff above the cords [30].

10. Endotracheal tube exchanger in ICU

10.1. Indications

- Mostly due to a cuff leak.
- The need for a different endotracheal tube (ETT) size as when smaller one is needed in patients with vocal cord edema or larger ETT for flexible bronchoscopy procedure.
- Change of special types of ETT like reinforced or double lumen to ordinary ETT.

10.2. Complications

However, exchanging the ETT may be life-threatening and lead to

- Esophageal intubation.
- Loss of the airway.
- Severe hypoxia.
- Cardiac arrest.

The risk may be more in those with a difficult airway or those with poor cardiopulmonary reserve.

10.3. Techniques

The ideal way for ETT exchange has not yet been studied. Experienced team with advanced airway skills should be consulted priorv to ETT replacement.

The ETT placement can be done under direct laryngoscopy or indirect laryngoscopy with or without a Bougie guide. The initial airway assessment by direct laryngoscopy will determine which tool should be used. When a good laryngeal view is obtained by direct laryngoscopy, ETT can be introduced safely; however, in difficult laryngeal view, video laryngoscopy should be sought. Intubation medications are recommended to be used as well in tube exchange. Video laryngoscopy has been shown, compared with historical controls, to reduce the number of attempts at ETT exchange, with fewer complications including hypoxemia, esophageal intubation, bradycardia, and need for rescue airway device intervention [31].

11. Virtual endoscopy and 3D reconstruction of airway

Virtual endoscopy (VE) (**Figure 5**) is a noninvasive technology by which two-dimensional (2D) or three-dimensional (3D) images are reconstructed by computer software from high-resolution computed tomography (CT) scan (**Figure 6**). Virtual bronchoscopy was initially reported in 1993, but it was modified in 1996 to be used in virtual laryngoscopy. The virtual images reconstructed by software have comparable quality of fiberoptic views with sensitivity of 100% to detect upper airway lesions [32, 33]. The novel application of virtual laryngoscopy is eminent in the assessment and staging of upper airway lesion, comprehensive preoperative airway assessment, and planning of complex reconstructive upper airway surgeries. The "fly-through" reconstructions provided accurate and comparable images to fiberoptic bronchoscopy, which provided valuable information for the evaluation of the airway passages in a step forward prior to going to the difficult airway management (**Figure 5**). The utilization of the 3D imaging package is now commercially available within the workstation delivered by the different vendors worldwide, to obtain 3D models of the airway. This approach will be the added value and advantage that most anesthetists and intensive care physician would be able to use this technology to construct VE images of the airway from existing CT images and find them easy to interpret (**Figure 7**).

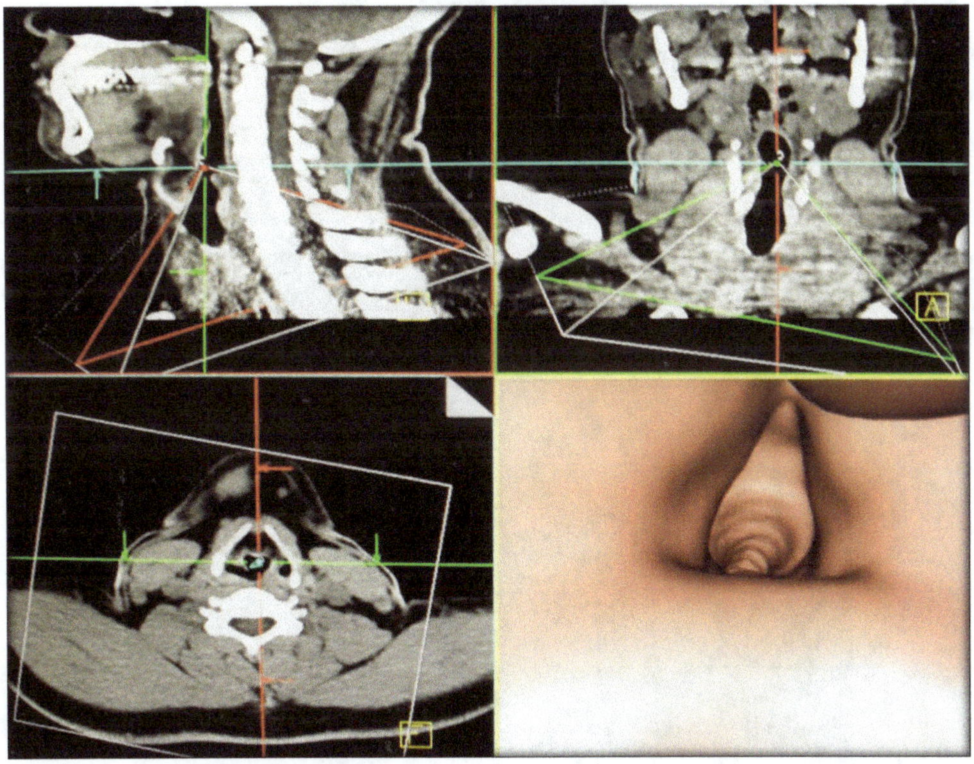

Figure 5. Virtual endoscopic evaluation of the air way. The vocal cords are well demonstrated. The accompanied reference images in axial, coronal, and sagittal planes with the virtual endoscope are noted, and its apex represents the eyepiece while the base represents the virtual lens.

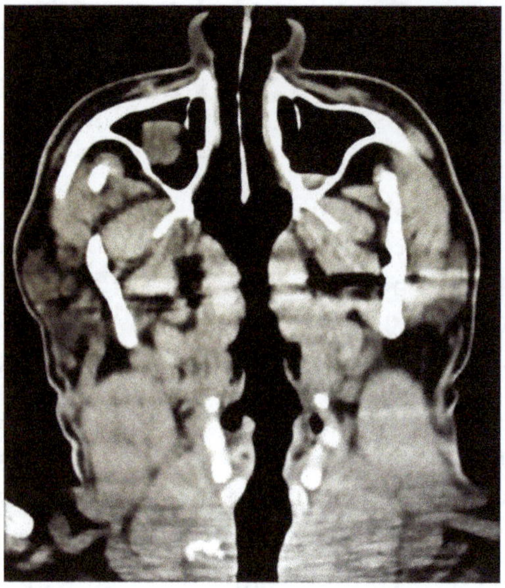

Figure 6. Curved MPR multi-planar reconstruction of the airway showing the entire airway in single plane from the nares down to the trachea allowing accurate measurement and orientation of the airway caliber at the different levels.

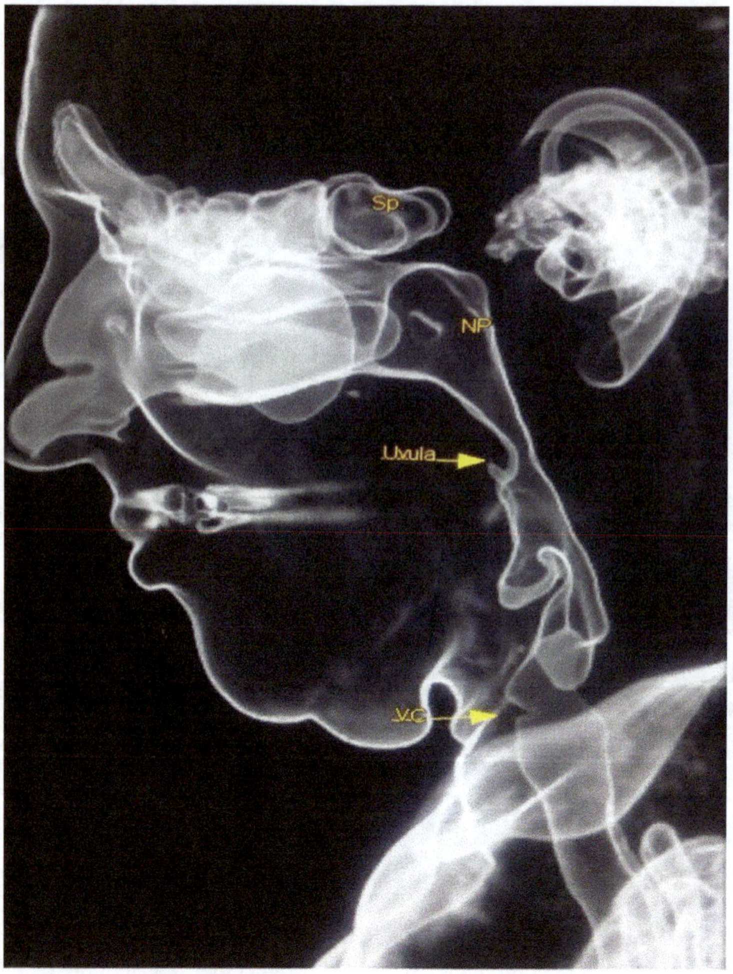

Figure 7. Lateral projections of the SSD-shaded surface display using volume-rendering techniques for the airway. SP: sphenoid sinus; NS: nasopharynx; VC: vocal cord.

This state-of-the-art technology has a promising future value in airway management for both anesthesiologists and intensivists as they will be able to easily interpret the airway images by noninvasive way (**Figure 8**).

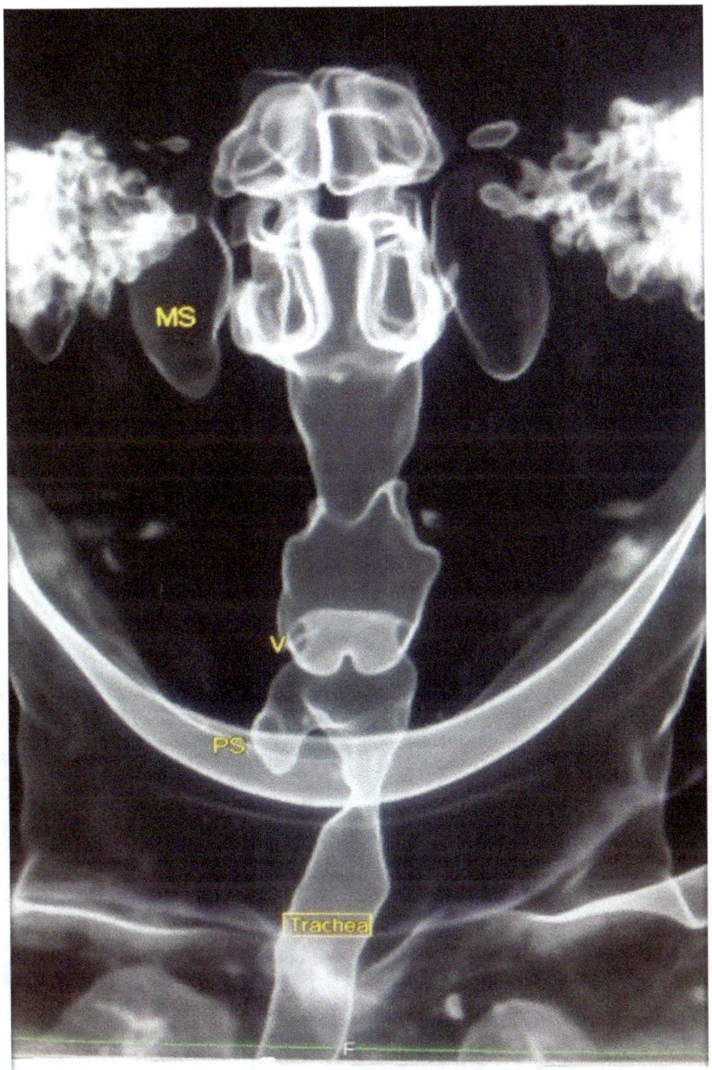

Figure 8. Antero-posterior (AP) curved MPR multi-planar reconstruction of the airway showing the entire airway in single plane from the nares down to the trachea allowing accurate measurement and orientation of the airway caliber at the different levels. **MS**: maxillary sinus; **V**: vallecula; **PS**: piriform sinus.

12. Ultrasound in airway management

12.1. Introduction

Ultrasound (US) examination of the upper airway in critically ill patients supplies a number of attractive advantages compared with competitive traditional imaging techniques or endoscopy. It is widely available, portable, repeatable, relatively cheap, pain-free, safe, and bedside machine in every operating theater and ICU suite.

12.2. Uses in airway management

- Locate the anatomy of major vessels and the thyroid gland in relation to tracheostomy site [34].
- Localize tracheal rings and cricothyroid membrane (**Figure 9**).
- Identify midline, puncture site for percutaneous tracheostomy.
- Checking of endotracheal intubation and detection of esophageal intubation [34].
- Estimation of gastric content [35].
- Recognize the air-tissue border from tongue to mid-trachea and at the pleural level [36].
- Localize the trachea by combining palpation of the sternal bone with US.
- Identify the "string of-pearls" sign that identifies the tracheal rings and mark the cricothyroid membrane as part of difficult airway management skills [34].
- Recognize sonographic evidence of lung movement during respiration and exclude a pneumothorax [34].
- Recognize endobronchial intubation and one-lung ventilation [36].

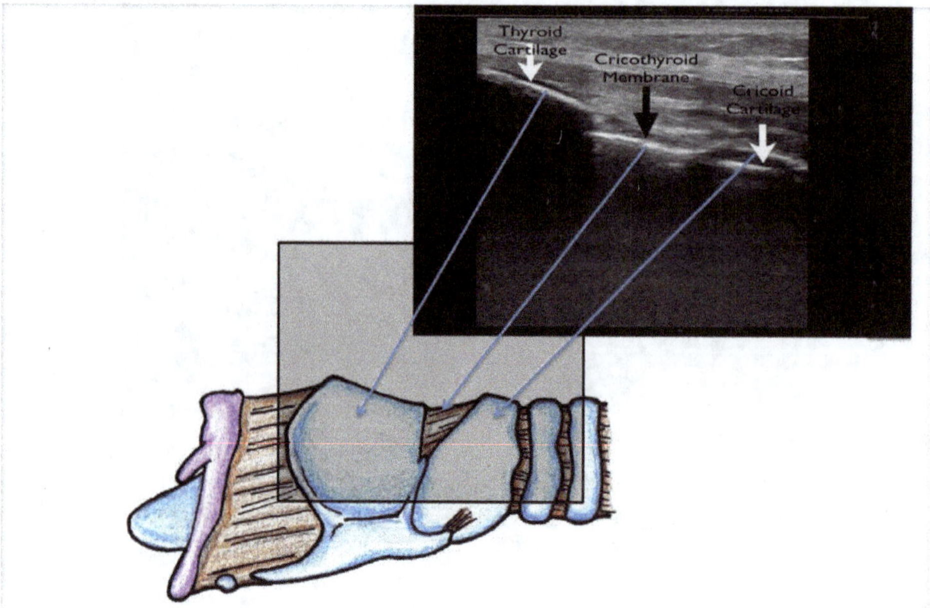

Figure 9. Ultrasound images of larynx and trachea rings.

13. Recommendations

The airway competence in ICU should be coping with the rapidly evolving advances in airway management. Therefore, efforts should be focused on the three pillars of airway mastery: airway providers as intensivists or critical care physicians, equipment, and operational plans. Not all institutions can afford all airway equipment in the market; however, they should make sure that critical care providers have a full access to the available tools and they are comfortable using it. Educational sessions and refresher courses should be tailored to meet the competence level of the ICU providers and equipment availability. Operational plan includes developing institutional airway protocols and implementing difficult airway guidelines. The protocols should consider different staffing models of ICU and make sure all the time at least one member of the team with the highest experience in airway should be always available.

14. Key points

- Airway management in intensive care patients may be lifesaving or life threatening.
- Maintenance of patent airway, adequate ventilation, and pulmonary gas exchange are very important in critically ill patients. Airway management in intensive care patients differs significantly from routine surgical procedures in the operating room.
- Critical care physicians should be familiar with the equipment and the techniques to maintain and secure the airway.

Competing interests

The authors declare that there are no competing interests.

Author details

Nabil Abdelhamid Shallik[1,2,3,4*], Mamdouh Almustafa[5], Ahmed Zaghw[5] and Abbas Moustafa[6,7]

*Address all correspondence to: nshallik@hamad.qa

1 Hamad Medical Corporation, Clinical Anesthesiology, Weill Cornell Medical College in Qatar, Doha, Qatar

2 Anesthesia and ICU Department, Tanta Faculty of Medicine, Tanta, Egypt

3 Anesthesia Section of Rumailah Hospital, Anesthesia, ICU and Perioperative Medicine Department HMC, Doha, Qatar

4 Medical Education and Qatar Robotic Surgery Center, HMC, Doha, Qatar

5 Department of Anesthesia, ICU and Perioperative Medicine, HMC, Doha, Qatar

6 Elminia University, Egypt

7 Radiology, HMC, Doha, Qatar

References

[1] Schwartz DE, Matthay MA, Cohen NH. Death and other complications of emergency airway management in critically ill adults. Anesthesiology. 1995;**82**:367-376

[2] Jaber S, Amraoui J, Lefrant JY, Arich C, Cohendy R, Landreau L, et al. Clinical practice and risk factors for immediate complications of endotracheal intubation in the intensive care unit: A prospective, multiple-center study. Critical Care Medicine. 2006;**34**:2355-2361

[3] Adnet F, Jouriles NJ, Le Toumelin P, Hennequin B, Taillander C, Rayeh P, et al. Survey of out-of-hospital emergency intubations in the French prehospital medical system: A multicenter study. Annals of Emergency Medicine. 1998;32:454-456

[4] Griesdale DE, Bosma TL, Kurth T, Isac G, Chittock DR. Complications of endotracheal intubation in the critically ill. Intensive Care Medicine. 2008;**34**:1835-1842

[5] Tagawa T, Sakuraba S, Okuda M. Pentax-AWS-assisted insertion of a transesophageal echocardiography probe. Journal of Clinical Anesthesia. 2009;**21**(1):73-74

[6] Roberts JR, Halstead J. Passage of a nasogastric tube in an intubated patient facilitated by a video laryngoscope. The Journal of Emergency Medicine. 2011;**40**(3):330

[7] El-Tahan M, Doyle DJ, Khidr AM, Hassieb AG. Case report: Double lumen tube insertion in a morbidly obese patient through the non-channeled blade of the King Vision™ Videolaryngoscope. F1000 Research. 2014;**3**:129. DOI: 10.12688/f1000research.4481.3

[8] Kajekar P, Mendonca C, Danha R, Hillermann C. Awake tracheal intubation using Pentax airway scope in 30 patients: A case series. Indian Journal of Anaesthesia. 2014;**58**:447-451

[9] Shinohara H, Ishii H, Kakuyama M, Fukuda K. Morbidly obese patient with a huge ovarian tumor who was intubated while awake using airway scope in lateral decubitus position. Masui. 2010;**59**:625-628

[10] Hirabayashi Y, Fujita A, Seo N, Sugimoto H. A comparison of cervical spine movement during laryngoscopy using the Airtraq or Macintosh laryngoscopes. Anaesthesia. 2008;**63**(6):635-640

[11] Siu LW, Mathieson E, Naik VN, Chandra D, Joo HS. Patient- and operator-related factors associated with successful GlideScope intubations: A prospective observational study in 742 patients. Anaesthesia and Intensive Care Journal. 2010;**38**(1):70-75

[12] Maassen R, Lee R, Hermans B, Marcus M, van Zundert A. A comparison of three videolaryngoscopes: The Macintosh laryngoscope blade reduces, but does not replace, routine stylet use for intubation in morbidly obese patients. Anesthesia and Analgesia. 2009;**109**(5):1560-1565

[13] Platts-Mills TF, Campagne D, Chinnock B, Snowden B, Glickman LT, Hendey GW. A comparison of GlideScope video laryngoscopy versus direct laryngoscopy intubation in the emergency department. Academic Emergency Medicine. 2009;**16**(9):866-871

[14] Raja AS, Sullivan AF. Adoption of video laryngoscopy in Massachusetts emergency departments. The Journal of Emergency Medicine. 2012;**42**(2):233-237

[15] Diehl JL, El Atrous S, Touchard D, et al. Changes in the work of breathing induced by tracheotomy in ventilator-dependent patients. American Journal of Respiratory and Critical Care Medicine. 1999;**159**:383

[16] Lin MC, Huang CC, Yang CT, et al. Pulmonary mechanics in patients with prolonged mechanical ventilation requiring tracheostomy. Anaesthesia and Intensive Care. 1999;**27**:581

[17] Lim CK, Ruan SY, Lin FC, et al. Effect of tracheostomy on weaning parameters in difficult-to-wean mechanically ventilated patients: A prospective observational study. PLoS One. 2015;**10**:e0138294

[18] Mohr AM, Rutherford EJ, Cairns BA, Boysen PG. The role of dead space ventilation in predicting outcome of successful weaning from mechanical ventilation. The Journal of trauma. 2001;**51**:843.

[19] Fikkers BG, van Veen JA, Kooloos JG, et al. Emphysema and pneumothorax after percutaneous tracheostomy: Case reports and an anatomic study. Chest. 2004;**125**:1805.

[20] Koitschev A, Graumueller S, Zenner HP, et al. Tracheal stenosis and obliteration above the tracheostoma after percutaneous dilational tracheostomy. Critical Care Medicine. 2003;**31**:1574.

[21] Scalise P, Prunk SR, Healy D, Votto J. The incidence of tracheoarterial fistula in patients with chronic tracheostomy tubes: A retrospective study of 544 patients in a long-term care facility. Chest. 2005;**128**:3906

[22] Arola MK. Tracheostomy and its complications. A retrospective study of 794 tracheostomized patients. Annales Chirurgiae et Gynaecologiae. 1981;**70**:96

[23] Coplin WM, Pierson DJ, Cooley KD, et al. Implications of extubation delay in brain-injured patients meeting standard weaning criteria. American Journal of Respiratory and Critical Care Medicine. 2000;**161**:1530

[24] Thille AW, Boissier F, Ben Ghezala H, et al. Risk factors for and prediction by caregivers of extubation failure in ICU patients: A prospective study. Critical Care Medicine. 2015;**43**:61

[25] Nishimura M. High- flow nasal cannula oxygen therapy in adults. Journal of Intensive Care. 2015;**3**:15

[26] Patel A, Nouraei SAR. Transnasal Humidified Rapid-Insufflation Ventilatory Exchange (THRIVE): A physiological method of increasing apnoea time in patients with difficult airways. Anaesthesia. 2015;**70**:323-329

[27] Benumof JL, et al. Laryngeal mask airway and the ASA difficult airway algorithm. Anesthesiology. 1996;**84**(3);686-699

[28] Siddiqui S, Seet E, Chan WY. The use of laryngeal mask airway Supreme™ in rescue airway situation in the critical care unit. Singapore Medical Journal. 2014;**55**(12):205

[29] Brimacombe JR, Berry A. The incidence of aspiration associated with the laryngeal mask airway: A meta-analysis of published literature. Journal of Clinical Anesthesia. 1995;**7**(4):297-305

[30] Strametz R, et al. Laryngeal mask airway versus endotracheal tube for percutaneous dilatational tracheostomy in critically ill adult patients. The Cochrane Database of Systematic Reviews. 2014;**30**(6):CD009901

[31] Mort TC, Braffett BH. Conventional versus video laryngoscopy for tracheal tube exchange: Glottic visualization, success rates, complications, and rescue alternatives in the high-risk difficult airway patient. Anesthesia & Analgesia. 2015;**121**(2):440-448

[32] Finkelstein SE, Schrump DS, Nguyen DM, Hewitt SM, Kunst TF, Summers RM. Comparative evaluation of super high-resolution CT scan and virtual bronchoscopy for the detection of tracheobronchial malignancies. Chest. 2003;**124**:1834-1840

[33] Osorio F, Perilla M, Doyle DJ, Palomo JM. Cone beam computed tomography: An innovative tool for airway assessment. Anesthesia & Analgesia. 2008;**106**(6):1803-1807

[34] Drescher MJ et al. Ultrasound of Esophageal Intubation. Academic Emergency Medicine. 2000;**7**(6):722-725

[35] Perlas A, Mitsakakis N, Liu L, Cino M, Haldipur N, Davis L, Cubillos J, Chan V. Validation of a mathematical model for ultrasound assessment of gastric volume by gastroscopic examination. Anesthesia & Analgesia. 2013;**116**(2):357-363

[36] Singh M, Chin KJ, Chan VW, Wong DT, Prasad GA, Yu E. Use of sonography for airway assessment: An observational study. Journal of Ultrasound in Medicine. 2010;**29**:79-85.

9

Brain Death in Children

Eleni Athanasios Volakli, Peristera-Eleni Mantzafleri, Serafeia Kalamitsou, Asimina Violaki, Elpis Chochliourou, Menelaos Svirkos, Athanasios Kasimis and Maria Sdougka

Abstract

Brain death (BD) is a distinct mode of death in pediatric intensive care units, accounting for 16–23% of deaths. Coma, absent brainstem reflexes, and apnea in a patient with acute irreversible neurological insult should alarm the attending physician to start the appropriate actions to establish or refute the diagnosis for BD. BD diagnosis is clinical, starting with the preconditions that should be met, and based on the examination of all brainstem reflexes, including the apnea test. Apnea testing should be conducted according to standard criteria to demonstrate the absence of spontaneous respirations, in the case of an intense ventilatory stimulus, setting at increased $PaCO_2$ levels ≥60 and ≥20 mm Hg, compared to baseline. When elements of clinical examination and/or apnea test cannot be performed, ancillary studies to demonstrate the presence/absence of electrocerebral silence and/or cerebral blood flow are guaranteed. Two clinical examinations by qualified physicians at set intervals are required. Time of death is the time of second examination and ventilator support should stop at that time, except for organ donation. The use of check list in documentation of BD helps in the uniformity of diagnosis and fosters further trust from medical, family, and community personnel.

Keywords: brain death, pediatric intensive care unit, apnea testing, brainstem reflexes, coma

1. Introduction

The evolution of intensive care has led to circumstances that a human being could be artificially maintained in life through technological advancements even in the presence of an irreversible neurological damage. Brain death (BD) in most instances occurs when an acute insult to the brain causes a neuropathologic viscious cycle of brain edema, increases intracranial pressure (ICP), and decreases cerebral blood flow that compromise blood supply to the brain and results in ischemia, a situation which resembles to "total brain infarction" according to Swedish Committee on defining death [1]. Severe traumatic head injury, infections, tumors, cerebral vascular accidents, or acute global anoxic/ischemic injury following severe respiratory failure, shock, or cardiac arrest are the main causes of BD in children [2]. Rarely, acute toxic neuronal injury as happened in fulminant hepatic failure or other metabolic diseases are the reasons, or cellular dysoxia, which prevents extraction or utilization of oxygen, as is the case in cyanide poisoning.

Brain death is a distinct mode of death both in adult and pediatric population; it is estimated that BD accounts for approximately 16–23% of deaths in the pediatric intensive care unit (PICU), while the corresponding values for adults are quite similar and depending on the nature of the unit, rising from 15% in multidisciplinary units up to 30% in neurocritical units [3–6]. Most research about BD involves adults; however, not all principles regarding BD could be transferred to children. The pediatric brain is immature; the development, plasticity, and maturation of central nervous system (CNS) ends by the 2 years of age according to the majority of researchers, while others believe to continue beyond the first decade of life [7]. Moreover, resilience to certain forms of injury could be found, due to the open fontanelles in infancy and the presence of certain forms of diseases that result in hydranencephalia and cerebral atrophy, and/or wide craniectomy, that could hasten the progress of intracranial hypertension. The above should be considered when interpreting diagnosis and confirming BD in infants and children [8].

The first effort to define BD as a new criterion for death was made in 1968 by a consensus report of the Ad Hoc Committee of the Harvard Medical School, without specific recommendations with respect to age [9]. Irreversible coma was defined as unresponsiveness to external stimuli, absent movements or breathing, absent reflexes, and a flat electroencephalograph (EEG).Later on, in 1975, on a review of the Harvard criteria by the American Academy of Neurology (AAN), they question the applicability of the consensus criteria to children stating that the above criteria may be inapplicable for children under 5 years of age since there are indications that the immature nervous system can survive significant periods of electrocerebral silence. In an effort to set a standard national definition on BD, in 1981, in the USA, the Uniform Determination of Death Act was adopted as part of the President's Commission [10]. Death was determined in accordance with accepted medical standards either as an irreversible cessation of circulatory and respiratory functions of a person, or irreversible cessation of all functions of the entire brain, including the brain stem. Age-specific guidelines were again not provided and medical standards were not described, and the commission recommended caution in applying neurological criteria to determine death in children younger than 5 years.

In 1995, the Quality Standards Subcommittee of the AAN published the practice parameters for determining brain death in adults to delineate the medical standards for the determination of BD in patients older than 18 years. The document emphasized the three cardinal clinical findings necessary to confirm irreversible cessation of all functions of the entire brain, including the brainstem: *coma or unresponsiveness* (with known cause), *absence of brainstem reflexes*, and *apnea*. Future research in apnea testing, and the need for validation of confirmatory tests was recommended [11]. However, despite the published parameters, considerable practice variations were recorded, which led to the 2010 update that sought to use evidence-based methods to answer questions historically related to variations in BD determination, to promote uniformity in diagnosis [12].

The irreversible cessations of all functions of brain, including the brainstem, are not universally accepted; the definition of BD in each nation depends on jurisdiction. In the USA, Australia, and New Zealand for example, a whole brain death definition is accepted. On the contrary, in the UK, India, and Canada a brainstem-based definition of death is in place and the term "death by neurological criteria" (DNC) is adopted [13–16]. In the UK, the most recent definition for DNC was published in 2008 by the Academy of Medical Royal Colleges (AoMRC) in the code of practice for the diagnosis and confirmation of death. Consciousness and breathing capacity were recognized as essential characteristics of life and the irreversible loss of them were regarded equal to death [13]. The applicability of the criteria in infants younger than 2 months were questioned, in agreement with a report presented by the British Paediatric Association (BPA) in 1991, which stated also that the criteria of DNC cannot be applied in infants younger than 37 weeks of gestation [17]. Caution was relieved by the guidelines issued in 2015 by the Royal College of Paediatrics and Child Health (RCCHD) considering the diagnosis of DNC in infants from 37 weeks corrected gestation (postmenstrual) to 2 months (postterm) of age. RCCHD stated that the 2008 criteria of death could be applied to this population with precautionary measures regarding the apnea test due to immaturity of the newborn infant's respiratory system [18].

The first specific pediatric guidelines on BD were issued in 1987 by the American Academy of Pediatrics (AAP) to solve questions and give answers for this special topic. These guidelines were a consensus opinion regarding necessary clinical history, physical examination criteria, observation periods, and ancillary laboratory tests required to determine brain death in children[19]. An update followed in 2011, with emphasis given to two different age populations: the one from newborn 37 weeks gestation to 30 days of life and the other from 31 days of life to 18 years [20]. These guidelines could serve as a basis for the development of national guidelines at each nation, taking into account legal, cultural, and religious differences, and will be analyzed in this chapter, enriched by the experience of a single centre and the discussion of relevant references.

BD in most occasions is intertwined to organ harvesting and transplantation, and much research in the field has been done through national organ procurement databases [21, 22]. Nevertheless, the declaration of BD should be done by the patient physicians only, according to local national and institutional guidelines, irrespective from the transplantation team [23, 24]. The priority of the medical system is to save lives rather than to obtain organs and the public must feel confident that they would become organ donors only after all reasonable attempts to save their lives have failed. Maintenance of public trust is essential for the functioning of organ transplantation systems around the world [24]. BD is still a controversial issue for some physicians, and civilians as well, who deny the conceptual basis for equating an irreversibly nonfunctioning brain with a dead human being [25]. Though, the ethical, psychosocial, and philosophical approach of BD is beyond the scope of this chapter which will concentrate on the biological and clinical approach only of pediatric patients dying from BD.

2. Dying from BD in the PICU

Regardless some terminology differences between the most widely USA definition of BD as the death of the whole brain, and the UK definition of death by DNC as the death of the brain-stem, the concept that is universally accepted is that *the patient dying from BD suffered an acute irreversible CNS insult that resulted to coma, absent brainstem reflexes, and apnea* [7]. Although cases of confirmation of BD in children have been described outside the PICU, the proper place where the patients should be treated and diagnosis takes place is the PICU [22–24]. Frequently, the first indication by the bedside nurse is the lack of spontaneous awakening periods, the absence of cough during suctioning, and the fixed dilated pupils, which should alarm the attending physician that the patient deteriorates, and may be is going to BD. All sedative medications, including antiepileptic drugs and neuromuscular blocking agents, should stop at that time, the patient should continue to receive the maximum supportive intensive care treatment to preserve homeostasis, and the preparations should begin to establish or refute the diagnosis of BD. The diagnosis of BD is confirmed by clinical examination criteria only, based on the absence of neurologic function with a known irreversible cause of coma. Ancillary studies are not required except in cases where the clinical examination and apnea test cannot be completed [13, 14, 20].

3. Management of critically ill children dying from BD

For the better understanding of the evolution to BD in children, we will present the sequence of the events that happen in pediatric patients treated in a PICU after a severe neurological insult, step by step, in a timely manner. Our data were obtained from a retrospective study regarding all deaths that occurred between January 2011 and April 2016, in a multidisciplinary eight-bed PICU of Northern Greece. Among 275 deaths, 44 (16%) were defined as BD. The incidence was higher in boys (28/44 patients, 63.6%). Mean age was 68.75 ± 44.04 months (range 2 months to 13 years) and mean severity of illness as estimated with the pediatric risk of mortality (PRISM III-24 h) score at admission was 21.67 ± 9.98. Head injury was the most frequent cause of BD (29.41%) followed by CNS infection (23.52%), hypoxic/ischemic insults (23.52%), CNS tumors (11.76%), and intracranial bleeding (11.76%).

The management of the patients was done under the relevant for the diagnosis international protocols, under sedation, mechanical ventilation, chemoprophylaxis, gastric ulcer prophylaxis, and artificial nutrition. At admission, 88.6% of patients were already on mechanical ventilation and almost half of them (52.3%) were in shock. Central venous catheters and arterial lines were inserted in all patients. Nine patients (20.5%) had intracranial pressure (ICP) monitoring. Almost all received osmotherapy with either NaCl 3% (37 patients, 84.1%) and/or mannitol 20% (36 patients, 81.8%). Sedation was achieved with midazolam at mean max dose of 0.93 ± 0.56 mg/kg/h and remifantanil at max dose of 0.09 ± 0.05 mcg/kg/min. Cis-attracurium was administered for neuromuscular blocking at a bolus dose of 0.2 mg/kg, as needed before interventions, e.g., suctioning to avoid inadvertent increase in ICP. Sodium thiopental at a max dose of 5 mg/kg/h was administered in 18 patients (40.9%) and four patients (9.1%) were treated with craniectomy, as a third tier therapy to refractory intracranial hypertention [26]. Diabetes insipidus was recorded in 33 patients (75%), and high sugar levels needed insulin therapy in 19 patients (43.2%). The higher serum Na and sugar levels that were recorded were 165 ± 15.39 mmol/l and 281 ± 159.07 mg/dl, respectively. During their stay, the majority of the patients (79.5%) needed inotropic and/or vasopressor support to preserve an acceptable hemodynamic status.

The clinical suspicion on BD was set on 3.59 ± 5.46 day through dilated unreacted pupils. Mean pupil size at admission was 4.07 ± 2.06 mm which was increased to the final size of 6.28 ± 1.13 mm. Following that all the prerequisites of BD were fulfilled, two clinical examinations were performed by a panel of three doctors registered for at least 2 years; one anesthetist, one neurologist or neurosurgeon, and the attending physician (pediatrician or pediatric surgeon), according to the Greek law. Mean sedation time was 4.02 ± 3.03 days. The first tests were done in 9.88 ± 6.50 days after admission and the second in 11.28 ± 6.53 days. Mean time between tests was 27.54 ± 11.80 h. Apnea testing was prepared according to national BD protocol, with preoxygenation with 100% oxygen for at least 10 min, and baseline mechanical ventilation aimed at 40 mmHg of $PaCO_2$ [11]. Oxygenation during apnea was done through a catheter tailored to endotracheal tube (ETT) size (size in CH doubled the ID size of ETT in mm), inserted in the endotracheal tube at a length corresponded to tracheal carina, with a flow of 1 l/min/age in years, initially, according to acute pediatric life support (APLS) recommendation for apneic oxygenation [27]. If oxygenation was inadequate, a gradually increase in O_2 flow in increments of 1 l/min up to max 12 l/min was performed [12]. For this purpose, we used a simple suction catheter of appropriate size as described above, with the valve occluded, and connected to an oxygen flow source, preferably a low pressure one (capable of giving oxygen at driving pressure of 1–2 bar). In the case of acute respiratory distress syndrome (ARDS), hypoxia, and need for high positive end expiratory pressure (PEEP), apnea testing was performed on continuous positive airway pressure (CPAP) modality. Duration of apnea was 10 min if feasible, or earlier if signs of hypoxia and/or hypotension appeared. Apnea testing was considered positive for BD if no spontaneous respiration occurred when the $PaCO_2$ level was >60 and >20 mmHg compared to baseline, in accordance with international guidelines [11, 12, 14].

A total of 88 apnea tests were recorded. Incomplete data concerning the way of oxygenation during the apnea test were revealed in 50% of the tests, probably due to the retrospective data analysis and incomplete recordings. Thirty-six patients (81.81%) completed the test successfully. Eleven apnea tests (12.5%) were aborted, mainly due to hypoxia (8/11, 72.72%) and to a lesser degree due to shock (3/11, 27.27%). In detail, four patients did not manage to complete the first apnea test (three hypoxia, one shock), while seven patients aborted the second test (five hypoxia, two shock). The data of apnea testing are presented in **Table 1**. Ancillary study with magnetic resonance angiography (MRA) was carried out in eight patients (18.18%). Patients died 54.58 ± 59.64 h after the completion of the second apnea test. Three families (6.81%) gave consent for organ donation.

	Mechanical ventilation mode	FiO_2%	pH	PaO_2 (mmHg)	$PaCO_2$ (mmHg)
Baseline	IPPV (68.4%)	50.8 ± 20.6	7.44 ± 0.062	133.88 ± 33.90	33.36 ± 4.60
	PRVC (22.5%)				
	SIMV-PS (9.1%)				
A. prep.		100	7.33 ± 0.084	382 ± 97.59	45.46 ± 4.18
A. Apnea test	CPAP (20.4%)	100	7.10 ± 0.063	235 ± 107.18	84.15 ± 10.53
	Tracheal O_2 (29.6%)				
	NA (50%)				
B. Prep.		100	7.33 ± 0.073	354 ± 127	45.21 ± 5.20
B. Apnea test	CPAP (22.7%)	100	7.11 ± 0.063	223 ± 129.72	84.79 ± 13.99
	Tracheal O_2 (25%)				
	NA (52.3%)				

IPPV, intermittent postitive pressure ventilation; PRVC, pressure regulated volume control; SIMV-PS, synchronized intermittend mandatory ventilation-pressure support; CPAP, continuous positive airway pressure; Tracheal O_2, tracheal insufflation of oxygen at age-related flows of 1 l/min/age (max 12 l/min); NA, not applicable (lack of data).

Table 1. Data of apnea testing (n = 77) in pediatric BD patients (n = 44).

4. Guidelines for the determination of BD in infants and children

4.1. Definition of BD

In 2011, a multidisciplinary committee was formed by the Society of Critical Care Medicine (SCCM) and the AAP to update the 1987 Task Force Recommendations for the diagnosis of pediatric BD [12, 14, 20]. According to guidelines, *BD is a clinical diagnosis based on the absence of neurologic function with a known diagnosis that has resulted in irreversible coma.* Coma and apnea must coexist to diagnose DB. A complete neurologic examination is mandatory to determine BD with all components appropriately documented. An algorithm for the diagnosis of BD in children adapted from Ref. [20] is provided in Appendix 1.

4.2. Age definition

Two age definitions were set with an impact on the timing of first exam and the observation period between tests.

- Newborns 37 weeks gestation to 30 days of life.
- Infants 31 days of life to 18 years.

Because of insufficient data in the literature, recommendations for preterm infants less than 37 weeks gestational age were not included in this guideline.

4.3. Timing of first exam

- Twenty-four hours for patients aged from 37 weeks gestation to 30 days of life. Time is counted after birth, cardiac arrest with successful resuscitation or other severe neurological insult.
- Twelve hours for patients aged 31 days of life to 18 years. Time is counted after cardiac arrest with successful resuscitation or other severe neurological insult.

It is reasonable to defer neurologic examination to determine brain death for longer than 24 h, if dictated by clinical judgment of the treating physician. Neonates who probably suffered from hypoxic/ischemic insult during the neonatal period and had been put in therapeutic hypothermia deserve a longer observation time before the first examination. Hypothermia not only could interfere with brainstem reflexes interpretation but hastens drug metabolism as well. In addition, the first examination should be postponed beyond 24 h if residual drug effect is suspected. In general, the first examination cannot be performed unless all the preconditions of diagnosing BD are met.

4.4. Irreversible and identifiable cause of coma

A known and irreversible cause of coma should be established before the diagnosis of BD. In most instances, the evolution of a brain damage to BD is depicted with computed tomography (CT) or magnetic resonance imaging (MRI). Sometimes, neuroimaging if performed early enough in the course of the disease is without significant findings. Serial examinations in such occasions are helpful. CT and MRI are introductory studies and should not be relied on to make the determination of brain death. Additional data such as results from cerebrospinal fluid (CSF) analysis and/or other microbiological data are supportive [12]. In 2011 AAP guidelines, three major causes of coma were recognized: traumatic brain injury, anoxic brain injury, and known metabolic disorder. In cases that the cause of coma is not identifiable, the physician should specify the cause of coma as "Other." It is advisable to keep these major causes when recording BD, which will enable international comparisons, if needed.

4.5. Preconditions

The interpretation and validity of the clinical neurological examination and the apnea testing should not leave any space for concern. All the potentially influencing factors must be corrected in advance and the subsequent undeniable preconditions must be met:

- *Cardiovascular stability.* Mean or arterial systolic pressure should be normal for age (no less than two standard deviations from the mean age responding values). Inotropic and vasomotor support may be necessary for the treatment of shock. Direct arterial pressure measurement is strongly recommended, not only for the monitoring but for blood gases analysis and $PaCO_2$ evaluation as well, which is an integral part of the apnea testing that follow.

- *Normothermia.* Therapeutic hypothermia is increasingly used as an adjunctive therapy of the insulted brain and the physician should be aware of the potential hypothermia impact on the diagnosis of brain death. Hypothermia is a depressant to central nervous system activity and may lead to a false diagnosis of brain death. Metabolism and clearance of medications are retarded, which can interfere with brain death examination. Achieving normothermia with a core body temperature of 35°C (95°F) before the first exam and maintaining it throughout the observation period is essential.

- *Homeostasis.* The most common metabolic disturbance during BD is hypernatremia due to diabetes insipidus that should be corrected with the administration of antidiouretic hormone or desmopressin. Hyperglygemia is common too, and close monitoring of glucose levels and treatment with insulin when necessary is indicated. Hyponatremia, hypoglycemia, hypothyroidism, severe pH disturbances, severe hepatic or renal dysfunction or inborn errors of metabolism may also occur and cause a potentially reversible coma in pediatric patients. All the above should be excluded before moving on diagnostic tests for BD. A high index of clinical suspicion for metabolic disturbances should be especially raised in situations where the clinical history alone does not provide a reasonable explanation for the evolution of BD.

- *Neuromuscular blocking (NMB) agents.* Adequate clearance of these agents should be confirmed. In case there is a doubt for residual NMB action, a nerve stimulator with documentation of neuromuscular junction activity and twitch response should be used to demonstrate good neuromuscular activity with 4/4 responds in "train of four" testing [12, 23].

- *Drug intoxications.* Barbiturates, opioids, sedative and anesthetic agents, antiepileptic agents, and alcohols should be discontinued. Adequate clearance (based on the age of the child, presence of organ dysfunction, total amount of medication administered, elimination half-life of the drug and any active metabolites) should be allowed before the neurologic examination. Recommendations of time intervals before brain death evaluation for many of the commonly used medications administered to critically ill neonates and children are listed in Appendix 2 of 2011 AAP guidelines. Laboratory testing of drug levels should be performed if there is a concern regarding residual drug effect. Although there is evidence that therapeutic and subtherapeutic barbiturate levels (phenobarbital and pentobarbital at 15–40 ug/ml) did not interfere with the reliability of BD diagnosis, it is advised these drugs to be at the low to mid therapeutic range before neurological examination [28]. Unusual causes of coma such as neurotoxins and chemical exposure, e.g., organophosphates and carbamates, should be occluded in rare cases where an etiology for coma has not been established.

4.6. Physical examination: coma

The neurologic examination BD criteria in pediatrics have been adapted from 2010 American Academy of Neurology criteria for BD determination in adults [12]. Patients must exhibit complete loss of consciousness, vocalization, and volitional activity and should be in a profound state of coma. Flaccid tone is confirmed by passive range of motion in extremities given there are no limitations to performing such an examination, e.g., previous trauma, and the patient is observed for any spontaneous or induced movements. Noxious stimuli in the cranial nerve distribution (deep supraorbital and/or condylomandibular pressure) and all four limbs (deep bed nail pressure), and trunk (sternal rub) should be applied and the responses, if any, should be carefully evaluated. Central (in the territory of cranial nerves, e.g., facial area) responsiveness to central and peripheral (outside the territory of cranial nerves) noxious stimuli must be absent, apart from spinally mediated reflexes. Complete absence of motion would equate a Clasgow Coma Scale (GCS) of 3. Observations such as decerebrate or decorticate posturing, true extensor or flexor motor responses to painful stimuli and seizures are not compatible with BD. Any motor response within the cranial nerve distribution, or any response in the limbs in response to cranial nerve stimulation, *precludes determination of brain death*. Spinal reflexes should be suspected in cases of motor responses in a somatic distribution after noncranial, e.g., peripheral nerve stimulus and not after stimulus in the cranial nerve territory [14].

4.7. Brainstem reflexes

The absence of all brain stem reflexes must be confirmed by the physical examination. Afferent and efferent pathways of cranial nerves are given in parentheses:

- *Oculomotor reflex (afferent II, efferent III).* Pupils must be >4mm up to 9 mm with absent pupillary response to bright light in both eyes. Fixed midsized or fully dilated pupils are common. In cases of uncertainty, a magnifying glass could be used. Interpret with caution pupil size less than 4 mm. Small constricted pupils should be suspected for drug intoxication [12, 14].

- *Corneal reflex (afferent V, efferent VII).* Special care should be taken not to damage the cornea during the examination. The absence of eyelid movements must be documented after touching the cornea with a cotton swab, a piece of gauze, paper, or water squirts.

- *Absence of facial or bulbar musculature movement in noxious stimulus (afferent V, efferent VII).* Deep pressure on the condyles at the level of the temporomandibular joints and deep pressure at the supraorbital ridge should produce no grimacing or facial muscle movement.

- *Oculovestibular reflex (caloric reflex, afferent VIII, efferent III, VI).* Check for patency of the external auditory canal with otoscopic examination. The eardrum should be visible, or it should be cleared before the test. Oculovestibular reflex is tested by irrigating each ear with ice water (caloric testing) after the head is elevated to 30° to place the horizontal semicircular canal in a horizontal position [14]. Each external auditory canal is irrigated (one ear at a time) with >10–50 ml of ice water. Movement of the eyes should be absent during 1 min of observation. Both sides are tested, with an interval of several minutes.

- *Oculocephalic reflex (eye doll reflex).* The same pathways as in the case of oculovestibular reflex are tested. Not required any more in AAP 2011 and ANZICS 2013 guidelines due to the fact that it is not considered strong enough stimuli to elicit a response and the risk of exacerbating possible cervical spinal trauma [14].

- *Gag reflex (afferent IX, efferent X).* The pharyngeal or gag reflex is tested after stimulation of the posterior pharynx using a tongue blade or suction device. The sucking and rooting reflexes are sought in neonates and infants [20].
- *Cough—tracheal reflex (afferent X).* The tracheal reflex is most reliably tested by examining the cough response to tracheal suctioning. The catheter should be inserted into the trachea and advanced to the level of the carina followed by one or two suctioning passes. The efferent limbs for this reflex are the phrenic nerve and the thoracic and abdominal musculature. Therefore, it cannot be assessed in patients with high cervical cord injury [12].

4.8. Apnea test

Only if all the above reflexes are absent, proceed with testing for apnea. The apnea test should be conducted last so that a high $PaCO_2$ does not confound the testing of the other cranial nerves [14]. Apnea testing is the cornerstone for the diagnosis of BD both in adults and children and is conducted similar to adults. However, despite the consensus criteria published for adults and pediatrics, considerable variation has been described in performing the apnea test in both populations [2, 21, 22, 29]. In 1987 Task Force guidelines for pediatric BD is reported that apnea testing using standardized methods can be performed, but this is ordinarily done only after other examination criteria are met. Yet, the standardized methods are not described and the two associated references reported different ways of performing the apnea test. The former, by Outwaker and Rockoff, described apnea testing in 10 children aged 10 months to 13 years who met the conventional criteria for BD. In their study, oxygen 100% was provided for 5 min before the test, the ventilator rate was set to zero, and a continuous flow of oxygen was provided through the ETT. Arterial blood gases (ABG) were drawn at 0, 1, 2, 3, and 5 min. All patients completed the test successfully; mean $PaCO_2$ was 39.4 ± 7.4 mm Hg at the beginning and 59.5 ± 10.2 at the end of the test, with a mean rise of 4.0 ± 0.9 mm Hg/min [30]. The latter, by Rowland and coworkers, in 9 children aged 4 months to 13 years, mentioned that PCO_2 rise was faster than adults, and faster in the beginning of apnea test (4.4 ± 1.6, 3.4 ± 1.3 and 2.6 ± 1.2 mm Hg/min at 5, 10, and 15 min, respectively). $PaCO_2$ ranged from 60 to 116 mm Hg after 15 min of apnea. All apnea tests were accomplished uneventfully and no spontaneous respirations were observed in any of the patients after 15 min of apnea. The authors recommended that prevention of hypoxia can be reliably achieved with administration of 100% oxygen for 10 min before discontinuing ventilator support, and continuing oxygen (6 l/min) through a catheter into the length of the ETT for the duration of the test. An initial apnea test of 10 min was proposed, and if the desired levels of PCO_2 failed to achieve, then a repeated test with a longer duration of 15 min was advised. The study concluded that apneic oxygenation can be safely conducted in children as a component of the clinical evaluation of BD [31].

The above studies performed apnea testing differently. Even in the recent guidelines, there are no accurate instructions on how to perform a safe apnea test in children. Questions such as how much time is necessary for the preoxygenation period, which is the optimum baseline PCO_2 level, which is the best way for apneic oxygenation, how to prevent hypoxia and/or hypotention during the apnea test, which is the exact duration of apnea testing, remain blurred and left to the resolution of the attending physician. Physicians should always remember that *apnea testing is the last element in clinical diagnosis of BD in suspected BD children*. There are references of prospective, retrospective studies, and case reports, in suspected BD children, mentioning that occasionally patients developed spontaneous breathing during apnea testing [2, 32–35]. These references not at all blunt the validity of apnea; on the contrary they confirm the value of the test on establishing pediatric BD. Not all parts of pediatric brain die simultaneously, especially in patients with preexisting neurologic disease. In cases that apnea is not positive for BD the patient is returned back to full support, until a following apnea test can be performed or an auxiliary test is pursued to establish or refute the diagnosis. It is worth mentioning that almost in all the aforementioned reports, most children died ultimately shortly afterwards, by a second apnea test that confirmed BD diagnosis or spontaneous cardiac arrest. One patient, who never fulfilled apnea testing, and therefore BD, remained in severe neurological impairment, keeping in life technology dependent, through tracheostomy, home mechanical ventilation, and gastrostomy [34]. Brain recovery of children that met all adult BD criteria based on neurologic examination has not been confirmed so far. The apparent reversibility of brain death reported by some authors through spontaneous respirations during apnea testing is questionable; further review of these cases would reveal that those children could not had fulfilled strict brain death criteria by currently accepted medical standards. There is no documented case of a person who *fulfils the preconditions and criteria for brain death* ever subsequently developing any return of brain function [8, 14, 18, 20, 23].

4.9. Performing apnea testing

The rationale behind the apnea test is that an intense ventilator stimulus, such as hypercapnia/respiratory acidosis is needed, to stimulate respiratory drive centers in the medulla to start respiratory efforts. During this procedure, concomitant hypoxemia should be avoided by the administration of 100% O_2. The levels of PCO_2 sufficient to stimulate the respiratory drive (PCO_2 threshold) was set at 60 mm Hg, based on the study of Scafer and Caronna, which report that three comatose, apparently BD adults, started to breath at PCO_2 levels of 44–56 mmHg [36]. According to AAP 2011 guidelines, if no respiratory effort is observed from the initiation of the apnea test to the time the measured $PaCO_2$ is ≥60 and ≥20 mm Hg above the baseline, the apnea test is consistent with brain death. Patients with chronic respiratory disease and chronic hypercapnia may need a higher respiratory stimulus, and in this case, the limit of ≥20 mm Hg above baseline is more appropriate.

Apnea testing should not pose risk in the patients tested; it should be safe, accurate, and reproducible [29]. In the literature, there is evidence that approximately 10% of all apnea tests are aborted (12.5% in our study), mainly due to hypoxia and to a lesser degree due to hypotension [22]. A preparation period is necessary; a fluid bolus, e.g., R/L 20 ml/kg (iv), may be helpful in the case of volume depletion in the context of diabetes insipidus that may be present; and inotropes and vasopressors should be ready and connected in line, even if they are not needed before apnea testing. The effects of raised PCO_2 levels in the circulatory system can vary. There could be an increase in heart rate and blood pressure due to sympathetic stimulation, or blood pressure may start falling due to the vasodilatation caused by the rising

PCO_2 levels and the myocardial depression caused by the acidosis; arterial line is necessary for a beat to beat evaluation of blood pressure and drug titration. Oxygenation is mostly maintained by the preoxygenation with 100% O_2 for 10 min, and through the apneic oxygenation during the test with the oxygen-diffusion technique, e.g., with tracheal insufflation of oxygen at a rate suitable for the age of the child (as described previously in our study). The catheter administrating oxygen should not be cut, the size should be appropriate to permit escaping for the excess oxygen through the ETT and prevent air trapping, and the oxygen rate should be appropriate; if these precautions are not met, there is a risk for inadvertent high oxygen pressures. Cases of barotrauma with pneumothoraces and/or pneumomediastinum have been described during apnea testing and should be avoided [37, 38]. In the case of hypoxia, CPAP could be applied through the application of the suitable valve in the T-piece. A Mapleson anesthesia bag attached to the ETT could also be used. There are reports of successfully performing the apnea test through a T-piece attached to the ET only; however, a question is arising if oxygen flowing simply at the end of ETT is capable of reaching the trachea to diffuse in the alveoli. Accomplishing apnea testing with the patient connected to ventilator should be avoided because all modern ventilators have built in apnea back up modes that do not allow zeroing the respiratory rate for a long time. Moreover, cardiac beating could trigger the ventilator if strong enough, and a false indication of spontaneous respiratory effort may appear. Maintenance of the homeostasis is of paramount importance for the safe and successful performance of the apnea test:

- Regular arterial blood gas (ABG) analysis should ensure normalization of the pH and $PaCO_2$; maintenance of core temperature above 35°C and normotension for age should be confirmed, even through dose adjustment of inotropic and vasopressor agents. Still in hemodynamic stable patients before the test, these drugs should be ready and connected to line for immediate hemodynamic support, in case hypotension occurs.

- Preoxygenation using 100% oxygen, aiming at nitrogen removal and oxygen enrichment, should be applied for at least 10 min [12]. Mechanical ventilation parameters could be modified as well at the same time, it is advisable to keep tidal volume and PEEP at the same level to avoid derecruitment and decrease only the respiratory rate aimed at eucapnia with baseline PCO_2 level of 35–45 mm Hg. This could facilitate the rise in $PaCO_2$ to the desired levels for a positive apnea testing [11, 12, 14].

- Intermittent mandatory mechanical ventilation is discontinued once the patient is well oxygenated and a normal $PaCO_2$ around 40 mm Hg has been achieved. Oxygenation should be accomplished with the apneic oxygenation method through the ETT as described earlier. The patient could also be changed to a T-piece attached to the ETT, or a self-inflating bag such as a Mapleson circuit connected to the ETT, or CPAP in cases of hypoxemia.

- Cardiac beating, blood pressure, and oxygen saturation should be continuously monitored while observing carefully for spontaneous respiratory effort (any respiratory muscle activity that results in abdominal or chest excursions or activity of accessory respiratory muscles) throughout the entire procedure [14].

- If the patient is well oxygenated ($SpO_2 > 85\%$) and hemodynamic stable, keep apnea duration to 10 min and then draw ABG for analysis. The longer the apnea times the more the possibilities for a positive apnea test. AAP 2011 guidelines suggest serial follow up ABG to monitor the rise in $PaCO_2$ while the patient remains disconnected from mechanical ventilation [20].

- Apnea test is consistent with brain death if no respiratory effort is observed for 10 min or the time (if earlier) that values of measured $PaCO_2$ ≥60 and ≥20 mm Hg above the baseline level are achieved. The patient should be placed back on mechanical ventilator support and medical management should continue until the confirmation of BD is completed by the second neurologic examination and the second apnea test.
- If oxygen saturations fall below 85% or hemodynamic instability limits completion of apnea testing draw ABG at this time, discontinue the test and return the patient to ventilator and full support. If $PaCO_2$ level of ≥60 and ≥20 mm Hg above the baseline has not been achieved at that time, another attempt to test for apnea may be performed at a later time, or an ancillary study may be pursued to assist with determination of brain death.
- Observation of any respiratory effort is inconsistent with brain death and the apnea test should be aborted.
- Use of a capnograph to detect spontaneous respirations through end tidal $EtCO_2$ fluctuations is desirable.

4.10. Inability to perform elements of clinical examination and/or apnea

Clinical neurological examination and/or apnea test cannot be performed under some circumstances, especially during trauma. Ocular trauma, severe maxilofascial injuries, skull base fractures that are running through the external ear canal, and ear drum rupture limit the ability to perform and evaluate many of the brainstem reflexes. Cervical spinal trauma with possible participation of phrenic nerve limits the spontaneous breathing ability during apnea testing. Flaccid tone in patients with high spinal cord injury or neuromuscular diseases poses further concerns about the validity of clinical examination.

Furthermore, apnea testing cannot be performed in cases of severe hypoxia, e.g., in ARDS patients even under CPAP conditions, and/or in patients with severe hemodynamic instability. When concerns about the potentials and validity of elements of clinical examination and/or apnea testing are arisen, then continued observation is recommended. A valid neurologic evaluation and apnea test could be performed at a later time, as soon as all issues are resolved. If this is not possible, then an ancillary study is indicated to establish BD diagnosis.

4.11. Ancillary studies

The 2011 AAP BD guidelines recommends that ancillary studies (electroencephalogram and radionuclide cerebral blood flow) are not required to establish brain death and are not a substitute for the neurologic examination. The term "ancillary study" is preferred to "confirmatory study" since these tests assist the clinician in making the clinical diagnosis of brain death. Ancillary studies are not common in places where the DNC concept, as the death of the brainstem, is accepted; on the contrary they are more common where the whole concept of BD, including the death of the brainstem, is acknowledged. Nevertheless, apart the above mentioned reasons that question the potential and safety of clinical examination, ancillary studies are sought also in suspected drug intoxication and to reduce the inter-examination observation period.

Before the use of ancillary studies, all the preconditions of BD that could be applied, and all parts of clinical examination, including apnea test, that could be performed, should be recorded. When an ancillary study supports the diagnosis of BD, a second clinical examination and apnea test must be done and components that can be completed must remain consistent with brain death. In this instance, the inter-examination observation interval may be shortened and the second clinical evaluation and apnea test (or all components that can be completed safely) can be performed and documented at any time thereafter for children of all ages [20].

4.11.1. EEG

Electroencephalograph (EEG) has been extensively studied in 485 suspected BD pediatric patients where signs of electrocerebral silence (ECS) were sought. In their first study, 76% of patients had ECS, which elevated to 89% in subsequent, if any, studies. Sixty-six patients had a second study that confirmed the ECS of the first study in 64/66 patients (97%). The two patients who showed EEG activity, in retrospect in depth analysis, would not have met the recent criteria for BD due to pharmacological agents present at the time of examination (a newborn with high phenobarbital levels of 30 μg/ml and a 5 years head trauma boy that received pentobarbital and pancuronium at the time of testing). In case that the first study showed EEG activity (85 patients), the second study showed ECS in 47/85 (55%) of patients. The rest 38/45 patients (45%), either did not have a second examination, or an ECG activity, as expected, were confirmed. It is worth mentioning that all the examined patients died (spontaneously or by withdrawal of support). Only one patient survived with severe neurological impairment from this entire group of 485 patients, the above-mentioned neonate with an elevated phenobarbital level, whose first EEG showed photic response [20].

4.11.2. CBF

Four-vessel cerebral angiography is the gold standard for determining the absence of cerebral blood flow (CBF). However, the technique is not always available, is very invasive and difficult to perform in young infants, and carry all the risk of transferring a potentially unstable patient outside the PICU. Thus, use of radionuclide CBF determinations to document the absence of CBF, with portable scanners where feasible, remains the most widely used methods to support the clinical diagnosis of brain death in infants and children. Evidence suggests that radionuclide CBF study can be used in patients with high dose barbiturate or other drugs therapy to demonstrate the absence of CBF. The classical appearance in a CBF scanning study positive for BD is the "hollow skull phenomenon" or "hot nose sign" due to the absence of circulation in the brain with relatively increased nasal region perfusion due to preserved external carotid artery flow [12, 20].

An extended study of CBF in 681 suspected BD patients showed that 86% of patients who met clinical BD criteria had absent CBF on first examination, a percentage that rose to 89% in case they had a following test. Among them, 26 patients had a second examination that confirm the absence of CBF in 24/26 patients (92%). The two exceptions with no flow in the first study that revealed some flow in the second study were two newborns. The first newborn had minimal flow on the second study and ventilator support was discontinued. The other newborn developed flow on the second study and had some spontaneous respirations and activity, and survived with severe neurologic impairment. Along with the 34 patients that had present flow in first study, 9/34 (26%) had no flow on the subsequent study, due to evolution to BD. The remaining 25/34 (74%) either had preserved flow or no further CBF studies were done, and all died (either spontaneously or by withdrawal of support). Interestingly, only one patient survived from this entire group (the one mentioned earlier) with severe neurologic deficit [20].

4.11.3. ECG versus CBF

There are 12 studies in the literature examining 149 suspected BD patients of any age with both initial EEG and CBF studies, which present special interest to compare one to another for their diagnostic yield. Data were stratified by three age groups: (i) all children ($n = 149$); (ii) newborns (<1 month of age, $n = 30$); and (iii) children aged >1 month to 18 years ($n = 119$). In the first EEG study, ECS was found in 70% in the whole cohort, 40% in newborns and 78% in older children. Similarly, the absence of flow in the first CBF study was documented in the same proportion in all age groups (70%), though performance was better in infants with absent flow in 63%, whereas in older children remained the same with absent flow in 71% of patients. Both studies were compatible with BD in 58% of all patients, only in 26% of newborns and 66% of older children. It seemed that for newborns, EEG with ECS was less sensitive (40%) than the absence of CBF (63%) when confirming the diagnosis of brain death, but even in the CBF group the yield was low. Performance was better for children older than 1 month of age and both of these ancillary studies remain accepted tests to assist with determination of brain death and are of similar confirmatory value. Radionuclide CBF techniques are increasingly being used in many institutions replacing EEG [20].

If the results of the ancillary study are equivocal, the patient cannot be pronounced BD. Observation under maximum supportive care is continued until a valid clinical examination and apnea testing is possible, or a subsequent ancillary study with definite results can be performed. A waiting period of 24 h is recommended before further radionuclide CBF study is performed, to allow for adequate clearance of Tc-99m. A waiting period of 24 h is reasonable and recommended before repeating EEG ancillary study as well.

There are reports of other newer ancillary studies performed in adults and children with suspected BD. Concerning the adult population, Transcranial Doppler is not included in adult AAN 2010 guidelines, whereas it is reported as a screening only test in ANZICS 2013 guidelines [12,14]. MRA angiography, CT angiography, somatosensory evoked potentials, and bispectral index are mentioned in adult 2010 guidelines but are not recommended due to insufficient evidence [12]. Correspondingly, pediatric AAP 2011 guidelines cannot recommend any of the above studies as ancillary studies to assist with the determination of BD in children [20].

4.12. Number of examinations

Two examinations, including apnea testing with each examination, separated by an observation period, are required. The examinations should be performed by different attending physicians involved in the care of the child, or as specified by national law. The first examination determines the child has met neurologic examination criteria for brain death. The second examination, performed by a different attending physician, confirms brain death, based on an unchanged and irreversible condition.

4.13. Number of examiners

According to AAP 2011 guidelines, two physicians (one each time) must perform two independent examinations separated by specific intervals. Apnea testing, as an objective test, could be performed by the same physician, preferably the attending physician who is managing ventilator care of the child. The committee recommends that these examinations be performed by different attending physicians involved in the care of the child. Physicians should have experience with neonates, infants, and children and have specific training in neurocritical care. They must be competent to perform the clinical examination and interpret results from ancillary studies. Pediatric intensivists and neonatologists, pediatric neurologists and neurosurgeons, pediatric trauma surgeons, and pediatric anesthesiologists with critical care training could serve as examiners for BD diagnosis in children. Adult specialists should have the appropriate neurologic and critical care training to diagnose brain death in children. Junior doctors, residents, and fellows should be encouraged to learn how to properly perform brain death testing by observing and participating in BD diagnosis performed by senior experienced attending physicians.

The exact number, specialty, and the required qualifications of the examiners vary according to national law; e.g., in Greece, three physicians (anesthetist, neurologist/neurosurgeon, and attending physician such as pediatrician/pediatric surgeon), who should be board registered for their specialty at least for 2 years, are required. The same panel of doctors is mandatory to perform the second examination at the set observation period. No one must be potentially involved in the organ donation and transplantation team.

4.14. Observation period

The recommended observation periods are as follows:

- 24 h for neonates (37 weeks gestation to term infants 30 days of age).
- 12 h for infants and children (>30 days to 18 years).

Observation period could be shortened in case of an ancillary study compatible with BD. On this occasion, the second neurologic examination and apnea test (or all components that can be completed safely) can be performed and documented at any time thereafter for children of all ages [20].

5. Special considerations for term newborns (37 weeks gestation to 30 days of age) by AAP 2011 guidelines

The younger the patient the greater the challenge of diagnosing BD in pediatric patients; the younger the patient the longer the observation period, unless clinical BD diagnosis is supported with ancillary studies whereas the observation period could be shortened [20]. Interestingly, the performances of ancillary studies which are supposed to help in the diagnosis are less accurate in very young infants. These reservations were recorded for the first time in AAP 1987 guidelines and are listed below for historical reasons [19]. Different diagnostic criteria were defined in those guidelines according three age categories starting from the 7th day of life; no recommendation was done then for neonates younger than 7 days of life due to insufficient data. Ancillary studies, especially EEG, were regarded an essential component of the diagnosis and were mandatory with different observation periods across age:

- Infants 7 days to 2 months: Two examinations and two EEG separated by at least 48 h.
- Children 2 months to 1 year: Two examinations and two EEG separated by at least 24 h. The second EEG was not necessary if a concomitant cerebral radionuclide scan or cerebral angiography demonstrated no flow or visualization of the cerebral arteries.
- Children older than 1 year: A shorter observation period of at least 12 h was recommended and ancillary testing was not required when an irreversible cause existed. However, with present ECS or absent CBF, the observation period in this age group could be further decreased.

In AAP 2011 guidelines, although some of the above precautions were revised, especially about the necessity of ancillary studies, there are still special considerations about the term newborns (37 weeks gestation to 30 days of life) in:

- *Clinical examination:* There is a concern about the maturation of brainstem reflexes on this age group and the difficulties arisen with the clinical examination. Therefore, a longer time of 24 h is recommended both before the initial evaluation for BD and for the observation period between tests. In cases of uncertainty, repeated clinical examinations are preferable to ancillary studies.
- *Apnea test:* Particularities of apnea testing in neonates are caused by the possibility that high oxygen pressures during preoxygenation may inhibit the potential stimulation of respiratory centers, and profound bradycardia may precede the gradual development of hypercapnia during apnea. The definition of a valid apnea test is the same as in older children.
- *Ancillary studies:* They are less sensitive in detecting brain electrical activity or cerebral blood flow than in older children. When both ancillary studies were conducted in 149 suspected BD neonates <1 month, absence of CBF (63%), although low, was more sensitive than demonstration of ECS (40%), which was even lower. Disparities were also recorded between studies; when the first examination showed ECS, the absence of CBF was confirmed in 66.7% of patients, while when the absence of flow was firstly recorded, ECS was present in only 42% of patients. Due to limitation of ancillary tests for this age, repeated clinical neurological examinations are indicated than relying on ancillary tests. However,

when ancillary tests are present and compatible with BD, the inter-examination interval could be shortened at the same way as happened to older children.

Similar recommendations for patients younger than 36 weeks to 1 month of age were issued by the ANZICS 2013 guidelines as well, stating that the initial evaluation for BD should defer for 48 h, with an interval of 24 h between the two tests [14].

6. Special considerations in patients younger than 2 months by RCCHD 2015 guidelines

Due to uncertainty about the validity of the 2008 AoMRC code of practice DNC criteria in young infants, in the UK, the RCCHD examined literature evidence for BD in very young patients from 37 weeks corrected gestation (postmenstrual) to 2 months postterm [18]. According to their guidelines, DNC is a clinical diagnosis with certain preconditions, and ancillary tests do not help in this diagnosis. They recommended that DNC for this age group should be made taking into account the following:

- *Preconditions:* The same preconditions are recommended as those detailed in the 2008 AoMRC code of practice and in the 1991 BPA report, with an additional prerequisite about the first clinical examination. Postasphyxiated infants or those receiving intensive care after resuscitation, having or not being treated with therapeutic hypothermia, should have a period of at least 24 h of observation. This observation period could be extended in the case of suspected residual drug-induced sedation.
- *Clinical diagnosis of DNC:* The same DNC clinical criteria are recommended as those used in the 2008 AoMRC code of practice for adults, children, and older infants, with special considerations on apnea. A stronger hypercarbic stimulus is used to establish respiratory unresponsiveness. Specifically, there should be a clear rise in $PaCO_2$ levels of >2.7 kPa (>20 mm Hg) *above a baseline of at least 5.3 kPa (40 mm Hg)* to >8.0 kPa (60 mm Hg) with no respiratory response at that level. Two clinical examinations are required with the same interval as in 2008 AoMRC code of practice.
- *Ancillary tests:* Ancillary tests were not found sufficiently robust to help confidently diagnose DNC in infants. They are required only in cases where a clinical diagnosis of DNC is not possible (for example because of extensive faciomaxillary injuries, or high cervical cord injury).
- *Examiners:* Two qualified pediatricians who have been registered for more than 5 years and are competent in the procedure are required. At least one should be a consultant. They should perform successfully two tests, including apnea.

7. Special considerations for premature newborns

Brainstem reflexes are not fully developed in premature babies, for example the pupillary response to light appears at 30 weeks, but is only consistently present at 32–35 weeks of gestation, and the central respiratory response to CO_2 is relatively poorly developed below 33 weeks of gestation. Due to the uncertainty surrounding this issue, there are not any international guidelines to address BD diagnosis in premature babies below 36–37 weeks postconceptual age [14, 20].

8. Declaration of death: documentation

Death is declared after the second neurologic examination and apnea test confirms an unchanged and irreversible condition. When there is a concern about the validity of the first clinical examination and ancillary studies are used, documentation of components from the second clinical examination that can be completed, including a second apnea test, must remain consistent with brain death. Documentation at each step of diagnosis is necessary, starting from the preconditions that should be met and finishing with the exact time of death, accompanied by the well written names and signatures of the responsible physicians. The use of a checklist provides standardized documentation to determine brain death ensuring that no step is missing and is highly recommended [20, 21, 24]. A checklist outlining essential examination and testing components is provided in Appendix 2.

The law, almost worldwide, recognizes that after DB declaration, preservation of technology-dependent life in modern ICUs is of no use, unless the patient is going to be an organ donor, whereas all the necessary actions should be undertaken. Time of clinical death after BD varies in different references according to national social, cultural, and religious preferences. In a preliminary announcement of our study, this time was approximately 2.74 days after the completion of the second apnea test, mainly attributed to the high emotional stress of the parents and the time needed by the family to accept the reality of BD for their children [39]. In one of the first relevant studies in children, it is reported that among 171 BD pediatric patients 47% had their ventilatory support withdrawn an average of 1.7 days after the diagnosis of BD, whereas in 46% support was continued until a cardiac arrest that happened an average of 22.7 days later [40]. The shorter period of 8.52 h is reported in Canada [2] and the longer period up to 4 years is recorded in Japan [7].

9. Parental support

The loss of a child is the most powerful emotional stress for a family. Moreover, there is evidence that parents cannot understand the concept of the brain death in a child that is apparently alive, connecting to ventilator with its heart beating. Good communication between the family and the medical team is necessary to make clear that, despite everything had been made for the recovery of their children, they will have a dismal outcome. The role of the bedside nurse who spent more time with the patients and the parents is fundamental in creating the trust to accept the reality of BD. From the very beginning of the admission of their child at the PICU, the parents should be fully informed of the disease, the treatments and the unfavorable prognosis. When parents are not well informed, they will take longer to understand the evolution to BD and accept the death of their child [7, 23].

Communication with families must be clear and concise, yet using a simple language without pompous medical terminology that they could not understand. Apart medical and nursing team, other medical workers could help families cope with the apparent death as well. The clerk and psychotherapists/psychologists may help them to take difficult end-of-life decisions and parents should be offered this possibility. The presence of family during the tests is questionable. Some families may find it helpful and relieving to see each diagnostic step and the complete loss of responsiveness, but a danger of severe emotional embarrassment lurks in case spinal reflexes are elicited [7]. The family must understand that after the confirmation of BD, their child meets legal criteria for death and continuation of medical therapies, including ventilator support, is no longer an option unless organ donation is planned [20].

10. Conclusions

Diagnosing BD in children is a challenging task and despite the existence of pediatric guidelines since 1987, great variation has been recorded. Strict adherence to published guidelines and medical standards for determining brain death is the minimum requirement for maintaining public trust. The neurological criteria, as outlined above, represent international practice in which the medical profession and the public can have complete confidence [16]. The use of checklist promotes the necessary documentation of each part of declaration of BD and is strongly recommended [2, 21, 24]. International guidelines should form a basis where national guidelines could be established, taking into account legal, ethical, cultural, and religious differences. Diagnosing BD is a medical duty and should be faced with the appropriate knowledge and responsibility.

Although it becomes more and more clear that BD is a clinical diagnosis, there are circumstances where ancillary studies are still necessary. Technology is rapidly evolving and newer methods assessing brain function are developed. Newer methods to assess CBF and neurophysiologic function comparing them to traditional ancillary studies is a forthcoming need, and they will be probably included in future guidelines to assist with determination of brain death in children. Additional information or studies are required to determine if a single neurologic examination is sufficient for neonates, infants, and children to determine brain death as currently recommended for adults over 18 years of age, by the 2010 AAN adult guidelines on BD [12, 20].

Appendices

Appendix 1. Brain death diagnosis algorithm (adapted from Ref. [20])

Appendix 2. Check list for determination of brain death (adapted from Ref. [20])

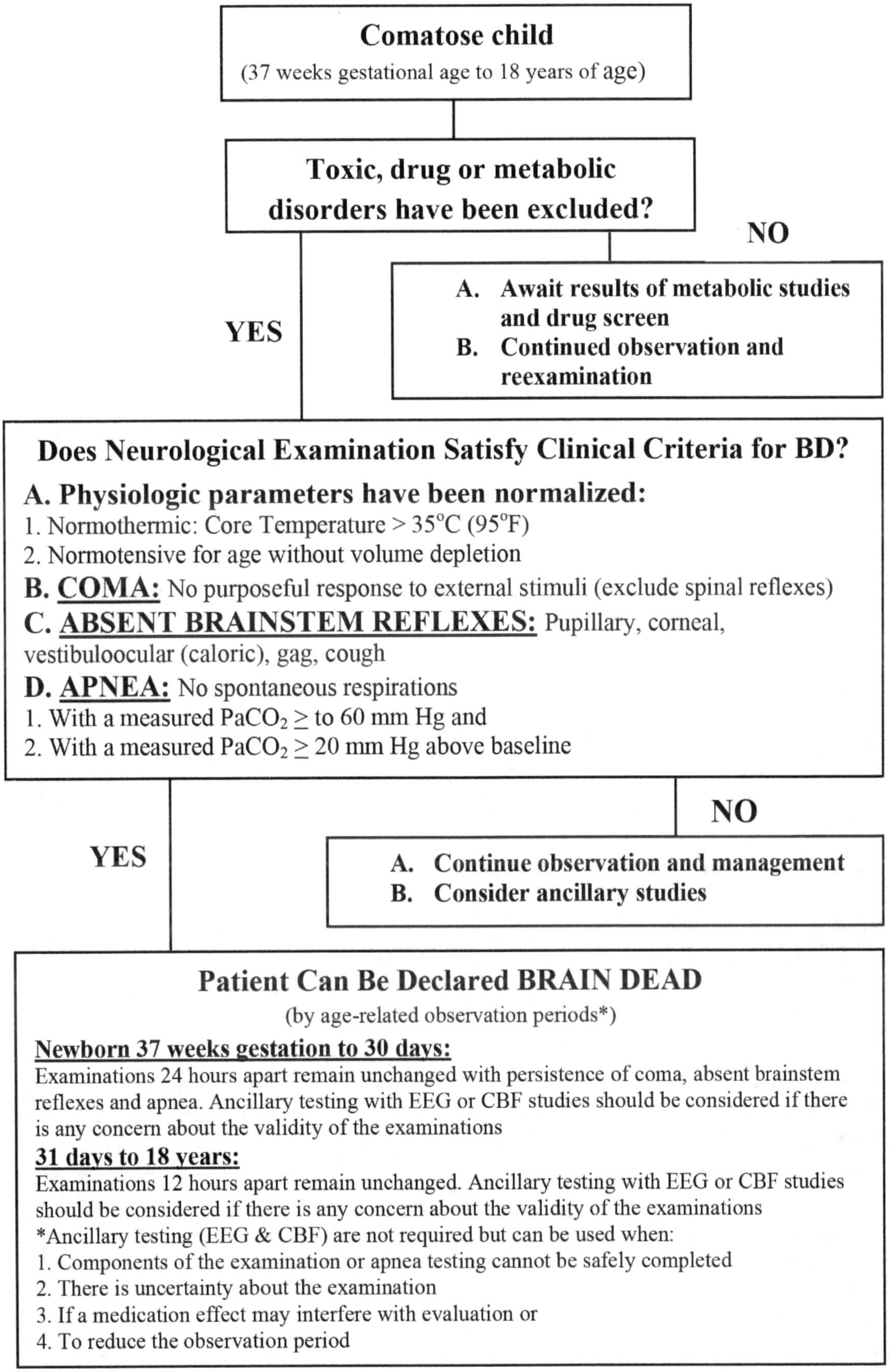
Comatose child
(37 weeks gestational age to 18 years of age)
Toxic, drug or metabolic disorders have been excluded?
NO
A. Await results of metabolic studies and drug screen
B. Continued observation and reexamination
YES
Does Neurological Examination Satisfy Clinical Criteria for BD?
A. Physiologic parameters have been normalized:
1. Normothermic: Core Temperature > 35°C (95°F)
2. Normotensive for age without volume depletion
B. COMA: No purposeful response to external stimuli (exclude spinal reflexes)
C. ABSENT BRAINSTEM REFLEXES: Pupillary, corneal, vestibuloocular (caloric), gag, cough
D. APNEA: No spontaneous respirations
1. With a measured $PaCO_2 \geq$ to 60 mm Hg and
2. With a measured $PaCO_2 \geq$ 20 mm Hg above baseline
NO
A. Continue observation and management
B. Consider ancillary studies
YES
Patient Can Be Declared BRAIN DEAD
(by age-related observation periods*)
Newborn 37 weeks gestation to 30 days:
Examinations 24 hours apart remain unchanged with persistence of coma, absent brainstem reflexes and apnea. Ancillary testing with EEG or CBF studies should be considered if there is any concern about the validity of the examinations
31 days to 18 years:
Examinations 12 hours apart remain unchanged. Ancillary testing with EEG or CBF studies should be considered if there is any concern about the validity of the examinations
*Ancillary testing (EEG & CBF) are not required but can be used when:
1. Components of the examination or apnea testing cannot be safely completed
2. There is uncertainty about the examination
3. If a medication effect may interfere with evaluation or
4. To reduce the observation period

Brain Death Examination for Infants and Children

Two physicians must perform independent examinations separated by specified intervals

Patient name and age	**Timing of first exam**	**Observation period**
Term newborn 37 wks gestational age and up to 30 days old	□ 24h after birth OR following CPR or SBI	□ At least 24h □ Shortened due to ancillary study consistent with BD
31 days to 18 years	□ 24h after CPR or SBI	□ At least 12h □ Shortened due to ancillary study consistent with BD

Section 1. PRECONDITIONS for brain death examinations and apnea test

A. IRREVERSIBLE AND IDENTIFIABLE CAUSE OF COMA

□Traumatic brain injury □Anoxic Brain injury □Known metabolic disorder □Other (specify)

B. CORRECTION OF CONTRIBUTING FACTORS	**Examination 1**		**Examination 2**	
a. Core Body Temperature > 35°C	□ Yes	□ No	□ Yes	□ No
b. Systolic blood pressure or MAP at acceptable range	□ Yes	□ No	□ Yes	□ No
c. Sedative /analgesic drugs excluded	□ Yes	□ No	□ Yes	□ No
d. Metabolic intoxication/abnormalities excluded	□ Yes	□ No	□ Yes	□ No
e. Neuromuscular/antiepileptic drugs excluded	□ Yes	□ No	□ Yes	□ No

□ *If ALL preconditions are marked YES, then proceed to the next section, OR*

□………………… *confounding variable was present. Ancillary study was performed to document BD.*

Section 2. PHYSICAL EXAMINATION ***Note: Spinal Cord Reflexes are Acceptable***	**Examination 1** **Date/time:**		**Examination 2** **Date/time:**	
a. Flaccid tone, unresponsive to deep painful stimuli	□ Yes	□ No	□ Yes	□ No
b. Pupils are midpositioned or fully dilated and non reactive	□ Yes	□ No	□ Yes	□ No
c. Corneal, cough, gag reflexes absent	□ Yes	□ No	□ Yes	□ No
Sucking and rooting reflexes absent (infants/neonates)	□ Yes	□ No	□ Yes	□ No
d. Oculovestibular (caloric) reflexes absent	□ Yes	□ No	□ Yes	□ No
e. Spontaneous respirations on ventilator absent	□ Yes	□ No	□ Yes	□ No

The …………………(specify) element could not be performed because of…………………………

□ *Ancillary study (EEG or radionuclide CBF) was therefore performed to document BD.*

Section 3. APNEA TEST *Aim to baseline eucapnia $PaCO_2 \geq 40$ mm Hg*	**Examination 1** **Date/Time:**	**Examination 2** **Date/Time:**
No spontaneous respiratory efforts were observed despite final $PaCO_2 \geq 60$ mm Hg and a ≥ 20 mm Hg increase above baseline (examinations 1 & 2)	Pretest $PaCO_2$: Apnea (min): Pretest $PaCO_2$:	Pretest $PaCO_2$: Apnea (min): Pretest $PaCO_2$:

Section 4. ANCILLARY TESTING	**Date/Time:**	
□ Elecroencephalogram (EEG) report documents electocerebral silence (ECS) OR	□ Yes	□ No
□ Cerebral Blood Flow (CBF) study report documents no cerebral perfusion	□ Yes	□ No

Section 5. Signatures

Examiner One

I certify that my examination is consistent with cessation of function of the brain and the brainstem. Confirmatory examination to follow.

(Printed Name)	(Signature)		
(Specialty)	(Lisence)	(Date mm/dd/yyyy)	(Time)

Examiner Two

□I certify that my examination □ and/or ancillary test report □confirms unchanged and irreversible cessation of function of the brain and the brainstem. **The patient is declared dead at this time.**

Date/Time of Death:

(Printed Name)	(Signature)		
(Specialty)	(Lisence)	(Date mm/dd/yyyy)	(Time)

CPR; Cardiopulmonary Resuiscitation, SBI; Severe Brain Injury

Author details

Eleni Athanasios Volakli*, Peristera-Eleni Mantzafleri, Serafeia Kalamitsou, Asimina Violaki, Elpis Chochliourou, Menelaos Svirkos, Athanasios Kasimis and Maria Sdougka

*Address all correspondence to: elenavolakli@gmail.com

Pediatric Intensive Care Unit, Hippokration General Hospital, Thessaloniki, Greece

References

[1] Swedish Committee on Defining Death. The Concept of Death. Summary. Stockholm: Swedish Ministry of Health and Social Affairs; 1984. p. 38

[2] Joffe AR, Shemie SD, Farrell C, Hutchison J, McCarthy-Tamblyn L. Brain death in Canadian PICUs: Demographics, timing, and irreversibility. Pediatric Critical Care Medicine. 2013;**14**:1-9

[3] Burns PJ, Sellers ED, Meyer CE, Lewis-Newby S, Truog RD. Epidemiology of death in the pediatric intensive care unit at five U.S. teaching hospitals. Critical Care Medicine. 2014;**42**(9):2101-2108

[4] Lee KJ, Tieves K, Scanlon CM. Alterations in end-of-life support in the pediatric intensive care unit. Pediatrics. 2010;**126**:e859-e864

[5] Volakli AE, Chochliourou E, Dimitriadou M, Violaki A, Mantzafleri P, Samkinidou E, et al. Death analysis in pediatric intensive care patients. Critical Care. 2016;**20**(Suppl 2):P451

[6] Spanish Society of Intensive and Critical Care and Units Coronary. Transplants: Percentage of Patients Diagnosed with Brain Death. NQMC:008518; 2011 March. Available from: http://www.qualitymeasures.ahrq.gov/summaries/summary/43713/...[Accessed: November 10, 2016]

[7] Shemie SD, Pollack MM, Morioka M, Bonner S. Diagnosis of brain death in children. The Lancet Neurology. 2007;**6**(1):87-92

[8] Koszer S, Moshe LS, Kao A, Riviello JJ. Determination of Brain Death in Children [Internet]. Available from: http://www.emedicine.medscape.com/article/1177999-Updated Oct 5, 2016. [Accessed: November 10, 2016]

[9] Ad Hoc Committee of the Harvard Medical School. A definition of irreversible coma. Report of the Ad Hoc Committee of the Harvard Medical School to examine the definition of brain death. The Journal of the American Medical Association. 1968;**205**(6):337-340

[10] President's Commission. Guidelines for the determination of death. Report of the medical consultants on the diagnosis of death to the President's commission for the study of ethical problems in medicine and biomedical and behavioral research. The Journal of the American Medical Association. 1981;**246**(19):2184-2186

[11] Wijdicks FME. Determining brain death in adults. Neurology. 1995;**45**:1003-1011

[12] Wijdicks EFM, Varelas NP, Gronseth SG, Greer MD. Evidence-based guideline update: Determining brain death in adults. Neurology. 2010;**74**:1911-1918

[13] Academy of Medical Royal Colleges. A Code of Practice for the Diagnosis and Confirmation of Death [Internet]. 2008. Available from: http://www.aomrc.org.uk/doc_details/42-a-code-ofpractice-for-the-diagnosis-and-confirmation-of-death [Accessed: January 20, 2017]

[14] Australian and New Zealand Intensive Care Society. The ANZICS Statement on Death and Organ Donation (Edition 3.2). Melbourne: ANZICS; 2013

[15] Shemie SD, Ross H, Pagliarello J, et al. Brain arrest: The neurological determination of death and organ donor management in Canada: Organ donor management in Canada: Recommendations of the forum on medical management to optimize donor organ potential. Canadian Medical Association Journal. 2006;**174**:S13

[16] Gardiner D, Shemie S, Manar A, Opdam H. International perspective on the diagnosis of death. British Journal of Anaesthesia. 2012;**108**(S1):i14-i28. DOI: 10.1093/bja/aer397

[17] British Paediatric Association. Diagnosis of brain stem death in children. A Working Party Report; 1991

[18] Marikar D. The diagnosis of death by neurological criteria in infants less than 2 months old: RCPCH guideline 2015. Archives of Disease in Childhood Education and Practice Edition. 2016;**101**(4):186. DOI: 10.1136/archdischild-2015-309706. Epub 2016 Mar 9

[19] Task Force for the Determination of Brain Death in Children. Guidelines for the determination of brain death in children. Task force for the determination of brain death in children. Archives of Neurology. 1987;**44**(6):587-588

[20] Thomas A. Nakagawa, Stephen Ashwal, Mudit Mathur, Mohan Mysore, and the society of critical care medicine, section on critical care and section on neurology of the american academy of pediatrics, and the child neurology society. Clinical report—Guidelines for the determination of brain death in infants and children: An update of the 1987 Task Force recommendations. Pediatrics. 2011;**128**:e720-e740

[21] Mathur M, Petersen LC, Stadtler M, Rose C, Ejike JC, Petersen F, et al. Variability in pediatric brain death determination and documentation in Southern California. Pediatrics. 2008;**121**:988

[22] Wijdicks EFM, Rabinstein AA, Manno ME, et al. Pronouncing brain death: Contemporary practice and safety of the apnea test. Neurology. 2008;**71**:1240

[23] Paul B. Diagnosis and management of brain death in children. Current Paediatrics. 2005;**15**:301-307

[24] Shore PM. Following guidelines for brain death examinations: A matter of trust. Pediatric Critical Care Medicine. 2013;**14**:98-99. DOI: 10.1097/PCC.0b013e31826775bb

[25] Zielinski PB. Brain death, the pediatric patient, and the nurse. Pediatric Nursing. 2011; **37**(1):17-21

[26] Kochanek PM, Carney N, Adelson PD, et al. American Academy of Pediatrics-Section on Neurological Surgery; American Association of Neurological Surgeons/Congress of Neurological Surgeons; Child Neurology Society; European Society of Pediatric and Neonatal Intensive Care; Neurocritical Care Society; Pediatric Neurocritical Care Research Group; Society of Critical Care Medicine; Paediatric Intensive Care Society UK; Society for Neuroscience in Anesthesiology and Critical Care; World Federation of Pediatric Intensive and Critical Care Societies. Guidelines for the acute medical management of severe traumatic brain injury in infants, children, and adolescents. Pediatric Critical Care Medicine. 2012;**13** Suppl 1:S1-S82. DOI: 10.1097/PCC.0b013e31823f437e

[27] Practical procedures: Airway and breathing. In: Samuels M, Wieteska S, editors. Advanced Pediatric Life Support. 5th ed. Wiley-Blackwell, Atrium, Southern Gate, Chichester, West Sussex, UK; 2010. pp. 210-211

[28] La Mancusa J, Cooper R, Vieth R, Wright F. The effects of the falling therapeutic and sub-therapeutic barbiturate blood levels on electrocerebral silence in clinically brain-dead children. Clinical Electroencephalography. 1991;**22**(2):112-117

[29] JScott JB, Gentile AM, Bennett NS, Couture MA, MacIntyre RN. Apnea testing during Brain Death Assessment: A review of clinical practice and published literature. Respiratory Care. 2013;**58**(3):532-538

[30] Outwaker KM, Rockoff MA. Apnea testing to confirm brain death in children. Critical Care Medicine. 1984;**12**(4):357-358

[31] Rowland TW, Donnelly JH, Jackson AH. Apnea documentation for determination of brain death in children. Pediatrics. 1984;**74**(4):505-508

[32] Riviello JJ, Sapin JI, Brown LW, et al. Hypoxemia and hemodynamic changes during the hypercarbia stimulation test. Pediatric Neurology. 1988;**4**(4):213-218

[33] Paret G, Barzilay Z. Apnea testing in suspected brain dead children: Physiological and mathematical modeling. Intensive Care Medicine. 1995;**21**(3):247-252

[34] Vardis R, Pollack MM. Altered apnea threshold in a pediatric patient with suspected brain death. Critical Care Medicine. 1998;**26**(11):1917-1919

[35] Brilli RJ, Bigos D. Threshold in a child with suspected brain death. Journal of Child Neurology. 1995;**10**(3):245-246

[36] Schafer JA, Caronna JJ. Duration of apnea needed to confirm brain death. Neurology. 1978;**28**:661

[37] Bar-Joseph G, Bar-Lavie Y, Zonis Z. Tension pneumothorax during apnea testing for the determination of brain death. Anesthesiology. 1998;**89**(5):1250-1251

[38] Burns JD, Russell JA. Tension pneumothorax complicating apnea testing during brain death evaluation. Journal of Clinical Neuroscience. 2008;**15**(5):580-582

[39] Mantzafleri PE, Volakli E, Violakli A, Chochliourou E, Svirkos M, Kasimis A, et al. Incidence and management of brain death in a Greek PICU. European Journal of Pediatrics. 2016;**175**(11):1393-1880:E-poster 1105

[40] Ashwal S, Schneider S. Brain death in children: Part I. Pediatric Neurology. 1987;**3**(1):5-11

10

Severe Acute Pancreatitis and its Management

Arshad Chanda

Abstract

Severe acute pancreatitis (SAP) is a severe form of acute pancreatitis, which requires often intensive care therapy. The common aetiology varies with geographic locations. In Middle East, biliary pancreatitis is the commonest type. Initial phase of the disease is due to profound release of the proinflammatory marker, then the organ dysfunction takes over. It mainly divided into three types depending upon the pathological changes that are oedematous, necrotic and haemorrhagic. The common clinical presentation is typical abdominal pain radiating to the back and relieved by typical positioning i.e. sitting or leaning forwards. Raised pancreatic amylase and lipase with imaging will help to diagnose the SAP. The outcome of SAP is dictated by various criteria and scores. The commonly used scoring systems are Ranson's and Glasgow scores, whereas the local complication is diagnosed and predicted by the Balthazar's score. The management of SAP is mainly analgesia, prevention of complications and supportive care. Initially, laparotomy was recommended routinely for SAP complicated by necrosis of the pancreas and continuous lavage, but nowadays, minimal invasive image guided drainage is the recommended modality. The most common complications of concern are the abdominal compartment syndrome, Acute respiratory distress syndrome (ARDS), and infection of the pancreatitis necrosis. SAP has a high mortality rate (up to 40%), but initial aggressive supportive management will improve the outcome.

Keywords: analgesia, Balthazar score, Glasgow score, image guided drainage, Ransom Score, severe acute pancreatitis

1. Introduction

Acute pancreatitis is an inflammatory condition of the pancreas with a wide spectrum of pathological and clinical manifestations. It ranges from mild and self-limiting condition to severe pancreatitis with multiorgan failure with high mortality [1, 2].

It was one of the most frequent gastrointestinal causes of hospital admissions in the United States with a total of 275,000 admissions in 2009. In the United Kingdom, hospitals serving a population of 300,000–400,000 people admit about 100 cases each year. Patients with severe acute pancreatitis need ICU admission and multidisciplinary team approach for treatment. It increases the health care cost enormously, and those survive will live with pancreatic endocrine and exocrine dysfunction.

This chapter will focus mainly on severe acute pancreatitis.

2. Definition

Acute pancreatitis is an acute inflammatory process of the pancreas. It is an acute condition presenting with abdominal pain and is usually associated with raised pancreatic enzyme levels in the blood or urine as a result of pancreatic inflammation. It is a disorder of the exocrine pancreas and is associated with acinar cell injury with local and systemic inflammatory responses [3].

3. Classification

There is a wide range of classifications for acute pancreatitis. The Revised Atlanta Classification in 2012 classified acute pancreatitis according to the severity of the disease, morphology and temporal relation [1, 3].

3.1. Classification according to the severity of pancreatitis

Acute pancreatitis is classified into three forms based on the severity [3].

1. Mild acute pancreatitis, which is characterized by the absence of organ failure and local or systemic complications.
2. Moderately severe acute pancreatitis, which is characterized by transient organ failure (resolves within 48 hours and without persistent organ failure >48 hours) and/or local or systemic complications.
3. Severe acute pancreatitis, which is characterized by persistent organ failure that may involve one or multiple organs.

3.2. Classification according to the phases of pancreatitis

Temporally, two phases of acute pancreatitis are as follows:

(i) Early-first week

Only clinical parameters are important for treatment planning and are determined by the systemic inflammatory response syndrome (SIRS), which can lead to organ failure.

(ii) Late-after the first week

Morphologic criteria based on CT findings combined with clinical parameters determine the care of the patient [4].

3.3. Classification according to the morphology of pancreatitis:

Morphologically, there are three types of acute pancreatitis as follows:

(i) Acute oedematous (interstitial) pancreatitis

(ii) Acute necrotizing pancreatitis

(iii) Haemorrhagic

Usually, the necrosis involves both the pancreas and the peripancreatic tissues, less commonly the peripancreatic tissues alone and rarely the pancreatic parenchyma alone [1].

The commonest cause in the western world is gallstones (50%) and alcohol (25%). Rare causes (<5%) include drugs (for example, valproate, steroids, and azathioprine), endoscopic retrograde cholangiopancreatography, hypertriglyceridaemia or lipoprotein lipase deficiency, hypercalcaemia, pancreas divisum and some viral infections (mumps and coxsackie B4). About 10% of patients have idiopathic pancreatitis, where no cause is found [5]. The aetiological factors are enumerated in **Table 1**.

Aetiology of Acute Pancreatitis	
Toxic Alcohol	Methyl alcohol Smoking Organophosphates Scorpion bite, certain spiders, Gila monster lizard
Mechanical obstruction/duct damage	Biliary pancreatitis—Cholelithiasis, Biliary sludge Malignancy—pancreatic, ampullary, cholangiocarcinoma Parasitic infections—ascariasis Periampullary diverticulum Penetrating duodenal ulcer, Duodenal obstruction
Trauma	Abdominal trauma—duct disruption
Metabolic	Hyperparathyroidism Hypertriglyceridemia Hypercalcaemia Diabetic ketoacidosis End-stage renal failure Pregnancy Post-renal transplant
Vascular	Necrotising vasculitis—SLE, Thrombotic thrombocytopenia Atheroma Shock
Immune-related—Auto-immune pancreatitis	Vasculitis—SLE, polyarteritis nodosa

Drugs	Corticosteroids, furosemide, tetracyclines, thiazides, oestrogen, valproic acid, Metronidazole, pentamidine, nitrofurantoin, erythromycin, methyldopa, ranitidine 5-ASA/salicylates, azathioprine/6-MP, didanosine, pentamidine, L-asparaginase
Infections	
Viral: Mumps, varicella-zoster, coxsackie, HSV, HIV	
Bacterial: Mycoplasma, Leptospira, Legionella	
Parasitic: Toxoplasma, cryptosporidium	
Fungal: As pergillus	
Miscellaneous/Idiopathic	Post-ERCP pancreatitis Pancreas divisum in some patients Ischaemia, hereditary pancreatitis is a rare familial condition

Table 1. Aetiology of acute pancreatitis.

4. Pathophysiology

The exact pathogenesis of acute pancreatitis is unknown, and there is an ongoing research at the molecular level. There are many pathophysiological hypothesis put forward to explain the processes. These hypotheses are based on the aetiology and risk factors. The final result of the pathophysiological process is activation of proteolytic enzymes (intra-acinar activation of trypsinogen) leading to breakdown of the junctional barrier between acinar cells and leakage of pancreatic fluid and enzymes into the interstitial space causing autophagy and autodigestion of acinar cells [2, 3]. **Diagram 1** depicts the hypothetical aetiopathogenic process of acute pancreatitis.

Three different phases can be seen during the pathogenesis of acute pancreatitis. The first phase is the acinar cell damage and death. The second phase is local inflammation of the pancreas. The third and final phase is the SIRS. The first two phases take place in the pancreas itself, while in the third phase causes the distant organ damage and extrapancreatic symptoms.

Pancreatic ductal obstruction and hypersecretion have been mentioned as factors that contribute to the initiation of the inflammatory process. Different pathophysiological mechanisms have been proposed for ethanol-induced pancreatitis. Explanations like ethanol-induced direct toxicity to the acinar cell, sphincter of Oddi dysfunction, hypertriglyceridaemia, free oxygen radical formation, and protein deposition within the pancreatic duct, which favours retrograde flow of enzymatic. These processes lead to activation of inflammation and membrane destruction. Newer hypotheses include ischaemia/reperfusion injury and enzymatic co-localisation. Post-endoscopic retrograde cholangiopancreatography (ERCP) pancreatitis: 1–3% develops pancreatitis, probably due duct disruption and enzyme extravasation. Patients at the risk of developing post-ERCP pancreatitis have sphincter of Oddi dysfunction or a history of recurrent pancreatitis, those who undergo sphincterotomy or balloon dilatation of the sphincter.

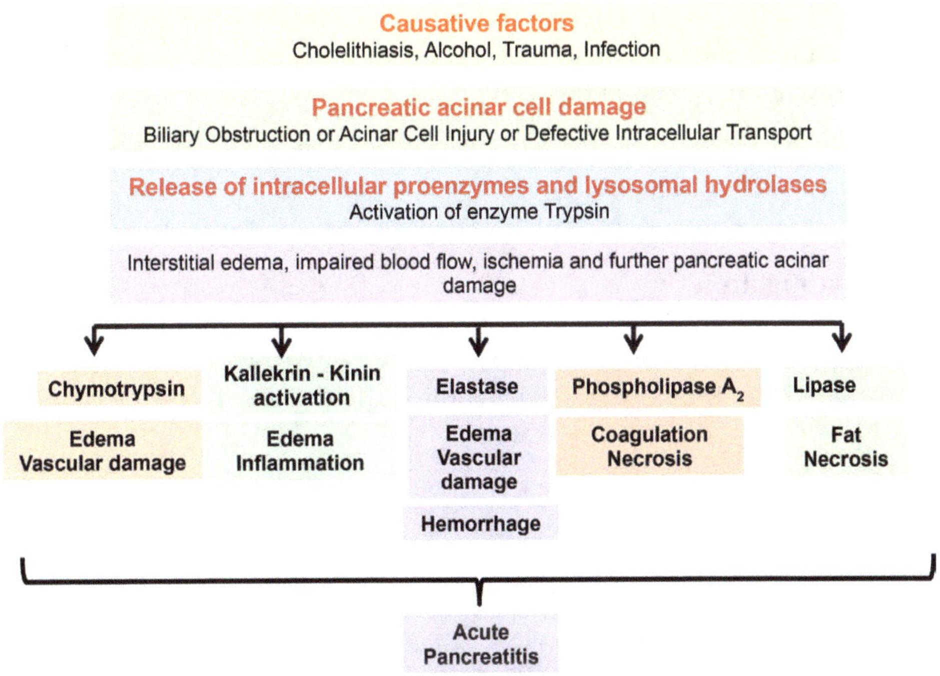

Diagram 1. Aetiopathogenesis of acute pancreatitis.

Systemic inflammatory response syndrome (SIRS) due to acute pancreatitis is because of the acinar cell death which releases activated pancreatic enzymes. This sets up a local inflammatory response which then activates systemic inflammatory response by release of cytokines, tumour necrosis factor, activation of immunocytes and the complement system activation [2–5].

5. Diagnosis of severe acute pancreatitis

5.1. Clinical presentation

Symptoms of acute pancreatitis are sudden onset of severe, persistent epigastric pain with or without radiation to the back. Radiation to the back is seen in about 50% of patients. It may be relieved by sitting or leaning forwards. Some patients complain of right upper quadrant pain. Pain is usually associated with nausea and vomiting.

5.2. Physical examination

Signs vary according to the severity of the disease. It ranges from mild epigastric tenderness to a diffusely tender abdomen.

Tachypnoea, tachycardia, and hypotension may be present. Fever due to inflammatory response. Acute swinging pyrexia suggests cholangitis. Icterus may be seen in biliary pancreatitis. Cullen sign, i.e. ecchymotic discoloration in the periumbilical area and Grey Turner sign, i.e. ecchymotic discoloration along the flanks due bleeding into the fascial planes, but these signs are not specific for acute pancreatitis. Abdominal distension due to ileus, guarding in the upper abdomen, free fluid may elicit shifting dullness. Pleural effusion is present in 10–20% of patients. Acute confusion due to metabolic derangement and hypoxaemia. Tetany is seen in some patient because hypocalcaemia [6, 7]

Perforated peptic ulcer, acute myocardial infarction, and cholecystitis should be rule out in differential diagnoses for acute pancreatitis.

5.3. Laboratory investigation

Serum amylase and lipase are both elevated in acute pancreatitis. The rise can be within 4–12 hours. The rise of >3 times the normal upper limit is the threshold for the diagnosis of acute pancreatitis [6, 7].

5.3.1. Serum amylase

It is an enzyme that hydrolyses the starch. The principal sources of amylase are the pancreas, salivary glands and fallopian tubes. Amylase has a shorter half life of 10 hours and returns to normal within 3–5 days. Hyperamylasaemia is seen in many other conditions. It may be increased in a number of other conditions like intestinal ischaemia and perforation, parotitis and acute renal failure, it is a less specific marker in acute pancreatitis. Its levels begin to rise 6–12 hours after the onset of acute pancreatitis, and they return to normal in 3–5 days. It has a high sensitivity (>90%) but a low specificity (as low as 70%) for the diagnosis of acute pancreatitis. Normal serum amylase level will not exclude acute pancreatitis if the patients present late to hospital [1, 6, 7].

5.3.2. Serum lipase

It a pancreatic enzyme that hydrolyses triglycerides. Its level increases within 4–8 hours of the onset and peaks at 24 hours and then returns to normal after 8–14 days. The rise in levels should be >3 times the upper limit of normal. It has excellent sensitivity in acute alcoholic pancreatitis. It is more specific than serum amylase for the diagnosis of acute pancreatitis. It has a sensitivity and specificity of 80–100% for acute pancreatitis. The principal sources of lipase are pancreas. The other sources are the tongue, liver, and intestine. These enzymes are useful in diagnosis of acute pancreatitis, but daily levels of these enzymes add no advantage in management. The levels are not useful in assessment of the severity of pancreatitis or decreasing levels are not marker of improvement. Simultaneous estimation of amylase and lipase levels does not improve accuracy [1, 6, 7].

5.3.3. Other lab data

In other laboratory investigations which help in etiological diagnosis are liver function test and serum triglycerides. Elevated liver enzymes, especially levels alanine transaminase Alanine Aminotransferase (ALT), level >150 U/L, it has a positive predictive value of 85% for gallstones. It will aid in diagnosis of acute biliary pancreatitis. Liver Function Test (LFT) should be done in all patients acute pancreatitis, patients within 24 hours of admission. C reactive Protein (CRP) levels will help in assessment of the severity of the disease process [5–7].

5.3.4. *Imaging*

The most commonly used imaging modalities in acute pancreatitis are transabdominal ultrasound, endoscopic ultrasound, dynamic contrast enhanced CT scan and Magnetic Resonance Cholangiopancreatography (MRCP). Imaging studies are not indicated for diagnosing acute pancreatitis as it does not predict disease severity at the time of presentation to emergency department. Imaging studies are indicated when there is diagnostic dilemma due to non-conclusive biochemical tests or because of the severity clinical condition or unexplained MODS, which warrants to rule out other intra-abdominal pathologies like gastrointestinal tract perforation and peritonitis.

It also helps in rule out other conditions during the differential diagnosis of acute pancreatitis. The role of CT scan and magnetic resonance imaging (MRI) lies in the detection of complications of acute pancreatitis, such as pancreatic necrosis, peripancreatic fluid collections or pseudocysts; the presence of these complications can also be used to predict the severity of the disease [6].

5.3.5. *Ultrasonography*

5.3.5.1. *Transabdominal ultrasound*

Transabdominal ultrasound is less sensitive and less useful to visualize the inflamed or necrotic pancreas. The distended abdomen because of the gas-filled bowel obscures the pancreatic view. It cannot assess the extent of necrosis.

It helps in detection of gall stones, which are found in about 50% patients with acute pancreatitis or dilatation of biliary tract secondary to obstruction.

Only indication of US scanning abdomen on presentation to emergency department is to rule out cholelithiasis as a cause for pancreatitis. Transabdominal ultrasound in later stages can help diagnosis of infection and therapeutic intervention-like guiding aspiration [6, 7].

5.3.5.2. *Endoscopic ultrasonography*

It is a combination of ultrasonography and endoscopic simultaneously. It is comparatively less invasive than endoscopic retrograde cholangiopancreatography (ERCP). It has a high sensitivity when compared to transabdominal ultrasound, especially in detecting the common bile duct microlithiasis and biliary sludge. It has a diagnostic yield of up to 88%. It helps in identifying patients who might benefit from endoscopic retrograde cholangiopancreatography and its therapeutic interventions. The added advantage of endoscopic ultrasonography is that it can be performed beside in unstable ICU patients, pregnant women where CT is contraindicated, and patients with metallic implants where MRCP is contraindicated [6, 7].

5.3.5.3. *CT scan*

Contrast-enhanced computed tomography is the gold standard to detect necrosis and to grade the severity of acute pancreatitis. This imaging modality also helps detecting local complication. CT scan findings range from localized oedema, pancreatic tissue inflammation (**Figure 1**), necrosis to extensive peripancreatic fluid collections (**Figure 2**).

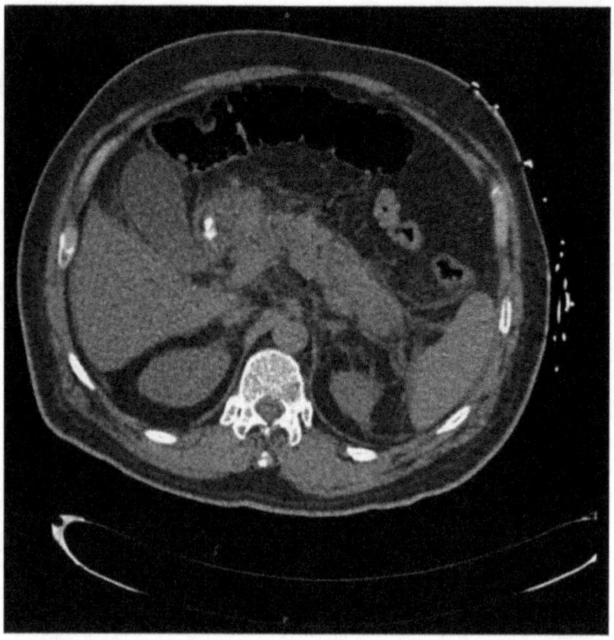

Figure 1. Oedematous pancreatitis.

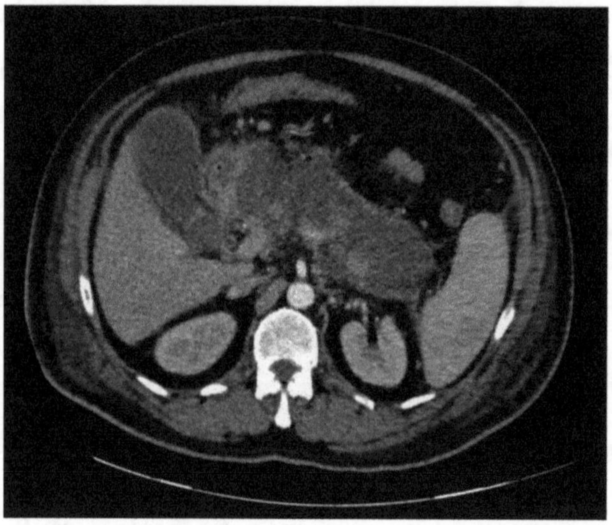

Figure 2. Pancreatitic necrosis.

CT findings of acute pancreatitis are diffuse or segmental enlargement of the pancreas due to interstitial oedema and irregular contour. Contrast non-enhancement represents pancreatic necrosis which is heterogeneous in appearance, peripancreatic fluid collection. Whole pancreatic necrosis is rare, multifocal areas are common. Necrosis is seen seen after 96 hours from the start of symptoms. CT scan performed before 72 hours will underestimate the degree of necrosis. The necrosis pancreas is variable involving the periphery with preservation of the core or involving the head, body, or tail separately or in combination. The outcome depends on the part of the pancreas involved. Necrosis of the entire pancreas has a relatively better outcome when compared to the head of pancreas involvement. Necrosis of the head of pancreas causes obstruction of the pancreatic duct there by an increase in pancreatic duct pressure causing to damage to acinar cells and leakage of destructive enzymes. Necrosis only in the distal portion of the pancreas has a favourable outcome and fewer complications [8]. **Figure 2** shows the CT image of pancreatic necrosis.

5.3.5.4. Efficacious use of computed tomography scanning in suspected acute pancreatitis

- **(i)** Patients in whom the clinical diagnosis is in doubt
- **(ii)** Patients with hyperamylasaemia and severe clinical pancreatitis **Figure 3** abdominal distension, tenderness, high fever (>39°C), and leucocytosis
- **(iii)** Patients with Ranson's score >3 or the acute physiology and chronic health evaluation (APACHE) II >8
- **(iv)** Patients showing lack of improvement after 72 hours of initial therapy,
- **(v)** Acute deterioration following the initial clinical improvement [8].

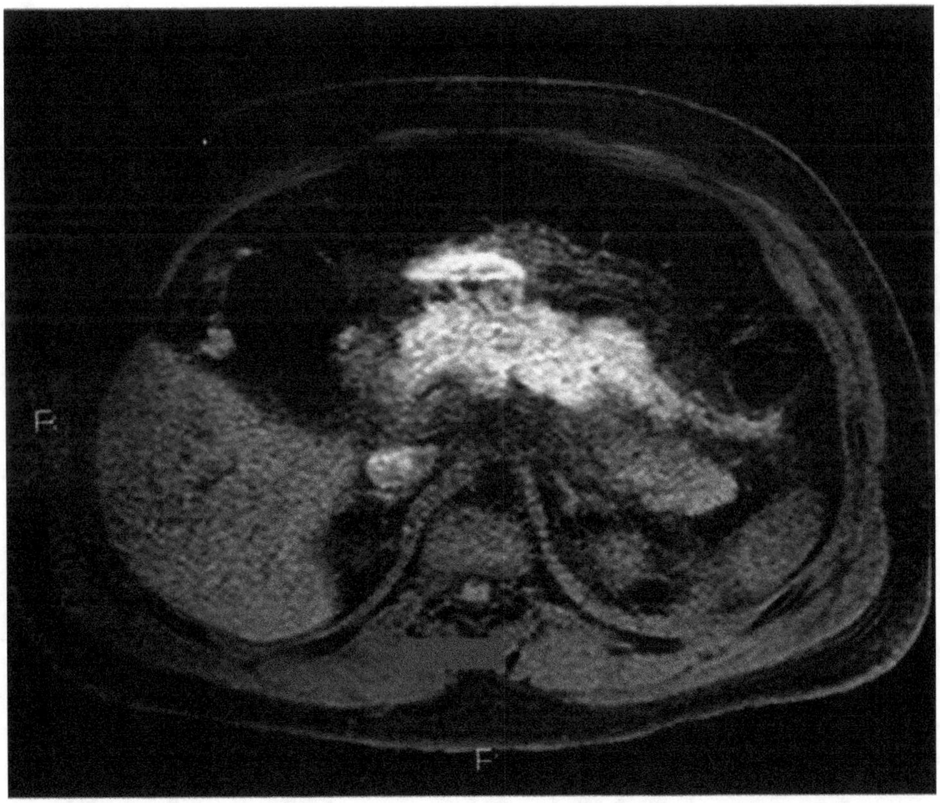

Figure 3. Haemorrhagic pancreatitis.

5.3.5.5. CT severity index

The modified CT severity index is a modification of the original CT severity index developed by Balthazar and colleagues in 1994. **Table 2** enumerates the details of the evaluation of Balthazar's computed tomography scoring system for acute pancreatitis.

The two factors that are useful in grading the severity of pancreatitis by CT are the extent pancreatic necrosis and the degree of peripancreatic inflammation. CT finding of necrosis and peripancreatic fluid collection strongly correlates with the complications (morbidity) and mortality [6, 7, 9, 10].

5.3.5.6. Grades of peripancreatic inflammation

(a) Normal pancreas

(b) Focal or diffuse pancreatic enlargement

(c) Pancreatic gland abnormalities associated with peripancreatic inflammation

(d) Single fluid collection

(e) Two or more fluid collections and/or gas present in or adjacent to the pancreas [10].

Inflammatory process	Grade	score
Normal	A	0
Focal or diffuse enlargement	B	1
Contour irregularity		
Inhomogeneous attenuation		
Grade B plus peripancreatic haziness/ Mottled densities	C	2
Grade B, C plus one ill-defined peripancreatic fluid collection	D	3
Grade B, C plus two ill-defined peripancreatic fluid collection or gas	E	4
Necrosis		
None	0	0
<30%	0	2
50%		4
>50%		6

Notes: Total score: Total points are given out of 10 to determine the grade of pancreatitis and aid treatment:
0–2: mild
4–6: moderate
8–10: severe.

Table 2. Evaluation of Balthzar's computed tomography scoring system for acute pancreatitis.

Repeat scanning is only indicated if there is any deterioration in clinical condition to rule out/ diagnose pancreatic necrosis, abscess or pseudocyst, haemorrhage, or bowel ischaemia or perforation.

5.3.5.7. Magnetic resonance imaging (MRI)

Magnetic resonance imaging (MRI) and MRCP are non-invasive imaging modalities. It has several advantages over CT, like no risk from radiation, can detect pancreatic duct continuity and parenchymal changes. It helps diagnose acute pancreatitis and identifying the aetiology of acute pancreatitis. MRI can accurately differentiate between necrotic and non-necrotic tissue.

5.3.5.8. Magnetic resonance cholangiopancreatography

It is especially useful to visualising the pancreatic duct and detecting lithiasis. MRCP is performed when ERCP has failed. The advantage of MRCP over CT scan is that iodinated contrast agents can be avoided and thereby avoid the risk for acute kidney injury.

Disadvantages of MRI and MRCP is transportation of critically ill patients to the MRI suite are limited access to patient during the acquisition of images and longer time to complete the study.

6. Assessment of severity

6.1. Why to assess the severity of the acute pancreatitis

1. To classify the disease process.
2. To predict the level of care needed, ICU or HDU for monitoring and supportive care.
3. To predict the outcome depending the severity of the acute pancreatitis, especially the mortality.
4. Select patients for specialised interventions as therapy to improve the outcome.
5. If patients are managed by the nonspecialist clinicians, then the scoring system will help them identify patients who need consultation and transfer to specialist centre.
6. For comparisons of severity within and between patient series.
7. In research for rational selection of patients for inclusion in trials.
8. It helps in intra-, inter-departmental and patient and patient family communication—using the same language.

Severity assessment should be carried out within 48 hours of diagnosis of acute pancreatitis. Patients with a body mass index over 30 are at higher risk of developing complications.

6.2. How to assess the severity of the acute pancreatitis

There are various scoring systems in vogue, using the clinical data, laboratory markers and radiological findings to assess and grade the severity of the acute pancreatitis. The scoring systems are of two types: one that correlates clinical features and lab indices and the other being the use of non-specific physiological scoring, namely, APACHE II and III. The commonly used scoring systems are the Ranson's criteria, Glasgow (Imrie) scoring systems, the APACHE II and III scoring systems (mainly used in ICU), the Simplified acute physiology score, bedside index of severity in acute pancreatitis (BISAP) scoring system, and the CT severity index. None of the scoring systems have a high sensitivity, specificity, positive predictive value or negative likelihood ratio. The scoring systems used at present are often inadequate in patients with severe Acute necrotizing pancreatitis (ANP), which is characterised by rapidly progressive multiple-system organ dysfunction [3, 4, 10].

6.3. Ranson's criteria

The Ranson's criteria were introduced in clinical practice in the early 1970s. It is the most widely used scoring system. Note that, 11 criteria are taken into account. **Table 3** enumerates the Ranson's criteria for assessment severity of acute pancreatitis. They were designed after analysis of 100 patients with alcohol-induced pancreatitis. It makes use of a combination of

Ranson's Criteria
Severity assessment
On admission
• Age > 55 years
• WBC > 16,000/μL
• Glucose > 11 (200 mg/dL)
• Lactate dehydrogenase (LDH) > 400 IU/dL
• AST > 250 IU/dL
After 48 hours
• Haematocrit fall > 10%
• Increase in urea > 1.8 mmol/L (>5 md/dL)
• Calcium < 2 mmol/L
• PaO_2 < 8 kPa (60 mmHg)
• Base deficit > 4 mmol/L
• Fluid deficit > 6 L
Risk factors mortality rate 0–2 < 1% 3–4 ≈ 15% 5–6 ≈ 40% >6 ≈ 100%

Table 3. Ranson's criteria for assessment severity of acute pancreatitis.

clinical and biochemical parameters obtained at admission and during the first 48 hours after admission. It reflects the extent of metabolic derangement and estimates the risk for mortality.

Drawbacks of the scoring system are that the study was only for alcoholic pancreatitis, do not take into consideration the ongoing treatment and predicts high mortality which is not the case in today's practice.

The Ranson's criteria have a sensitivity 74%, specificity 77%, positive predictive value 49% and negative predictive value 91% [3, 4, 10].

6.4. Modified Glasgow criteria (Imrie score)

A decade after the Ranson's criteria were introduced, a re-evaluation of those criteria was done and found that the eight of the criteria were most predictive of the severity and outcome. **Table 4** enumerates the modified Glasgow criteria (Imrie score) for assessment severity of acute pancreatitis.

Those eight criteria were renamed as Glasgow criteria or Imrie score. It's use is limited in Emergency department (ED) as some of the variables are only evaluated at 48 hours. The criteria excluded from the Ranson's criteria are Lactate dehydrogenase (LDH), base deficit, and fluid deficit, and these were found to be least contributory in assessment of severity and outcome [9, 10].

The Glasgow (Imrie) criteria are valid for both alcohol induced and biliary pancreatitis. A scores 3 or more after 48 hours of presentation indicates severe acute pancreatitis.

6.5. Other markers of severity

6.5.1. C-reactive protein

It is an acute phase reactant. It should be done after 48 hours of presentation. It can be used both for the assessment of severity and monitoring the progress of the disease. Levels more than 100 mg/L late in the first week after presentation indicate that patient is developing pancreatic

Modified Glasgow criteria
On admission
• Age > 55 years
• WBC > 15,000/ μL
• Glucose > 10 ((no history of diabetes)
• PaO_2 < 8 kPa (60 mmHg)
After 48 hours
• Calcium < 2 mmol/L
• Serum albumin <32 g/L
• Lactate dehydrogenase (LDH) > 600 IU/dL
• AST/ALT > 600 IU/dL

Table 4. Modified Glasgow criteria (IMRIE SCORE) for assessment severity of acute pancreatitis.

necrosis. Procalcitonin will help identifying the pancreatic infection. IL-6, trypsinogen activation peptide, polymorphonuclear elastase, and carboxypeptidase B activation peptide can also be used for assessing the severity and monitoring the progress of the disease, but these are either used as a research tool or not yet routinely available.

Persistent high haematocrit is also an indicator of pancreatic necrosis and organ failure. If initial resuscitation is inadequate, then haemoconcentration is not a useful marker [3, 4, 10].

6.6. The acute physiology and chronic health evaluation (APACHE) II scoring system

The acute physiology and chronic health evaluation (APACHE) II is (Knaus et al.) used to quantify the severity of the illness in ICU patients. It contains 12 continuous variables, the age and the pre-morbid conditions (which reflect a diminished physiological reserve). Patients with an APACHE II score >8 have severe acute pancreatitis and are likely to develop organ failure. It can be used in monitoring the patient's response to therapy throughout the patient's hospital stay unlike Ranson's and Glasgow, which is assessed in the first 48 hours. Hence, it can assess both the severity and progress/deterioration. Disadvantages being that it is complex to perform and has been evaluated prospectively only in first 24–48 hours after the onset of pancreatitis. In criteria used, factors with most predictive value for mortality include advanced age, presence of renal or respiratory insufficiency and presence of shock. It has a sensitivity of 65%, specificity of 76%, positive predictive value of 43% and negative predictive value of 89%. APACHE III is also been used in predicting the severity of pancreatitis [10].

6.7. Bedside index of severity in acute pancreatitis (BISAP) score

BISAP score is a beside scoring system with fewer variables than Ranson's criteria. The data sued in scoring are the basic data recorded during the time of admission or taken from the first 24 hours of the patient's evaluation. **Table 5** enumerates the criteria of bedside index of severity in acute pancreatitis (BISAP) score for assessment severity of acute pancreatitis. It is a prognostic scoring system that predicts the mortality, whereas Ranson's score predicts

Bedside index of severity in acute pancreatitis (BISAP) score		
	Scores	
	1	**0**
BUN >25 mg/dL (8.9 mmol/L)	>25 mg%	<25 mg%
Abnormal mental status with a Glasgow coma score <15	Present	Absent
Evidence of SIRS (systemic inflammatory response syndrome)	2/4	Absent
Patient age	>60 years old	<60 years old
Imaging study reveals pleural effusion	Present	Absent

Table 5. Bedside index of severity in acute pancreatitis (BISAP) score for assessment severity of acute pancreatitis.

persistent organ failure. BISAP scores have the advantages over Ranson's and Glasgow scores of being calculated within 24 hours of admission, use fewer variables. BISAP score is higher in patients having SIRS, in older patients and in patients with altered mental status. It has the disadvantage that it cannot easily distinguish transient from persistent organ failure [3, 4, 10].

Patients with a score of zero predict a mortality of less than 1 whereas patients with a score of 5 predict a mortality rate of 22%. The way forward may be to use a combination of the Ranson's score, the radiological scoring systems and a descriptive organ failure score such as the sepsis-related organ failure assessment.

7. Management

Management of acute pancreatitis should be aggressive and begins early in the emergency department once the diagnosis is made. Initial resuscitation can affect the outcomes of acute pancreatitis significantly.

The treatment can be divided into three major parts as follows:

1. ICU admission and management
2. Treatment of the local complications
3. Treatment of the aetiology [2, 3, 8]

7.1. ICU/HDU admission

ICU/HDU admission is needed in patients with severe acute pancreatitis for close monitoring, organ support, and follow up. It is difficult to decide which patient is a candidate for ICU/HDU admission at the time of presentation. There is a lack of early and adequate predictors of impending organ dysfunction. But the patients present with signs of organ dysfunction like hypotension, respiratory insufficiency, coagulopathy (including Disseminated intravascular coagulation (DIC), and acute kidney injury are definite candidates for ICU/HDU admission. Other than organ dysfunction patients with severe metabolic derangements like hyperglycaemia, severe hypocalcaemia and patients with comorbidities like heart failure, chronic kidney disease where the acute on chronic organ dysfunction may develop are the candidates for ICU admission [10]

7.2. Monitoring

Monitoring a patient with acute severe pancreatitis can be divided into the following:

1. Monitoring of vital signs: Heart rate, blood pressure, respiratory rate, oxygen saturation, urinary output and level of consciousness
2. Biochemical evaluation of organ function: Blood gases, lactic acid, renal function test, coagulation profile, haematocrit, blood glucose and serum electrolyte levels, especially calcium,

magnesium, and liver function test. These test may alert impending organ dysfunction, improvement or worsening of the organ function

3. Development of local complications like pancreatic necrosis and infection, which are associated with increased morbidity and mortality.
   a. Pancreatic necrosis is detected by contrast enhanced CT scan
   b. Pancreatic infection needs repeated contrast enhanced CT scan with CT/US guided fine needle aspiration
4. Intra-abdominal pressure (IAP): Intra-abdominal hypertension (IAH) is related to the development of complications, especially necrosis and infection, bowel oedema. High IAP is one indication for intervention like aspiration or surgery [6, 7, 10].

7.3. Organ support

7.3.1. Cardiovascular dysfunction: hypotension and early fluid resuscitation

Hypotension is one of the most common presentations with acute pancreatitis. It is a sign of impending organ dysfunction. The hypotension is due to the third space loss secondary to the inflammatory response, this contributes to hypoperfusion and end organ perfusion dysfunction. Aggressive fluid resuscitation and rapid restoration of intravascular volume are the main stay of the treatment. It requires several liters of fluids. Both crystalloids and colloids can be used as resuscitation fluids. There is no evidence that colloids have any added benefit over crystalloids. Among the crystalloid, use of 0.9% sodium chloride is to be avoided. As it causes hyperchloraemic metabolic acidosis, which is associated with renal impairment, infections and activation of trypsinogen in a pH-dependent manner. Lactated Ringer's solution is a cystalloid, it is a balanced salt solution, It is fluid of choice it has been found to be less incidence of SIRS compared to normal saline. Both under resuscitation as well as over resuscitation can lead to adverse outcomes, hence very close monitoring is recommended. Over resuscitation can lead interstitial oedema, bowel oedema, Acute respiratory distress syndrome (ARDS) which can lead to organ dysfunction. Monitoring of fluids status should be done by physical examination (clinical condition, vital signs and urine output), volume responsiveness and dynamic parameters by sonography or invasive or semi invasive haemodynamic parameters. Metabolic indicators like serial measurements of blood urea nitrogen and haematocrit [11, 12].

7.3.2. Pulmonary dysfunction

Pleuropulmonary abnormalities are commonly associated with pancreatitis, respiratory dysfunction is rarely seen at the time of presentation to Emergency department (ED) but usually develops after fluid resuscitation. It manifests as acute lung injury or acute respiratory distress syndrome. It is one of the major components of multiple organ system dysfunction syndromes. Other manifestations are bilateral infiltrates, pleural effusion, pulmonary hypertension, and decreased thoracic compliance [11, 12].

7.3.2.1. *Pulmonary management*

Patients with acute severe pancreatitis should be monitored closely for early detection of failure. Respiratory support usually initiated by supplemental oxygen and mechanical ventilation is often required depending on the severity of respiratory dysfunction. Nasogastric decompression will decrease the distension and improve the compliance and prevent aspiration. Non-invasive ventilation is poorly tolerated in most of the patients because of abdominal distension and reduced functional residual capacity, careful selection of patient is warranted. Non-invasive ventilation is good choice to start with as it may avoid endotracheal intubation. Acute lung injury and Acute respiratory distress syndrome (ARDS) secondary to acute severe pancreatitis is similar to any other condition using lung protective strategies. Pleural effusion may need ultrasound-guided drainage. Good analgesia will help in chest physiotherapy, early physiotherapy will prevent atelectasis and related complications [11, 12].

7.3.3. *Pain relief*

Pain is one of the symptoms of acute severe pancreatitis. It causes discomfort and heightened sympathetic activity, impairment of oxygenation due to restriction of abdominal wall movement. Effective analgesia can be provided by the use of opioids and parenteral route, i.e. intravenous route is the preferred route. Analgesia may improve pulmonary dysfunction. In the past, morphine was supposed to exacerbate acute pancreatitis by promoting contraction of the sphincter of Oddi and increase pressure in the sphincter of Oddi dysfunction, but there is no good supportive evidence. Another modality of pain management is use of drugs like local anaesthetics through in epidural route [13, 14].

7.3.4. *Nutrition support in acute pancreatitis*

Acute pancreatitis is a catabolic and hypermetabolic pathophysiological condition. This disease process increases protein demand and the calorie requirements. This altered metabolic state is further deranged by poor oral intake due to pain, ileus or partial obstruction of the duodenum from pancreatic oedema. There are increased protein losses locally in the retroperitoneum due to inflammation and through pancreatic fistulae. These features may be compounded by the pre-existing malnutrition, e.g. in alcohol abuse [11, 12, 13].

If malnutrition and a prolonged negative nitrogen balance are not taken care, it may result in poor pancreatic healing, increased risk of infection, impaired immunity, gut dysfunction leading to translocation of bacteria. Nutritional care and therapy along with other therapeutics measures will results in faster recovery and better outcome.

Feeding during severe acute pancreatitis may be challenging. The questions to address during the initiation of the nutritional support are when? How? and what?

Earlier concept of feeding in acute pancreatitis: the pathogenesis of pancreatitis is assumed to be perpetuation of premature enzymatic activation. 'Resting the pancreas' the approach to avoid stimuli to exocrine secretion from the pancreas was thought to be most physiological method to treat the pancreatitis. Hence, parenteral nutritional was the preferred option to avoid stimulation of the inflamed pancreatic gland. The other hypothesis is that systemic inflammatory response syndrome is caused by the absorption of the pancreatic endotoxins and ultimately leads to multiorgan failure. If the gut mucosal barrier is maintained, then it reduces the absorption of endotoxin. The present concept of nutritional support in acute pancreatitis: the preferred route of nutritional support is 'enteral route', it should be initiated as early as possible within 24–48 hours of presentation. Parenteral route is second choice, especially if the presentation is severe and it is unlikely to start oral intake within the next 5–7 days. The advantages of the enteral feeding are improved gut blood flow, maintenance of mucosal integrity and barrier function there by reduction in microbial translocation and pancreatic infection, and better glycaemic control, avoidance of central venous access-related complications are benefits of enteral nutrition. There benefits are translated in lower incidence of infections, multiorgan failure and outcome, i.e. mortality and length of stay when compared to parenteral nutrition [11–13].

7.3.5. Route of enteral nutrition

If nutritional support is supplemented by the enteral route, then it is usually delivered by tube feeding. There is a controversy about nasogastric versus nasojejunal feeding. But there is not much evidence to support any one over the other. Though traditionally nasojejunal feedings (to be delivered distal to the ligament of Treitz) have been preferred with the concept of less stimulation of the exocrine pancreas, cholecystokinin (CCK) cells that are present in the distal third part of the duodenum get stimulated when food passing through duodenum. It releases CCK that stimulates the pancreas and increased volume of pancreatic enzymes and bicarbonate secretion. This may worsen the course of the disease. Nasogastric tube feedings have now been shown to as safe as the jejunal feeding. Nasogastric insertion can be at bedside. Fluoroscopy endoscopic (endoscopically placed guide wire) and specialist help is not needed. With the Nasogastric (NG) feeding, the standard precautions of aspiration like elevation of head end of bed should be followed.

The indication for nasojejunal feeds is when patients cannot tolerate gastric feeding due to ileus and slow bowel transit time. Nasojejunal (NJ) tube placement needs fluoroscopy, endoscopic, and specialist help. NJ tube may get displaced back into the stomach. Prokinetics and right-lateral positioning pass the tube through the into-duodenum. The correct positioning of the tube should be ascertained regularly by radiography [2, 7, 13].

7.3.6. Enteral nutritional supplements

No specific enteral nutrition supplement or immunonutrition formulation had any advantage. Low fat formulas with medium-chain triglycerides should be used enteral because it helps in better assimilation by direct absorption into the portal vein as there is lipase deficiency.

7.3.7. Complications of nutritional therapy

The common complications are metabolic and splanchnic. They are as follows:

Hyperglycaemia: Beta-cell death, peripheral insulin resistance irrespective of the route of feeding, needs monitoring of serum glucose and use IV insulin.

Hypertriglyceridemia is usually due to overfeeding. Monitor serum triglyceride level and titrate fat content.

Feed intolerance: Monitor abdominal pressure, bowel distension, residual volume and diarrhoea. Displacement of NJ tube [2, 9].

8. Pathogenesis of pancreatic infection and antibiotic prophylaxis

Infection is common in pancreatic necrosis, it occurs in approximately 40–70% of patients. Infection causes an increase in morbidity and mortality. There are various theories proposed for the mechanisms of infection in severe acute pancreatitis, namely bacterial translocation from the colon, via the biliary tree, especially in biliary pancreatitis, bacterial migration through the pancreatic duct from the lumen of the duodenum and haematogenous spread from bacteraemia due to other causes like infected central venous lines [5, 9, 10].

8.1. Role of antibiotic prophylaxis in severe acute pancreatitis

Prophylactic antibiotics in severe acute pancreatitis have been a topic of debate in the last 4–5 decades. Pancreatic necrosis more than 30% increases the chances of infection. The right choice of antibiotics is very important, those which have high penetration into pancreatic tissue. Carbapenems are both broad spectrum and excellent pancreatic penetration properties. Other antibiotics, which penetrate well in the pancreatic tissue, are cephalosporin, ureidopenicillins, fluoroquinolones, metronidazole and imipenem. Aminoglycosides have a poor penetration ability. Patients with mild pancreatitis do not benefit from antibiotics. In a meta-analysis by Sharma et al. [16], use of prophylactic antibiotics has shown mortality benefit in patients with Acute necrotizing pancreatitis (ANP) confirmed by contrast-enhanced CT (21–12.3%). Ref. [15, 16] prophylactic antibiotics use has not shown to decrease the need for interventional and surgical management but no effect on mortality.

8.2. Prophylactic antifungal therapy

Fungal infection in severe acute pancreatitis is associated with high morbidity and mortality.

It has been noted that the incidence depends on the severity of the disease, extent of necrosis and use of broad spectrum antibiotic administration. Prophylactic use of fluconazole has shown to be effective in decreasing the morbidity but not the mortality [10].

9. Treatment of local complications

9.1. Pancreatic necrosis and abscess

The presence of non-viable tissue in the pancreatic parenchyma, which is detected by the non-enhancement on the contrast-enhanced CT, is called as pancreatic necrosis. It can be focal or diffuse with associated peripancreatic involvement. It can be sterile necrosis or get infected in approximately 70% of the cases. The diagnosis of infection of the necrotic pancreas is difficult. Infected necrosis is diagnosed in the patients who show no signs of improvement, signs of sepsis (leukocytosis and fever are confounded by the SIRS), worsening of clinical condition, especially after improvement. The lab data to confirm the infection of the necrotic pancreatic tissue are not reliable. Biomarker like CRP is usually high in severe acute pancreatitis, but procalcitonin can be used as a marker, but still it is not specific because in patients who are critically ill, there are other infection like Central Line-associated Bloodstream Infection (CLABSI), Ventilator-Associated Event (VAE) (Ventilator-Associated pneumonia (VAP)), Catheter-associated Urinary Tract Infections (CAUTI), etc. wherein procalcitonin is raised.

The best method to confirm the diagnosis of infected pancreatic necrosis is CT/US guided fine needle aspiration, Gram's staining, and culture. Multiple samples from all pockets should be taken or sampling needs to be repeated. Pancreatic abscess is a collection of pus in close proximity to pancreatic necrosis, which develops as a local infection of the necrotic pancreatic tissue after severe acute pancreatitis.

9.2. Management of sterile pancreatic necrosis

Sterile pancreatic necrosis is usually managed conservatively (non-operatively). Earlier in the 1990s, all necrotic pancreatitis use to undergo necrosectomy. Surgical intervention in sterile pancreatic necrosis may increase the risk of infection and thereby an increase in the mortality. Patients with sterile pancreatic necrosis need close observation for evidence of infection. In selected patients with extensive necrosis may need surgical intervention if they do not improve for more than 6–8 weeks [3, 8, 11, 12].

9.3. Management of infected pancreatic necrosis pancreatic necrosis and abscess

Infected necrotic pancreatitis requires debridement and there is a consensus on surgical intervention in such cases. There is still a controversy about the best approach for debridement of the infected necrotic pancreatic tissue.

The aim of the intervention is removal of the infected necrotic substance. To achieve this goal, there are several techniques suggested. It ranges from drainage, debridement, lavage laparoscopy to laparotomy and packing.

9.4. Percutaneous drainage

- Anterior
- Retroperitoneal

This can be done when there are infected fluid collections or pus. It will be difficult to drain if it is just infected necrotic tissue or fluid/pus is too viscous. It has to be done CT/US guided and needs expertise. Complications are rare in expert hands. Usual complications with percutaneous drainage are bleeding, viscous perforation, fistula formation and super infection [3, 11, 12].

9.5. Surgical debridement/necrosectomy

- Minimally invasive
- Open surgical

These procedures can be performed transperitoneal or retroperitoneal which is decided on the location of necrosis and collections. Some patients need multiple sitting and planned relaparotomies. The open surgical approach carries higher risk of morbidity and mortality when compared to laparoscopic technique. There is higher risk of bleeding, perforation multiple organ failure, enterocutaneous fistula, incisional hernia, and new-onset diabetes mellitus [13, 14]

9.6. Management of the etiological factor

There is very few or nothing to do for the etiological management other than biliary pancreatitis. The treatments depend on the severity of the pancreatitis. In severe pancreatitis, there is no role of surgery. Surgery increases the morbidity and mortality. ERCP (endoscopic retrograde cholangiopancreatography) with sphincterotomy is indicated in patients with acute cholangitis. This will help in decreasing the pressure in pancreatic duct and lessens the severity of the disease. ERCP with sphincterotomy decreases the morbidity but not the mortality [13, 14].

10. Prevention of acute pancreatitis

Change in dietary habits and consumption of balance diet will prevent the gall stone formation, earlier cholecystectomy will prevent the recurrence of pancreatitis. Regular exercise, avoiding the high caloric intake, regular use of low fat diet will control the serum triglyceride levels and early introductions of statins will help in preventing the hyperlipidaemia associated pancreatitis. Moderation in alcohol intake will reduce the incidence of alcoholic pancreatitis [13, 14].

Author details

Arshad Chanda

Address all correspondence to: drarshadchanda@yahoo.com

Hamad General Hospital, Doha, State of Qatar

References

[1] Working Group IAP/APA Acute Pancreatitis Guidelines. IAP/APA evidence-based guidelines for the management of acute pancreatitis. Pancreatology. 2013;**13**:e1-e15

[2] Johnson CD, Besse MG, Carter R. Acute pancreatitis. British Medical Journal. 2014; **349**:4859. DOI: 10.1136/bmj.g4859

[3] Nirula R. Chapter 9: Diseases of the pancreas. In: High Yield Surgery. Philadelphia, PA: Lippincott Williams & Wilkins; 2000

[4] Clinical Practice and Economics Committee. AGA institute medical position statement on acute pancreatitis. Gastroenterology. 2007;**132**:2019-2021

[5] Ignatavicius P, Vitkauskiene A, Pundzius J, Dambrauskas Z, Barauskas G. Effects of prophylactic antibiotics in acute pancreatitis. HPB. 2012;**14**:396-402

[6] Wang GJ, Gao CF, Wei D, Wang C, Ding SQ. Acute pancreatitis: Etiology and common pathogenesis. World Journal of Gastroenterology. 2009;**15**(12):1427-1430

[7] Quinlan JD. Acute pancreatitis. American Family Physician. 2014;**90**(9):632-639

[8] Wu BU, Johannes RS, Sun X, et al. The early prediction of mortality in acute pancreatitis: a large population-based study. Gut 2008;**57**:1698.

[9] Banks PA, Bollen TL, Dervenis C, et al. Classification of acute pancreatitis—2012: Revision of the Atlanta classification and definitions by international consensus. Gut. 2013;**62**:102-111. DOI: 10.1136/gutjnl-2012-302779

[10] Ince AT, Baysal B. Pathophysiology, classification and available guidelines of acute Pancreatitis. The Turkish Journal of Gastroenterology. 2014;**25**:351-357

[11] Thoeni RF. The revised Atlanta classification of acute pancreatitis: Its importance for the radiologist and its effect on treatment. Radiology. 2012;**262**:751-764

[12] Suvarna R, Pallipady A, Bhandary N, Hanumanthappa. The clinical prognostic indicators of acute pancreatitis by Apac he II scoring. Journal of Clinical and Diagnostic Research. 2011;**5**(3):459-463

[13] Vincent JL, Abraham E, Moore FA, Kochanek PM, Fink MP. Text Book of Critical Care. 6th ed. Elsevier Saunders. Philadelphia, PA 19103-2899: 2011. pp. 804-813

[14] Bersten AD, Soni N. Oh's Intensive Care Manual. 6th ed. Butterwoth, Heinemann, Elsevier Oxford. pp. 479485

[15] Knaus WA, Draper EA, Wagner DP, Zimmerman JE (1985). "APACHE II: a severity of disease classification system". Critical Care Medicine. **13**(10):818-29.

[16] Sharma VK, Howden CW. Prophylactic antibiotic administration reduces sepsis and mortality in acute necrotizing pancreatitis: a meta-analysis. Pancreas 2001;**22**(1):28-31.

11

Haemodynamic Monitoring in the Intensive Care Unit

Mainak Majumdar

Abstract

Monitoring is a cognitive aid that allows clinicians to detect the nature and extent of pathology and helps assessment of response to therapy. The cardiovascular system is the most commonly monitored organ system in the critical care setting. It helps identify the presence and nature of shock and guides response to resuscitation by detection of cardiac rate and rhythm, evaluation of volume state, cardiac contractility and systemic vascular resistance. Newer technologies allow greater assessment of oxygen delivery to vulnerable tissues. We discuss the nature, history, modalities and interpretation of the most commonly available haemodynamic monitoring methods in clinical use currently.

Keywords: monitoring, arterial pressure, pressure transduction, oscillometry, plethysmography, volume state, central venous pressure, pulmonary artery occlusion pressure, stroke volume variation, cardiac output, pulmonary artery catheter, transpulmonary dilution, Fick principle, oesophageal Doppler, echocardiography, pulse contour analysis, tissue perfusion, lactate clearance, arteriovenous PCO_2 gradient, mixed venous saturation, central venous saturation, gastric tonometry

1. Introduction

The verb 'monitor' is derived from the Latin word monere- to warn. While there is little conclusive evidence that any one modality of monitoring changes patient outcomes significantly [1], all forms of critical care monitoring should be considered cognitive aids providing information beyond conventional physical examination. Synthesising this added information in the patient's individual context to improve clinical decision-making, thus enabling early aggressive manipulation of patient physiology is key to the management of critically unwell patients.

Monitoring is an integral part of critical care practice and is essential to the daily care of the critically ill patient. The goal of all resuscitation is prevention or treatment of organ dysfunction and cellular injury by optimisation of tissue oxygen delivery according to the metabolic need. Manipulation of the macro-circulation to defend capillary autoregulation and micro-circulatory oxygen delivery relies heavily on the advanced haemodynamic monitoring to optimise volume state and cardiac function. Critical care monitoring and end points of resuscitation are now integrated into many resuscitation pathways and best practice guidelines [2, 3].

Invasive haemodynamic monitoring is now ubiquitous in critical care practice. Invasive monitoring assists both in the diagnosis and assessment of response to therapy in shock states and helps distinguish hypovolemic, cardiogenic, obstructive and distributive shock states.

It is incumbent on the critical care practitioner not only to be familiar with the commonly used modalities of haemodynamic monitoring but also to understand the physical principles underlying the monitoring equipment, allowing competent interpretation of haemodynamic data for use in clinical practice, identification of artefacts and effective troubleshooting of equipment.

2. Haemodynamic monitoring standards for critical care units

Patients admitted to critical care units in general show evidence of (single or multiple) organ failure or are at risk of such organ failure. Haemodynamic instability, leading to mismatch between tissue oxygen delivery and demand, is a major contributing factor for organ failure. All critically unwell patients should be monitored, but the degree of monitoring may vary depending on the severity of organ dysfunction [4].

The minimum standards of monitoring in a critical care environment are specified by the College of Intensive Care Medicine and they are as follows [5]:

- Continuous electrocardiography
- Non-invasive arterial pressure monitoring
- Pulse oximetry
- Central and cutaneous temperature monitoring
- End tidal capnography (to confirm tracheal placement of endotracheal or tracheostomy tubes and to monitor all patients receiving ventilatory support)
- Continuous monitoring of ventilation
- Endotracheal cuff monitoring
- Pressure monitoring–continuously and simultaneously display arterial, central venous and at least one other pressure
- Where indicated, monitoring and display of other physiologic variables such as cardiac output

Patients in or at high risk of respiratory or circulatory failure should have, at the very least, an arterial line for continuous invasive blood pressure monitoring and regular sampling of arterial blood gases and serum lactate.

Delivery of most pressors and inotropes necessitates central access. While the role of central venous pressures in estimating 'volume state' has been questioned repeatedly in literature, it does allow opportunity for central venous pressure monitoring.

Where indicated, further monitoring to monitor cardiac output, pulmonary artery pressures, volume state and tissue-oxygen extraction, may need to be instituted.

3. Physical principles of pressure transduction

Pressure transduction is in widespread use in the critical care environment, with pressure indices being measured for a variety of invasive haemodynamic variables such as arterial pressure, central venous pressure, pulmonary artery pressure and the like.

The basic transducer system is common to all means of invasive pressure monitoring. It consists of a fluid-coupled strain gauge system.

A cannula directly inserted into the lumen of the vessel whose pressure is being measured is connected through sterile plastic tubing containing fluid at high pressure to a strain gauge.

The strain gauge system itself, in modern clinical practice, is a semiconductor strain gauge integrated into a silicon diaphragm. The pressure wave transmitted through the fluid coupling system deforms the crystal lattice structure of the silicon, changing the resistance. Most modern transducers have four such piezoresistors within the diaphragm area (see **Figure 1**), with two being subject to tangential and two to radial stress [6].

The resistors are connected in a four-arm configuration and provide an output such that

$$V_{\text{out}}/V_{\text{supplied}} = \Delta R/\Omega \quad (1)$$

where V_{out} = measured output voltage; $V_{supplied}$ = supply voltage (known); Ω = base resistance of resistor (known) and ΔR = change in resistance with applied pressure.

The output current is shielded from AC power supply pickup and displayed on the monitor. Commercially available transducers are individually calibrated and have a high level of accuracy.

The transducer is initially zeroed to ambient air pressure and then connected to the patient's circulation in a circuit as shown in **Figure 2**.

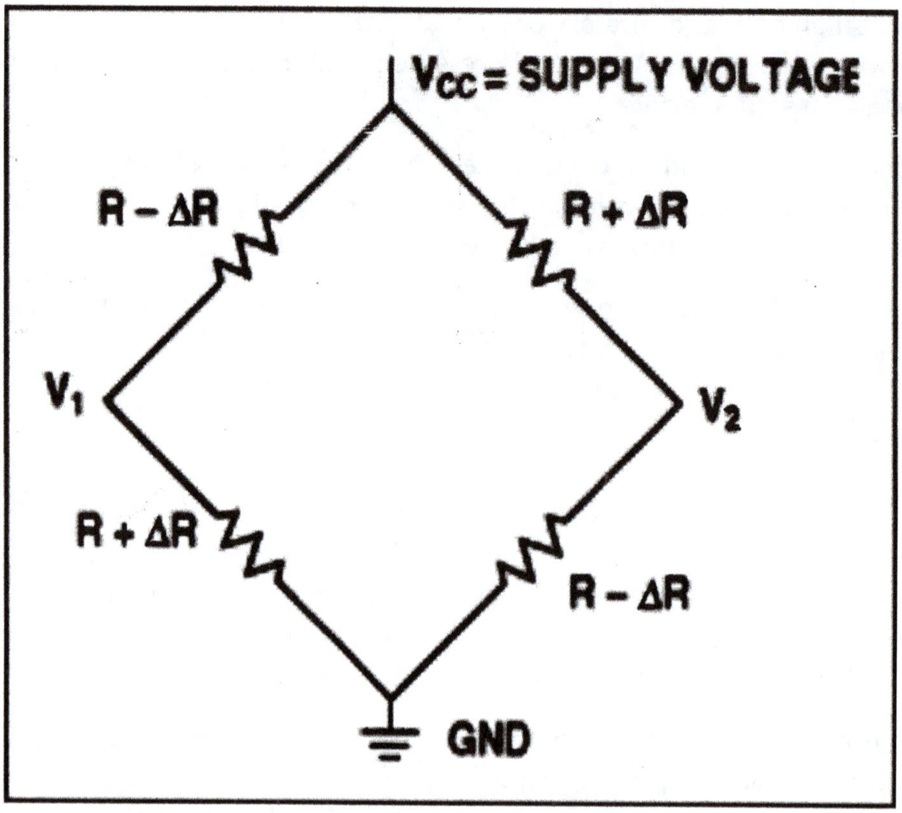

Figure 1. Piezoresistive integrated semiconductor pressure sensors incorporate four piezoresistors in the diaphragm. When the diaphragm is deflected, two resistors are subjected to tangential stress and two to radial stress. The four are connected to a four-element bridge.

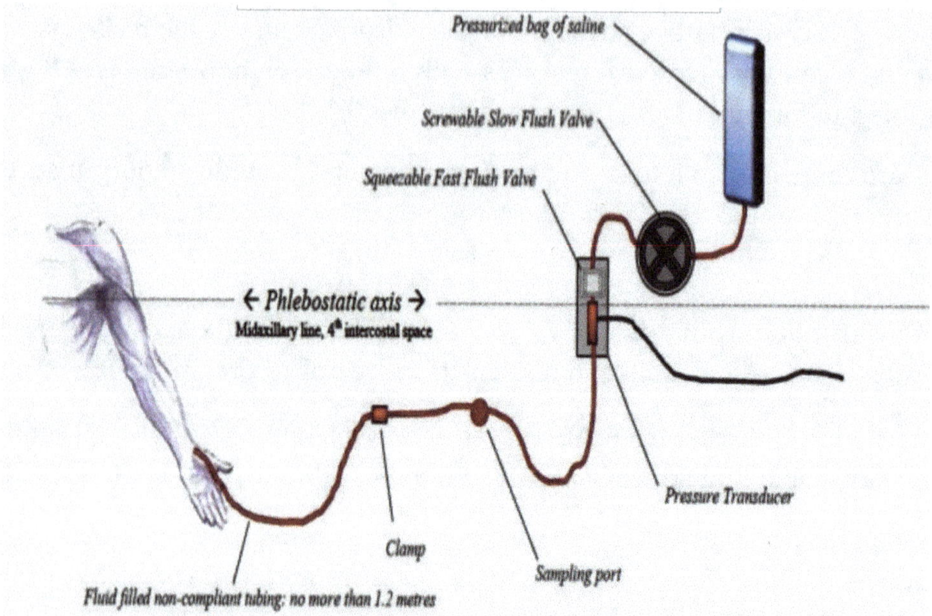

Figure 2. Standard fluid-coupled transducer set up for pressure monitoring.

4. Continuous electrocardiography

Continuous electrocardiography is a common way of monitoring both cardiac rate and rhythm in critical care units and almost ubiquitously applied in regular critical care practice.

Adequate information can be gained from a three-lead single-channel display although it is often conventional to use a five-lead dual-channel display.

If there are specific concerns regarding evolving cardiac ischemia, most modern monitoring systems permit the use of conventional 12-lead continuous display. The need for on-going continuous 12-lead views is rarely necessary. As part of routine practice in most units, though, it is conventional to monitor 12-lead ECGs at least daily and serially where indicated (e.g. evolving myocardial ischaemia).

Critical care units involved with significant volumes of cardiothoracic surgical care and/or cardiology should use equipment that can accurately detect pacing activity and represent it on the continuous electrocardiography display.

5. Arterial pressure monitoring

Arterial blood pressure monitoring, whether by direct or indirect means, forms an essential part of any cardiovascular assessment and is one of the vital signs routinely assessed in every patient.

In 1733, Stephan Hales was the first to describe the measurement of 'the force of blood' in animal experiments using a water manometer in *Haema Staticks*.

5.1. Non-invasive blood pressure monitoring

In 1896, Scipione Riva Rocci described the use of a pneumatic cuff using Vierordt and von Basch's adaptation of Poiseuille's mercury manometer. His technique, first published as *'Un nuovo sfigmomanometro'* in *Gazetta Medical do Torino*, of inflating a rubber pneumatic cuff cased in a non-expansile material wrapped circumferentially round the arm to occlude the radial pulse, letting the air escape and measuring the pressure at which the pulse reappears (the systolic blood pressure), is still used in clinical practice worldwide.

In 1905, Nikolai Korotkoff described systolic and diastolic blood pressure measurement by auscultation. He combined Riva Rocci's cuff technique with a binaural stethoscope. Like Riva Rocci, he inflated the arm cuff till the pulse was occluded. He then auscultated the brachial artery, measuring both the pressure at which the brachial pulse became audible (systolic blood pressure) and then became inaudible again (diastolic blood pressure) as the cuff was slowly deflated [7].

Blood pressure measurement became widespread in clinical practice at the instigation of John Harvey Cushing. It is now standard of care to measure blood pressure in most healthcare settings and it is recognised as a vital sign.

Thus, simple non-invasive indirect arterial blood pressure management entered routine cardiovascular assessment as a measure additional to the classic palpation of rate, rhythm, volume and character of peripheral and central pulses described by Galen and Celsus—a practice dating back to ancient times and described in medical textbooks from India, China, Egypt and Greece.

All non-invasive measures of arterial pressure rely on the detection of blood flow. Over the latter half of the twentieth century, automated techniques of non-invasive blood pressure measurement were developed and refined. Oscillometry and finger plethysmography are currently the most commonly used techniques in Australasia.

Oscillometry is essentially an automated refinement of the Korotkoff technique. Oscillations at the cardiac frequency are high pass filtered out and plotted into an oscillometry envelope. Oscillations in the cuff pressure increase in amplitude as the cuff pressure falls between systolic and mean arterial pressures. The point of maximum oscillation amplitude corresponds closely with the mean arterial blood pressure. The amplitude of oscillations then falls between mean and diastolic blood pressure. The exact point on the oscillometry envelope used to determine systolic and diastolic blood pressure remains controversial and commercially available oscillometric systems use proprietary algorithms that are not available for public scrutiny. Overall, mean arterial pressures measured by oscillometry closely approximate invasive mean arterial pressures [8].

Since Jan Penaz first described the volume clamp technique of determining blood pressure using continuous finger plethysmography in the 1960s (based on the previous work of Karel Wesseling), various devices have been developed that provide arterial pressure tracings and continuous non-invasive measures of blood pressure using cuff-based finger plethysmography. Commercially available systems vary from the Finapres$_{TM}$ (Finapres Medical Systems BV, Netherlands) to the recently released ClearSight$_{TM}$ (Edwards Lifesciences, USA), which combines finger plethysmography with pulse contour analysis to estimate continuous cardiac output.

Ultrasound detection of arterial wall motion using devices like Puritan Bennett's Infrasonde$_{TM}$ [9] and photometric wave velocity measurement (pulse transit time bears an approximately inverse ratio to systolic blood pressure) has been described [10].

5.2. Invasive blood pressure monitoring

Invasive arterial pressure monitoring is standard of care in most modern critical care units. It consists of percutaneous insertion of a cannula into a peripheral artery identified either by palpation or under ultrasound guidance.

The common sites for arterial cannulation include radial, ulnar, brachial, axillary, femoral and dorsalis pedis arteries. Cannula sizes usually vary between 18 and 22 gauge.

The arterial cannula is attached to a fluid-coupled pressure transducer system as described above and provides accurate beat-by-beat measurement of arterial pressure besides providing a sampling port for arterial blood gases and blood tests.

There is little evidence that any one site is 'safer' than another for arterial cannulation. The shape, size or material of the catheter and the duration of insertion does not seem to influence the risk of complications. There is little evidence to support the utility of an Allen's test prior to radial artery cannulation [11]. The author prefers to avoid end arteries like the brachial.

Like all invasive procedures, arterial cannulation comes with potential risks including local haematoma formation, ischaemia of the distal limb, ischaemia of the overlying skin, retrograde embolisation, pseudo aneurysm, arteriovenous fistula formation and injury to surrounding structures. The sampling port remains an obvious source of infection, but, compared to central venous access devices, the risks of line-related sepsis are far lower from arterial catheters alone. Finally, it is good practice to clearly label the arterial line and its connections to minimise the risk of inadvertent retrograde injection.

In addition, technical factors associated with the fluid-coupled transduction system need to be taken into account. Specifically, it is important to verify that the transducer has been zeroed appropriately to ambient air pressure at the phlebostatic axis. It is vital to assess the pressure tracing itself to see if the dicrotic notch is visible and whether there is evidence of 'damping' (where there is an excess of compliance in the system, e.g. due to air in the fluid coupling, inadequately inflated pressure bag or excess length of transducer tubing) or 'ringing' (often noted as a spike or 'overshoot' of the systolic pressure trace caused by a poor compliant transduction system, and sometimes, due to resonance with reflected waves from the radial styloid process or similar anatomical structures).

5.3. Interpretation of arterial pressure monitoring data

Over the years, blood pressure monitoring has been used as a surrogate measure of overall cardiovascular function, with an abnormal blood pressure being a significant marker of haemodynamic dysfunction.

In essence, blood pressure is directly proportional to both cardiac output and systemic vascular resistance.

Thus, arterial hypotension may indicate decreased stroke volume due to hypovolaemia and decreased systemic venous return, poor myocardial contractility or cardiac outflow obstruction due to pulmonary embolus or tamponade. Equally, it may be due to vasodilation due to sepsis or systemic inflammatory response. Often, it may be a combination of more than one factor. In short, hypotension is an excellent, if sometimes late marker of circulatory dysfunction and/or impairment of tissue perfusion. However, it is only one of the many parameters a clinician needs to assess the aetiology of circulatory dysfunction and distinguish between hypovolemic, distributive, cardiogenic and obstructive shock.

Significant persistent hypotension is often associated with evidence of end organ compromise due to failure of autoregulation of blood supply through the tissue capillary beds, evidenced by poor peripheral circulation (with decreased peripheral and central capillary refill), altered levels of consciousness, renal dysfunction with oligoanuria and abnormal renal function markers in the serum, hepatic dysfunction (commonly a transaminitis with aspartate transaminase rising higher than alanine transaminase) and evidence of increasing anaerobic metabolism characterised by a rise in serum lactate. Similarly, resolution of these factors, together with return to baseline blood pressure or normotension, is a marker of successful resuscitation.

It is important to note that while the left ventricle generates pulsatile systemic blood flow, tissue capillary beds receive continuous blood flow at a constant pressure and most capillary beds are able to autoregulate the flow of blood within the organ at pressures between 55 and 110 mmHg. The aorta plays the vital role of converting pulsatile cardiac outflow into the steady blood flow perfusing the tissues. Thus, tissue perfusion relies on mean arterial pressure. The coronary circulation, on the other hand, relies on diastolic blood pressure for perfusion. Systolic blood pressure largely denotes the shear force of the pulsatile outflow on the elastic tissue of the aorta and the larger arteries. It is also important to remember that there are differences between pressures measured at different points in the arterial tree. The further out in the arterial tree the measurement is taken, the higher the measured systolic pressure and the lower the diastolic compared to pressures at the aortic root. The difference between systolic pressures measured in a proximal vessel (e.g. femoral artery) and a distal vessel (e.g. dorsalis pedis artery) is not clinically significant and the mean pressure, which determines tissue perfusion, is nearly identical regardless of the point of measurement.

With invasive measurement in an accurately zeroed and adequately damped transducer system, the measurement of systolic, diastolic and mean arterial pressure (defined as the area under the waveform-time curve divided by the time interval of the beat) is fairly accurate and reliable. The arterial waveform itself provides visual confirmation of the pulsatile blood flow in the vessel being transduced.

With non-invasive measures, the exact values of systolic and diastolic pressure vary depending on the technique and, to an extent, the operator. The mean arterial pressure may be approximated to diastolic pressure +1/3 (difference between systolic and diastolic pressure). The Riva Rocci palpatory technique does not measure diastolic pressure and there may be significant inter-observer variability with both the palpatory and auscultatory (Korotkoff) methods of blood pressure determination, especially in haemodynamically unstable patients. Mean arterial pressures measured by oscillometry are usually accurate. However, the measurement of diastolic and systolic pressures is based on proprietary algorithms and the determination of diastolic pressure, especially, is problematic. Finger plethysmography and photoelectric methods using peripheral pulse transit time rely on adequate peripheral blood flow. They are difficult to acquire reliably in shocked, peripherally shut down patients—the subset whose management benefits most from regular arterial pressure monitoring.

6. Measurement of cardiac output

Cardiac output is the volume of blood pumped by the heart per unit time. It is the product of heart rate and stroke volume. It can be manipulated by alterations to heart rate and rhythm, preload, contractility and afterload.

Measurement and optimisation of cardiac output ultimately is the best way to guide and facilitate tissue perfusion and oxygenation.

There are different methods of measuring cardiac output based on the Fick principle, thermo dilution, pulse contour analysis, Doppler and bio-impedance. Each method comes with its own advantages and disadvantages. The ideal mode of monitoring would be minimally or non-invasive, cost effective, continuous, reproducible and reliable in a variety of physiologic states with a fast response time [12].

6.1. Fick principle

This is the gold standard for cardiac output measurement. The Fick principle is based on the fact that the total uptake (or release) of a substance by the peripheral tissues is equal to the product of the blood flow to the tissue and the arterial-venous concentration difference of the substance.

In practice, the simplest way to measure this is in terms of oxygen consumption, i.e. the difference between inspired and expired oxygen. The cardiac output is calculated thus

$$CO = VO_2/(CaO_2 - CvO_2) \tag{2}$$

where CO = cardiac output; VO_2 = oxygen consumption; CaO_2 = arterial oxygen concentration; CvO_2 = venous oxygen concentration.

Accurate measurement of VO_2 outside of stringent physiology laboratory conditions is difficult and so this method is not commonly applied in clinical practice.

When used in clinical practice for ventilated patients, it is easier to estimate pulmonary capillary blood flow by measuring the volume of CO_2 produced, the alveolar and mixed venous CO_2 [13]. This is done by periodically introducing a dead space into the ventilator circuit and assuming pulmonary end capillary, arterial and end tidal CO_2 rise instantly but mixed venous PCO_2 does not. Cardiac output is estimated thus

$$CO = Q_{PCBF} = \Delta CO_2/(C_V CO_2 - C_A CO_2) \tag{3}$$

where CO = cardiac output; Q_{PCBF} = pulmonary capillary blood flow; ΔCO_2 = CO_2 excreted by lungs per minute = (expiratory flow) × (CO_2 fraction in expired air); $CvCO_2$ = mixed venous CO_2; C_ACO_2 = alveolar arteriolar CO_2 = (end tidal CO_2) × (slope of the CO_2 dissociation curve).

The available systems are limited in that they are designed for use in patients who are intubated and ventilated. Concerns have previously been expressed about using rebreathed CO_2 in the circuit, leading to raised E_TCO_2 and tachycardia, leading to an artefactually elevated cardiac output measurement [14]. Moreover, measured expired PCO_2 may not reflect change in pulmonary capillary and arterial PCO_2 and CO_2 may not have had a chance to reach a steady state within the limited sampling time. The actual slope of the CO_2 dissociation curve also varies with both haemoglobin content and PCO_2. Errors in measurement may be introduced in patients with significant V/Q mismatch or intracardiac shunt (where pulmonary blood flow may not represent total cardiac output), severe chest trauma and high cardiac output states with low minute ventilation.

6.2. Pulmonary artery catheterisation

Pulmonary artery catheterisation [15] and thermo dilution to measure cardiac output has been the gold standard in clinical practice. In the end expiratory phase, a known volume of injectate (usually saline or dextrose at room temperature or cooler) is injected rapidly (in less than 4 s) to rapidly lower the temperature of the pulmonary artery and the change in blood temperature over time is monitored. In essence, the rate of blood flow is in inverse proportion to the change in temperature and mean change in temperature is therefore inversely proportional to the cardiac output. The Stewart Hamilton equation is then used to derive the output.

$$\text{CO} = [V(T_b - T_i)]K1[K2/T(b)t\,dt] \tag{4}$$

where CO = cardiac output; V = volume of injectate; T_b = temperature of blood; T_i = temperature of injectate; K1, K2 = correction constants for specific heat and density of injectate and for blood and dead space volume; T(b)t dt = change in blood temperature as a function of time.

Instead of thermo dilution, dye dilution has also been used to measure cardiac output with pulmonary artery catheters. If a dye like indocyanine green is injected into the pulmonary artery, the change in its concentration is related to the rate of blood flow and can be calculated from the Stewart Hamilton equation thus

$$\text{CO} = I\int Ci\,dt \tag{5}$$

where CO = cardiac output; I = amount of indicator (in moles);

Ci dt = integral of indicator concentration over time.

There are commercially available cardiac output catheters capable of continuous cardiac output monitoring. These use intermittent heating of blood in the pulmonary artery through a heating filament integrated into the catheter and calculate the cardiac output by thermo dilution.

There is a significant margin of error of up to 15% in measurement of cardiac output by pulmonary artery catheter thermo dilution. There can be up to 10% variation in the measured output without significant change to the patient's clinical state.

Pulmonary artery catheters carry a significant risk of complications including catheter malposition, catheter migration, catheter knotting, pulmonary artery rupture, valve injury, arrhythmia, thrombus on catheter leading to embolisation, air embolus from balloon rupture, infection and haematoma. Failure to inject at end expiration, injection time of greater than 4 s, temperature sensor touching the vessel wall, severe tricuspid regurgitation, profound hypothermia, intracardiac shunts and infusions running rapidly in other ports of the catheter may all lead to inaccuracies in the measured thermo dilution cardiac output. In a randomised control trial, risks of catheter-related complications rose significantly from 0.7% associated with central venous catheters to 1.5% associated with pulmonary artery catheters, though there was no significant increase in mortality or hospital length of stay [16]. Later, the PAC-Man trial was unable to demonstrate significant benefit or harm with the use of pulmonary artery catheters [17].

6.3. Transpulmonary dilution techniques

Over the last two decades, various techniques have been described and entered clinical practice, using thermo dilution or dye/indicator dilution techniques. These are all based around the injection of a bolus into the right atrium via a central venous catheter and the detection of temperature change or dye/indicator concentration at a proximal artery (femoral, axillary or brachial). Using the Stewart Hamilton equation as above, cardiac output can be calculated by any of these techniques.

In addition, it is possible to calculate the mean transit time of the injectate from the dilution curve. Multiplying the mean transit time with the cardiac output allows calculation of the total intrathoracic thermal (in thermo dilution), water (using lithium injectate) or blood (using indocyanine green) volumes with these devices. Subtracting intrathoracic blood volume (measured by indocyanine green dye dilution) from total intrathoracic fluid volume (measured using thermo dilution or lithium) allows assessment of extravascular lung water.

Measurements of cardiac output using transpulmonary dilution (see **Figure 3**) correlate well with measurements using pulmonary artery catheter or using the Fick principle, with an estimated added margin of error of around 5%.

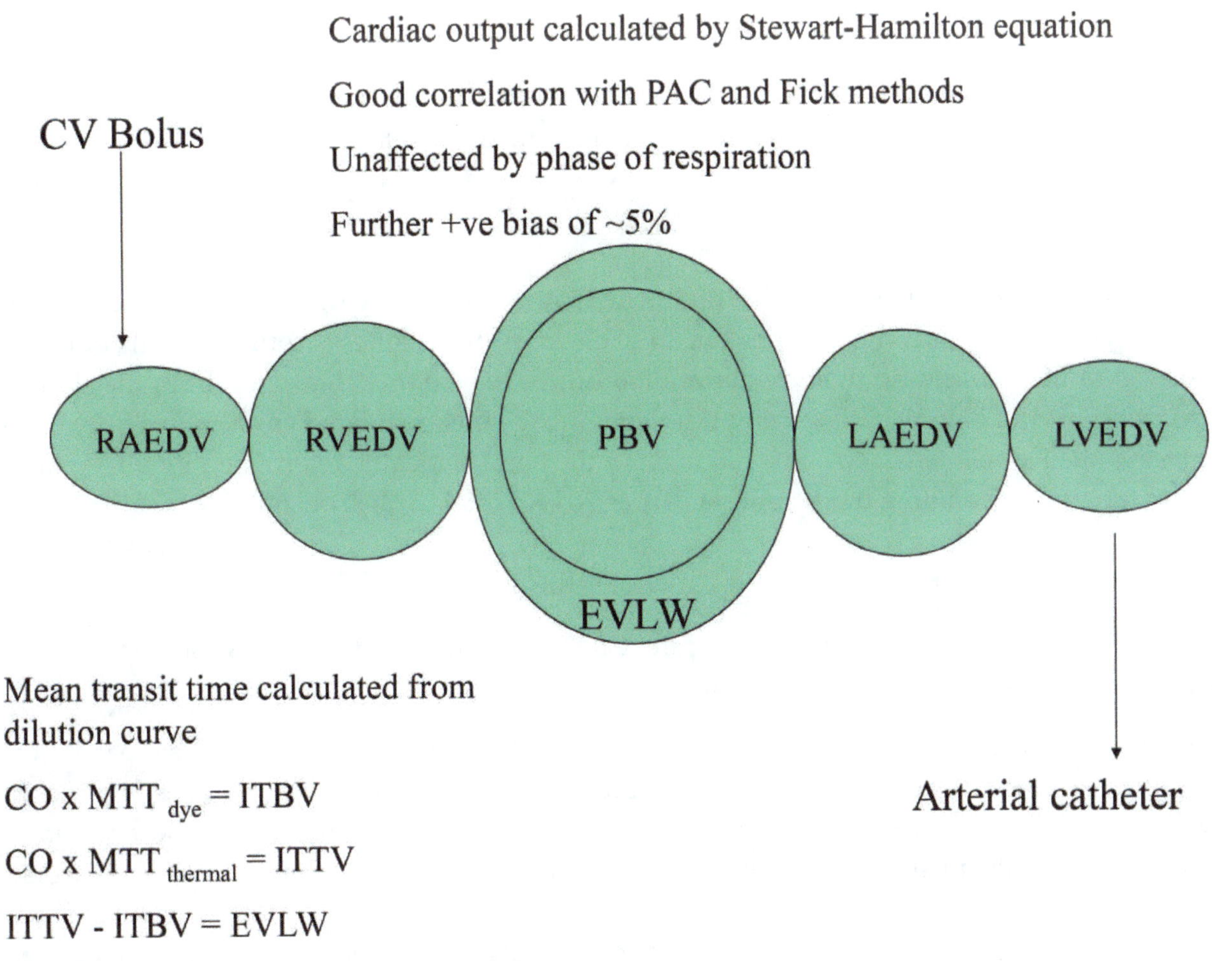

Figure 3. Schematic diagram for transpulmonary dilution technique for measurement of cardiac output.

While the risks of inserting catheters for transpulmonary dilution are identical to the individual risks of inserting arterial and central venous catheters, it is important to recall that the central venous catheter tip must lie as close as practicable to the right atrium. Femoral central venous catheters are not appropriate—the volumes measured include the variable contents of an extremely compliant capacitance vessel—the inferior vena cava!

6.4. Pulse contour analysis

Pulse contour analysis is predicated on the principle that the area under the systolic curve is proportional to the stroke volume. The arterial waveform (dP/dt) is analysed, and after calibration for arterial compliance, systemic vascular resistance and patient-specific calibration factors, the stroke volume is calculated.

Various monitors such as the LiDCO $Plus_{TM}$ (Cambridge, UK) and the $PiCCO_{TM}$ (Pulsion Medical System, Germany) use transpulmonary dilution to calculate the cardiac output and correlate this to pulse contour analysis to provide continuous cardiac output monitoring. The continuous cardiac output is recalibrated every 4–8 hours (depending on the manufacturer's specifications) to cardiac output derived from transpulmonary dilution.

Devices like the $FloTrac_{TM}$/$EV1000_{TM}$ system (Edwards Lifesciences, USA) allow pulse contour analysis of the arterial waveform acquired from any arterial catheter without the need to calibrate to other methods of cardiac output measurement. The $EV1000_{TM}$ monitor can also be combined with the $ClearSight_{TM}$ (Edwards Lifesciences, USA) probe, which uses a finger cuff-based volume clamp technique to acquire the arterial waveform.

6.5. Oesophageal Doppler

Oesophageal Doppler uses a flexible probe with a transducer at the tip that can be inserted like an orogastric tube into the oesophagus to a distance of 30–40 cm from the teeth oriented parallel to the descending thoracic aorta. Blood flow velocity is determined from the shift in frequency of red blood cells. Velocity time integral (VTI) is calculated from the velocity time curve of the Doppler envelope. The diameter of the aorta is ideally determined by ultrasound. Assuming the descending thoracic aorta carries 70% of total cardiac output

$$CO = HR.CSA.VTI/0.7 \tag{6}$$

where CO = cardiac output; HR = heart rate; CSA = measured aortic cross-section area; VTI = velocity time integral of the Doppler curve.

It is contraindicated with intra-aortic balloon pumps, anatomical anomalies such as coarctation of aorta or extrinsic compression of the descending aorta. In children, there is significant variation in the cross-sectional diameter during each beat and CSA cannot be accurately measured. Finally, in shock states, it is hard to know if the assumption that 70% of cardiac output goes to the descending aorta is true or not. Nevertheless, it is a simple device to use, with few contraindications or significant risks and the cardiac output measured with this device correlates well with pulmonary arterial catheter measurements.

6.6. Echocardiography

Australasian critical care practice has enthusiastically embraced the use of echocardiography and most practitioners have reasonable familiarity with the technique [18].

Using a transthoracic or transoesophageal probe, valuable information is gained not just about the global contractile function and filling state of the patient but also regarding regional wall motion abnormalities, pericardial or proximal aortic pathology and valvular abnormalities. The greatest advantage in clinical practice is the direct view of left ventricular function and its ability to directly measure volumetric indices (e.g. left ventricular end diastolic volume, LVEDV) than surrogate pressure indices (e.g. pulmonary artery occlusion pressures) as markers of volume state.

Two-dimensional echocardiography provides valuable information on systolic function including fractional shortening or fractional area change, which can then be approximated to left ventricular ejection fraction. It also provides valuable information on the filling state (e.g. no specific training is needed to interpret the 'kissing' left ventricular walls in severe hypovolaemia or the dilated inferior vena cava with no diameter change during forced inspiration). In experienced hands, subtle abnormalities in relaxation patterns give excellent clues to diastolic ventricular function. Finally, Doppler interrogation allows estimation of the more 'traditional' pressure indices such as pulmonary artery pressures from the tricuspid regurgitation jet.

The Doppler envelope of the left ventricular outflow tract (LVOT) allows calculation of the velocity time integral (VTI). Given that the LVOT itself is a relatively constant dimension and its diameter is easy to measure, this is an easy way to measure cardiac output at the aortic root.

$$(\pi d^2/4) \cdot \mathrm{HR} \cdot \mathrm{LVOT\ VTI} \tag{7}$$

where d = LVOT diameter; HR = heart rate; LVOT VTI = velocity time integral of blood flow at the left ventricular outflow tract.

One of the great advantages of transthoracic echocardiographic haemodynamic assessments is the fact that it is non-invasive. A full left ventricular study is rarely necessary in acute situations where it is being used to guide resuscitation and adequate clinical information can still be gathered from limited views. This has to be balanced against the fact that echocardiography is more time consuming and requires the presence of both equipment and a skilled operator at all times to be of meaningful use in assessing response to therapy. There is also an element of interobserver variability depending on the level of skill of the operator. Transthoracic views are more difficult in the supine positive pressure ventilated critically ill patient, and patients with thoracic trauma, cardiac surgery and pneumothoraces are notoriously difficult to acquire windows on. The problem is easily bypassed by adding transoesophageal echocardiography to the skill mix. On the other hand, this not only requires an additional skill set but also necessitates insertion of a probe into the oesophagus with the attendant risks of oesophageal injury or rupture. Moreover, transoesophageal probes cannot be left for long periods of time in the patient.

Echocardiography offers an accurate non-invasive series of haemodynamic snapshot views in the hands of a skilled operator and probably represents, where available, the best modality of cardiac monitoring to assess circulatory failure and guide resuscitation.

6.7. Other techniques

Various other devices using a variety of techniques are available for clinical use. These include:

- Thoracic bioimpedance
- Thoracic bioreactance: NICOM monitor (Cheetah medical, USA)
- Impedance plethysmography: ECOM monitor (ECOM medical, USA)
- Suprasternal portable Doppler ultrasound probes: USCOM (Australia)

Though initial studies in many of these devices has looked promising, they are not in common use currently and often suffer the drawbacks of both clinical unfamiliarity and limited validation data in critically ill patients.

7. Assessment of volume state

Much has been written over the years about estimation of preload. By definition, it is the amount of stretch in the muscle fibre just prior to contraction and is related to the length of the individual sarcomere just prior to contraction. As sarcomere length increases, the force of muscle contraction increases. Once maximal sarcomere length is reached, there is no further increase in contraction strength. In a section of muscle tissue, as increasing numbers of sarcomeres are maximally stretched, the strength of contraction plateaus. This is represented by the Frank Starling curve in **Figure 4**.

The practical aspect of this means that contractility and stroke volume of the left ventricle increases up to a point as systemic venous return increases. Beyond that point, stroke volume does not increase and there is tissue and pulmonary oedema with right ventricular stretching and poor collapsibility of the vena cava.

Since sarcomere length cannot be measured in clinical situations, the closest approximation available is the left ventricular end diastolic volume, either measured directly using echocardiography or indirectly by measuring the left ventricular end diastolic pressure or its surrogate pressures—pulmonary capillary occlusion pressure, right atrial pressure or central venous pressure using appropriately placed catheters. Transpulmonary dilution techniques allow measurement of intrathoracic blood volume or global end diastolic volume. It is important to remember that these are static measures of preload (see **Figure 5**).

From the practical point of view, contemplation of preload is less relevant than answering the question—'Is this patient fluid recruitable?' Multiple studies have suggested that only 50% of haemodynamically unstable patients respond to fluid challenge [19, 20].

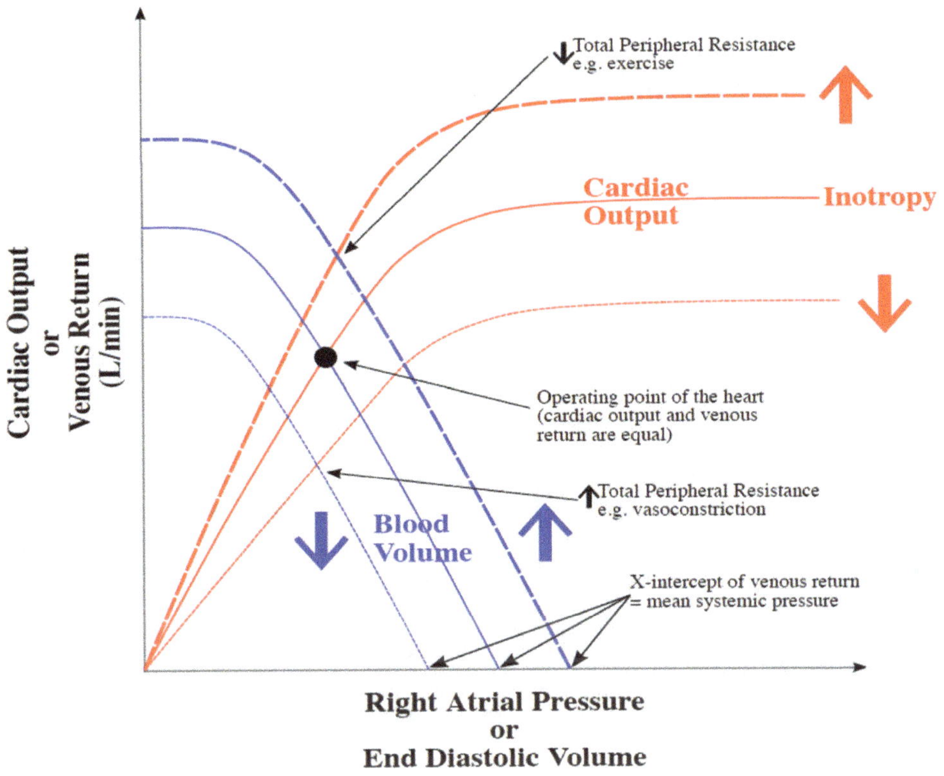

Figure 4. Frank Starling curve.

The most common static measure of preload used to answer this question is the central venous pressure. This correlates well with right atrial pressure and, in theory, is a reasonable pressure surrogate of right ventricular end diastolic volume. However, there is an extremely large body of literature demonstrating no correlation [21] between CVP and change in CVP and fluid responsiveness in a variety of clinical situations. Other measures of cardiac filling pressures like pulmonary artery occlusion pressure have also been shown to be poor predictors of volume responsiveness [22].

Increasingly, dynamic measures of preload estimation have been described and have entered clinical practice [19].

Passive leg raising to 45° in a supine patient provides the equivalent of a 500 mL fluid challenge in terms of increasing cardiac preload and the haemodynamic effects are detectable within minutes. Passive leg raise as a measure of volume responsiveness is well validated in critically unwell patients and may be considered a reversible autotransfusion.

Pulse pressure variation, derived from arterial waveform analysis, stroke volume variation (SVV) from pulse contour analysis and variation in the amplitude of the plethysmograph waveform in pulse oximetry have all been validated as measures of fluid responsiveness. Essentially, they reflect the changes to systemic venous return in hypovolemic patients as the intra-thoracic pressure changes during the respiratory cycle. SVV > 10% in positive pressure ventilated patients in sinus rhythm and a normally compliant chest wall is a sign of fluid recruitability.

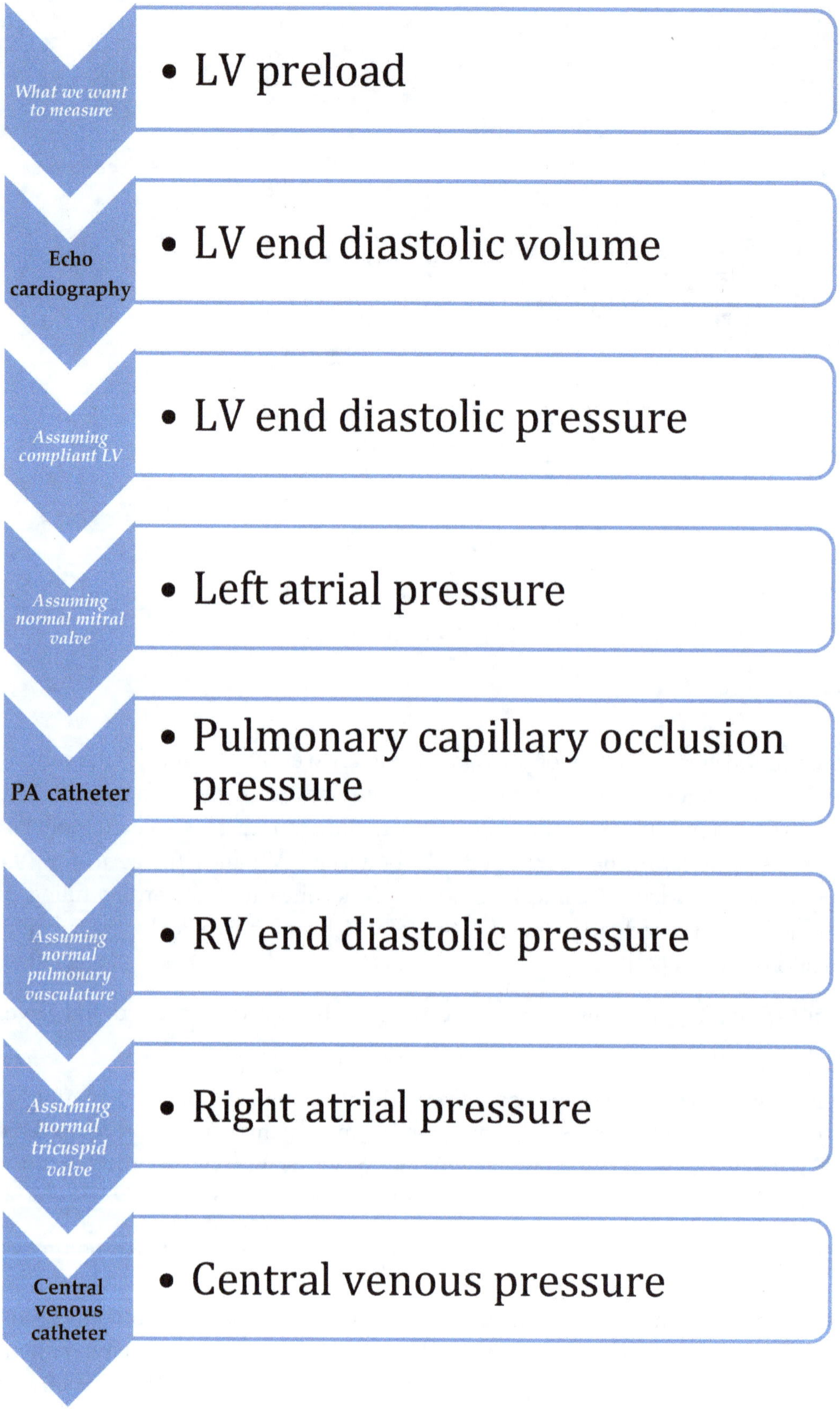

Figure 5. Static measures of LV preload.

Earlier work [23] using oesophageal tonometry suggests an increment of ≥10% in stroke volume after a volume challenge is a reasonable sign of fluid recruitability. In the end, the greatest measure of fluid responsiveness may be the administration of an empirical volume of fluid (the author prefers 250 mL aliquots) and monitoring haemodynamic changes resulting from the intervention.

8. Assessment of peripheral tissue perfusion

Shock is defined as 'inadequate tissue oxygen for aerobic cellular respiration'. Shock results from both macro-circulatory and micro-circulatory failure, leading to inadequate tissue perfusion. In addition, mitochondrial dysfunction may result in cellular oxygen misuse. Furthermore, stress and physiologic compensation can increase oxygen demand in situations of poor delivery. Thus, oxygen delivery and demand inadequacy can compound organ failure, resulting in death despite optimal management [24].

Shock resuscitation has been aimed at 'restoring' or 'maximising' oxygen delivery and tissue oxygenation. Kern and Shoemaker suggested that mortality decreased and oxygen delivery increased when management was guided by end points such as central venous pressure, mean arterial pressure, cardiac output, oxygen transport and mixed or central venous oxygen saturation [25]. Early goal-directed therapy advocated by Rivers and Nguyen [26] has found its echo in many resuscitation protocols, especially in the management of severe sepsis [3] and perioperative management of high-risk surgical patients. Ghaferi et al. described failure to identify and rescue patients with perioperative complications early as a potential reason for increased hospital mortality independent of case mix, patient characteristics and complication rates [27]. Combined with the global move towards rapid rescue and resuscitation teams for ward patients outside of critical care areas, this has moved goal-directed therapy outside of monitored critical care areas into the general ward population where invasive monitoring may not be safely accessible.

Yet, in situations like septic shock [28] and cardiac failure [29], despite optimisation of the macro-circulation with mean arterial pressure and cardiac output targets, micro-circulatory failure can result in persistent tissue failure [30]. Thus, it is important to monitor patients for evidence of micro-circulatory failure.

8.1. Lactate clearance

Glycolysis produces pyruvate, which either enters aerobic mitochondrial metabolism with a high ATP yield from the Krebs cycle or is processed anaerobically to lactate with a much lower ATP yield. Thus, in the absence of hypovolaemia and severe hepatic dysfunction, high circulating levels of lactate may represent high incidence of anaerobic metabolism due to lack of oxygen uptake, poor tissue perfusion or mitochondrial dysfunction. The Sepsis-3 guidelines acknowledge serum lactate >2 mmol/L to be a marker of septic shock [31].

Persistent hyperlactatemia is considered to reflect occult hypoperfusion and has been associated with poor outcomes in trauma [32], cardiac arrest [33] and high-risk surgery [34].

Modern blood gas sampling machines, easily accessible to critical care teams, provide a rapid and convenient method of quantifying and serially monitoring serum lactate as a marker of successful resuscitation.

8.2. Venous-arterial CO_2 gradient

Carbon dioxide is a by-product of oxidative metabolism and tissue production of CO_2 is related to its oxygen uptake.

Thus,

$$VCO_2 = R.VO_2 \tag{8}$$

where VCO_2 = tissue CO_2 production; VO_2= tissue O_2 uptake; R = respiratory quotient.

From the Fick principle (Eq. (2)), therefore

$$VCO_2 = CO(CaCO_2 - CvCO_2) \tag{9}$$

$$\text{i.e. } VCO_2 = CO.k.P(v - a)CO_2.$$

$$P(v - a)CO_2 = VCO_2/CO.k \tag{10}$$

where VCO_2 = tissue CO_2 production; CO = cardiac output; $P(v - a)CO_2$ = venous-arterial CO_2 gradient; K = coefficient of CO_2 concentration and partial pressure.

In other words, since k and R are constants, $P(v - a)CO_2$ is directly proportional to tissue CO_2 clearance and inversely proportional to cardiac output. Given its diffusible nature, CO_2 washout depends on tissue oxygen uptake and cardiac output.

Thus, $P(v - a)CO_2$ is dependent on cardiac output, tissue oxygen uptake and CO_2 washout. Thus, $P(v - a)CO_2$ will increase in low cardiac output states.

CO_2 washout is extremely flow-dependent and any decrease in local or regional capillary hypoperfusion will increase tissue stagnation of PCO_2 and a rise in diffusion of CO_2 to venous capillary beds with residual circulation, increasing $P(v - a)CO_2$. Thus, in the presence of normal measured cardiac output, high $P(v - a)CO_2$ may represent occult tissue hypoperfusion or impaired oxygen uptake.

In critically ill patients with normal cardiac index, $P(v - a)CO_2 > 6$ mmHg seems to be a good discriminator of occult hypoperfusion identified by persistent hyperlactatemia [35]. This has since been corroborated in septic shock [36] and high-risk surgical patients [37, 38] resuscitated with early goal directed therapy.

Thus, after optimisation of cardiac output in patients with circulatory failure, it seems reasonable to target $P(v - a)CO_2 < 6$ mmHg. How this is best achieved in clinical practice seems unclear.

8.3. Mixed venous saturation (SvO_2) and central venous saturation ($ScvO_2$): measures of global tissue oxygen extraction

Global tissue oxygen extraction is defined as the proportion of transported oxygen in the circulation taken up by the tissues. Thus,

$$ERO_2 = VO_2/TO_2 \tag{11}$$

where ERO_2 = extraction ratio of oxygen; VO_2 = tissue oxygen uptake; TO_2 =oxygen transported in the circulation = cardiac output × O_2 content of arterial blood.

By the Fick principle (Eq. (2))

$$ERO_2 = CO(CaVO_2 - CvVO_2)/TO_2 \tag{12}$$

Since,

$$TO_2 = CO.CaVO_2 \tag{13}$$

$$ERO_2 = 1 - (CvVO_2/CaVO_2) = 1 - SvO_2/SaO_2 \tag{14}$$

where SaO_2 = arterial O_2 saturation; SvO_2 = mixed venous saturation.

When SaO_2 is 100%,

$$ERO_2 = 1 - SvO_2 \tag{15}$$

Usual ERO_2 is 25–30% and is a function of metabolic demand, activity and mitochondrial activity. With increasing tissue oxygen consumption due to exercise, stress or sepsis, ERO_2 increases up to its maximum limit. Past ERO_2max, tissues are unable to take up further oxygen and anaerobic glycolysis resulting in lactate release occurs.

$ScvO_2$ is easier to sample and monitor through a central venous catheter than SvO_2 which necessitates insertion of a pulmonary artery catheter.

It is worth noting that a falling SvO_2 or $ScvO_2$ should trigger optimisation of TO_2 (increasing SaO_2, cardiac output, O_2 carrying capacity of blood, i.e. haemoglobin) before considering mitochondrial or tissue dysfunction. In essence, this forms the basis of goal directed therapy. While $ScvO_2$ directed inotrope therapy has been described to reduce mortality from septic shock [26], it is important to understand that SvO_2 and $ScvO_2$ cannot discriminate between reasons for increased VO_2 or decreased TO_2. A normal SvO_2 does not imply adequacy of oxygen demand and supply. Finally, once TO_2 has been optimised, it is unclear what therapies can be offered for mitochondrial dysfunction.

8.4. Gastric tonometry

Gastric tonometry has been described as a specific monitor for splanchnic perfusion, based on the phenomenon that early on in haemodynamic stress, there is diversion of blood flow away from splanchnic circulation.

Gastric luminal PCO_2 is equilibrated to the medium contained in a balloon at the end of a nasogastric probe and gastric mucosal pH is calculated using the Henderson-Hasselbach equation. Arterial HCO_3^- is measured as a surrogate for mucosal HCO_3^-. Mucosal-arterial PCO_2 gap >25 mmHg or splanchnic pH < 7.3 suggests poor splanchnic perfusion.

Unfortunately, in practice, it is limited by confounding factors such as enteral feeding and buffering of gastric acid by duodenal and oesophageal reflux.

8.5. Other techniques of micro-circulatory assessment

As discussed before, correction of macro-circulatory variables does not equate to successful oxygen supply at the tissue level.

Capillary blood flow can be visualised non-invasively at the bedside using sidestream dark field imaging in different capillary beds (e.g. sublingual, rectal, etc.) [39]. Currently, it is important to take multiple readings in several capillary beds for periods of 20 s or longer to eliminate measurement errors and inter-observer variability may exist. This technology shows promise and with refinement, may become a rapid, accurate and repeatable way of assessing capillary blood flow.

Tissue oxygenation in target tissue capillary beds (StO_2) can be measured non-invasively using near-infrared spectroscopy (NIRS). Unfortunately, there is little evidence behind 'normal' or 'target' values specific to capillary beds in critically unwell patients and this modality of monitoring, though promising, is still not common in clinical practice.

Sublingual tonometry provides a simple, non-invasive and inexpensive measure of adequacy of tissue perfusion [37, 40]. Further studies with this promising technology are needed to establish its clinical utility in everyday clinical care.

Acknowledgements

I like to acknowledge the input and encouragement of my critical care medical, nursing and technician colleagues. I thank my family for their patience and forbearance during the writing of this chapter. There are no conflicts of interest to declare in the writing of this chapter.

Author details

Mainak Majumdar

Address all correspondence to: mainak.majumdar@mh.org.au

Intensive Care Unit, Royal Melbourne Hospital, Parkville, VIC, Australia

References

[1] Bellomo R, Uchino S. Cardiovascular monitoring tools: Use and misuse. Current Opinion in Critical Care. 2003;**9**(3):225–229

[2] Brain Trauma Foundation September [Internet]. 2016. Guidelines available from: https://braintrauma.org/uploads/03/12/Guidelines_for_Management_of_Severe_TBI_4th_Edition.pdf [Accessed: 20 February 2017]

[3] Dellinger RP, Levy MM, et al. Surviving sepsis campaign: International guidelines for management of severe sepsis and septic shock: 2012. Critical Care Medicine. 2013;**41**(2):580–637. DOI: 10.1097/CCM.0b013e31827e83af

[4] Huygh J, Peeters Y, Bernards J, Malbrain MLNG. Haemodynamic monitoring in the critically ill: An overview of current cardiac output monitoring methods. F1000research. 2016;**5**(F100 Faculty Rev):2855. DOI: 10.12688/f1000research.8991.1

[5] Minimum Standards for Intensive Care Units (Professional Document IC-1), College of Intensive Care Medicine [Internet]. 2016. Available from: http://cicm.org.au/CICM_Media/CICMSite/CICM-Website/Resources/Professional%20Documents/IC-1-Minimum-Standards-for-Intensive-Care-Units_1.pdf [Accessed: 20 February 2017]

[6] Bicking RE. Fundamentals of Pressure Sensor Technology [Internet]. 1998. Available from: http://www.sensorsmag.com/sensors/pressure/fundamentals-pressure-sensor-technology-846 [Accessed: 20 February 2017]

[7] Booth J. A short history of blood pressure measurement. Proceedings of the Royal Society of Medicine. 1977;**70**(11):793–799

[8] Babbs CF. Oscillometric measurement of systolic and diastolic blood pressures validated in a physiologic mathematical model. Biomedical Engineering Online. 2012;**11**:56. DOI: 10.1186/1475-925X-11-56

[9] Zezulka AV, Sloan P, Davies P, Beevers DG. Oscillometric measurement of systolic and diastolic blood pressures validated in a physiologic mathematical model. Postgraduate Medical Journal. 1985;**61**:321–323

[10] Chung E, Chen G, Alexander B, Canneson M. Non-invasive continuous blood pressure monitoring: A review of current applications. Frontiers of Medicine. 2013;**7**:91. DOI: 10.1007/s11684-013-0239-5

[11] Slogoff S, Keats AS, Arlund C. On the safety of radial artery cannulation. Anesthesiology. 1983;**59**(1):42–47

[12] Mehta Y, Arora D. Newer methods of cardiac output monitoring. World Journal of Cardiology. 2014;**6**(9):1022–1029. DOI: 10.4330/wjc.v6.i9.1022

[13] Jaffe MB. Partial CO_2 rebreathing cardiac output- operating principles of the NICO system. Journal of Clinical Monitoring and Computing. 1999;**15**(6):387–401

[14] Eger EI. Cardiovascular effects of carbon dioxide in man. Anesthesiology. 1974;**41**(4): 341–349

[15] Swan HJ, Ganz W, Forrester J, Marcus H, Chonette D. Catheterisation of the heart in man with use of a flow directed balloon tipped catheter. New England Journal of Medicine. 1970;**283**:447–451

[16] Sandham JD, Hull RD, Brant RF, Knox L, et al. A randomised controlled trial of the use of pulmonary artery catheters in high risk surgical patients. New England Journal of Medicine. 2003;**348**:5–14

[17] Harvey S, Harrison DA, Singer M, Ashcroft J, Jones CM, et al. Assessment of the clinical effectiveness of pulmonary artery catheters in management of patients in intensive care (PAC-man): A randomised controlled trial. Lancet. 2005;**366**:472–477

[18] Statement on the Role of Echocardiography in Intensive Care Medicine (Professional Document IC-24), College of Intensive Care Medicine [Internet]. 2016. Available from: http://cicm.org.au/CICM_Media/CICMSite/CICM-Website/Resources/Professional%20Documents/IC-24-Statement-on-the-Role-of-Echocardiography-in-Intensive-Care-Medicine_1.pdf [Accessed 20 February 2017]

[19] Marik PE, Cavallazzi R, Vasu T, Hirani A. Dynamic changes in arterial waveform derived variables and fluid responsiveness in mechanically ventilated patients: A systematic review of the literature. Critical Care Medicine. 2009;**37**:2642–2647

[20] Boyd JH, Forbes J, Nakada T, Alley KR, Russell JA. Fluid resuscitation in septic shock: A positive fluid balance and elevated central venous pressure increase mortality. Critical Care Medicine. 2011;**39**(2):259–265

[21] Marik PE, Baram M, Vahid B. Does the central venous pressure predict fluid responsiveness? A systematic review of the literature. Chest. 2008;**134**:172–178

[22] Osman D, Ridel C, Ray P, Monnet X, Anguel N, Richard C, et al. Cardiac filling pressures are not appropriate to predict hemodynamic response to volume challenge. Critical Care Medicine. 2007;**35**(1):64–68

[23] Kuper M, Gold SJ, et al. Intraoperative fluid management guided by esophageal Doppler monitoring. British Medical Journal. 2011;**342**:d3016. DOI: 10.1136/bmj.d3016

[24] Kipnis E, Ramsingh D, Bhargava M, Dincer E, et al. Monitoring in the intensive care. Critical Care Research and Practice. 2012;**2012**:473507. DOI: 10.1155/2012/473507

[25] Kern JW, Shoemaker WC. Meta analysis of haemodynamic optimisation in high risk patients. Critical Care Medicine. 2002;**30**(8):1686–1692

[26] Rivers E, Nguyen B, Havstad S, et al. Early goal directed therapy in the treatment of severe sepsis and septic shock. New England Journal of Medicine. 2001;**345**(19):1368–1377

[27] Ghaferi AA, Birkmeyer JD, et al. Variation in hospital mortality associated with inpatient surgery. New England Journal of Medicine. 2009;**361**:1368–1375

[28] Sakr Y, Dubois MJ, De Backer B, Creteur J, Vincent, JL. Persistent micro circulatory alterations are associated with organ failure and death in patients with septic shock. Critical Care Medicine. 2004;**32**(9):1825–1831

[29] De Backer D, Creteur J, Dubois MJ, Sakr Y, Vincent JL. Microvascular alterations in patients with acute severe heart failure and cardiogenic shock. American Heart Journal. 2004;**147**(1):91–99. DOI: 10.1016/j.ahj.2014.04.022

[30] Siegenthaler N, Giraud R, Romand JA, Bendjelid K. Physiopathologic aspects of micro circulation in intensive care. Revue Medicale Suisse. 2008;**4**(183):2696–2701

[31] Singer M, Deutschmann CS, Seymour CW, et al. The third international consensus definitions of sepsis and septic shock (Sepsis-3). Journal of the American Medical Association. 2016;**315**(8):801–810. DOI: 10.1001/jama.2016.0287

[32] Claridge JA, Crabtree TD, Pelletier SJ, et al. Persistent occult hypoperfusion is associated with a significant increase in infection rate and mortality in major trauma patients. Journal of Trauma. 2000;**48**(1):8–14

[33] Kliegel A, Losert H, Sterz F, et al. Serial lactate determinations for prediction of outcome after cardiac arrest. Medicine. 2004;**83**(5):274–279

[34] Meregalli A, Oliviera RP, Friedman G. Occult hypoperfusion is associated with increased mortality in haemodynamically stable high risk surgical patients. Critical Care. 2004;**8**(2): R60–R65

[35] Mekontso-Dessap A, Castelain V, Anguel N, et al. Combination of venoarterial PCO_2 difference with arteriovenous O_2 content difference to detect anaerobic metabolism in patients. Intensive Care Medicine. 2002;**28**(3):272–277

[36] Vallee F, Vallet B, Mathe O, et al. Central venous to arterial carbon dioxide difference: An additional target for goal directed therapy in septic shock? Intensive Care Medicine. 2008;**34**(12):2218 2225

–

[37] Marik PE, Monnet X, Teboul JL. Haemodynamic parameters to guide fluid therapy. Annals of Intensive Care. 2011;**1**(1):1. DOI: 10.1186/2110-5820-1-1

[38] Futier E, Robin E, Jabaudon M, et al. Central venous O_2 saturation and venous to arterial CO_2 difference as complementary tools for goal directed therapy during high risk surgery. Critical Care. 2010;**14**(5):R193

[39] Boerma EC, Mathura KR, et al. Quantifying bedside derived imaging of microcirculatory abnormalities in septic patients: A prospective validation study. Critical Care. 2005;**9**(6): R601–R606

[40] Marik PE. Regional carbon dioxide monitoring to assess the adequacy of tissue perfusion. Current Opinion in Critical Care. 2005;**11**(3):245–251

Permissions

All chapters in this book were first published in IC, by InTech Open; hereby published with permission under the Creative Commons Attribution License or equivalent. Every chapter published in this book has been scrutinized by our experts. Their significance has been extensively debated. The topics covered herein carry significant findings which will fuel the growth of the discipline. They may even be implemented as practical applications or may be referred to as a beginning point for another development.

The contributors of this book come from diverse backgrounds, making this book a truly international effort. This book will bring forth new frontiers with its revolutionizing research information and detailed analysis of the nascent developments around the world.

We would like to thank all the contributing authors for lending their expertise to make the book truly unique. They have played a crucial role in the development of this book. Without their invaluable contributions this book wouldn't have been possible. They have made vital efforts to compile up to date information on the varied aspects of this subject to make this book a valuable addition to the collection of many professionals and students.

This book was conceptualized with the vision of imparting up-to-date information and advanced data in this field. To ensure the same, a matchless editorial board was set up. Every individual on the board went through rigorous rounds of assessment to prove their worth. After which they invested a large part of their time researching and compiling the most relevant data for our readers.

The editorial board has been involved in producing this book since its inception. They have spent rigorous hours researching and exploring the diverse topics which have resulted in the successful publishing of this book. They have passed on their knowledge of decades through this book. To expedite this challenging task, the publisher supported the team at every step. A small team of assistant editors was also appointed to further simplify the editing procedure and attain best results for the readers.

Apart from the editorial board, the designing team has also invested a significant amount of their time in understanding the subject and creating the most relevant covers. They scrutinized every image to scout for the most suitable representation of the subject and create an appropriate cover for the book.

The publishing team has been an ardent support to the editorial, designing and production team. Their endless efforts to recruit the best for this project, has resulted in the accomplishment of this book. They are a veteran in the field of academics and their pool of knowledge is as vast as their experience in printing. Their expertise and guidance has proved useful at every step. Their uncompromising quality standards have made this book an exceptional effort. Their encouragement from time to time has been an inspiration for everyone.

The publisher and the editorial board hope that this book will prove to be a valuable piece of knowledge for researchers, students, practitioners and scholars across the globe.

List of Contributors

Adel E. Ahmed Ganaw, Abdulgafoor M. Tharayil, Ali O. Mohamed Bel Khair, Saher Tahseen, Jazib Hassan, Mohammad Faisal Abdullah Malmstrom and Sohel Mohamed Gamal Ahmed
Department of Anesthesiology, ICU and Perioperative Medicine, Hamad Medical Corporation, Doha, Qatar

Melek Nihal Esin
Public Health Nursing Department, Florence Nightingale Nursing Faculty, Istanbul University, Istanbul, Turkey

Duygu Sezgin
Department of Nursing & Midwifery, Education & Health Sciences Faculty, University of Limerick, Limerick, Ireland

Massimo Baiocchi, Maria Benedetto, Marta Agulli and Guido Frascaroli
Anaesthesiology and Intensive Care Unit, Cardiothoracic and vascular Department, Policlinico S. Orsola University Hospital, Bologna, Italy

Syed Abdul Rahman, Arif Valliani and Arshad Chanda
Surgical Intensive Care Unit, Hamad Medical Corporation, Doha, Qatar

Abdulgafoor M. Tharayil, Adel Ganaw, Syed Abdulrahman, Zia M. Awan and Sujith M. Prabhakaran
Department of Anaesthesia, Hamad Medical Corporation, Doha, Qatar

Jose J. Zaragoza
Intensive Care Unit, Hospital Español, Mexico City, Mexico
Mexican College of Critical Care Medicine, Mexico City, Mexico

Faustino J. Renteria
Intensive Care Unit, Hospital Español, Mexico City, Mexico

Selim Öncel
Division of Pediatric Infectious Diseases, Department of Pediatrics and Child Health, Section of Internal Medical Sciences, Kocaeli University Faculty of Medicine, Kocaeli, Turkey

Nabil Abdelhamid Shallik
Hamad Medical Corporation, Clinical Anesthesiology, Weill Cornell Medical College in Qatar, Doha, Qatar
Anesthesia and ICU Department, Tanta Faculty of Medicine, Tanta, Egypt
Anesthesia Section of Rumailah Hospital, Anesthesia, ICU and Perioperative Medicine Department HMC, Doha, Qatar
Medical Education and Qatar Robotic Surgery Center, HMC, Doha, Qatar

Mamdouh Almustafa and Ahmed Zaghw
Department of Anesthesia, ICU and Perioperative Medicine, HMC, Doha, Qatar

Abbas Moustafa
Elminia University, Egypt
Radiology, HMC, Doha, Qatar

Eleni Athanasios Volakli, Peristera-Eleni Mantzafleri, Serafeia Kalamitsou, Asimina Violaki, Elpis Chochliourou, Menelaos Svirkos, Athanasios Kasimis and Maria Sdougka
Pediatric Intensive Care Unit, Hippokration General Hospital, Thessaloniki, Greece

Arshad Chanda
Hamad General Hospital, Doha, State of Qatar

Mainak Majumdar
Intensive Care Unit, Royal Melbourne Hospital, Parkville, VIC, Australia

Index

www.ingramcontent.com/pod-product-compliance
Lightning Source LLC
LaVergne TN
LVHW081028210926
848485LV00004B/974